Clinical Orthopaedic
Rehabilitation

Clinical Orthopaedic Rehabilitation

Editor

S. BRENT BROTZMAN, MD

Staff Orthopaedic Surgeon
  Spohn Hospital;
Chief of Foot and Ankle Service
  Orthopaedic Surgery and Sports Medicine Associates
Corpus Christi, Texas

with 342 illustrations

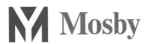 Mosby

St. Louis Baltimore Boston Carlsbad Chicago Naples New York Philadelphia Portland
London Madrid Mexico City Singapore Sydney Tokyo Toronto Wiesbaden

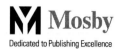

Mosby

Dedicated to Publishing Excellence

A Times Mirror
Company

Publisher: Anne S. Patterson
Editor: Kathryn H. Falk
Developmental Editor: Carolyn Malik
Project Manager: John Rogers
Production Editor: Cheryl Abbott Bozzay
Designer: Renée Duenow
Manufacturing Supervisor: Linda Ierardi

Printed in the United States of America
Composition by Clarinda Company
Printing/binding by Courier Companies, Inc.

Mosby–Year Book, Inc.
11830 Westline Industrial Drive
St. Louis, Missouri 63146

Library of Congress Cataloging in Publication Data

Clinical orthopaedic rehabilitation / S. Brent Brotzman, editor.
    p.   cm.
    Includes bibliographical references and index.
    ISBN 0-8151-1034-0
    1. Physically handicapped—Rehabilitation. 2. Orthopedics.
 I. Brotzman, S. Brent.
    [DNLM: 1. Orthopedics—methods. 2. Rehabilitation—standards.
WE 168 C6405 1995]
RD797.C55 1995
617.3—dc20
DNLM/DLC
for Library of Congress   95-42300
                                       CIP

95 96 97 98 99 / 9 8 7 6 5 4 3 2 1

Contributing Authors

KELLY AKIN, PT

Staff Physical Therapist
  Physical Therapy Department
  Campbell Clinic
Memphis, Tennessee

JAMES R. ANDREWS, MD

Clinical Professor of Orthopaedics and Sports Medicine
  University of Virginia School of Medicine;
Clinical Professor, Department of Orthopaedic Surgery
  University of Kentucky Medical Center;
Medical Director, American Sports Medicine Institute
  Birmingham, Alabama

MARYLYLE BOOLOS, PT, AT, C

Rehabilitation Hospital of the Mid-South
Memphis, Tennessee

JILL BRASEL, PT

Clinical Coordinator
  Physical Therapy Department
  Campbell Clinic
Memphis, Tennessee

S. BRENT BROTZMAN, MD

Staff Orthopaedic Surgeon
  Spohn Hospital;
Chief of Foot and Ankle Service
  Orthopaedic Surgery and Sports Medicine Associates
Corpus Christi, Texas

JAMES H. CALANDRUCCIO, MD

Instructor
  University of Tennessee–Campbell Clinic
  Department of Orthopaedic Surgery;
Staff Orthopaedic Surgeon
  Campbell Clinic
Memphis, Tenessee

HUGH U. CAMERON, MB, ChB, FRCS(C), FAAOS

Associate Professor
  Department of Surgery, Pathology, and Engineering
  University of Toronto;
Staff Orthopaedic Surgeon
  Orthopaedic and Arthritic Hospital
Toronto, Canada

ROBERT DONATELLI, PT, PhD

National Director of Sports Rehabilitation
  Physiotherapy Associates;
Instructor, Physical Therapy Department
  Emory University School of Rehabilitation Medicine
Atlanta, Georgia

DAVID GROH, PT

Staff Physical Therapist
  HealthSouth Sports Medicine and Rehabilitation Center
Birmingham, Alabama

PENNY HEAD, PT, AT, C

Sports Medicine Coordinator
  Physical Therapy Department
  Campbell Clinic
Memphis, Tennessee

FRANK W. JOBE, MD

Associate, Kerlan–Jobe Clinic;
Clinical Professor, Department of Orthopaedics
  University of Southern California School of Medicine;
Orthopaedic Consultant
  Los Angeles Dodgers
  PGA Tour
  Senior PGA Tour
Los Angeles, California

MARK T. JOBE, MD

Assistant Professor
　University of Tennessee–Campbell Clinic
　Department of Orthopaedic Surgery;
Staff Orthopaedic Surgeon
　Campbell Clinic
Memphis, Tennessee

ANA K. PALMIERI, MD

Orthopaedic Resident
　University of Tennessee–Campbell Clinic
　Department of Orthopaedic Surgery
Memphis, Tennessee

KAREN ROSS, PT

Executive Director
　Sports Physical Therapy
Corpus Christi, Texas

THOMAS A. RUSSELL, MD

Associate Professor
　University of Tennessee–Campbell Clinic
　Department of Orthopaedic Surgery;
Russell Orthopaedic Center;
Staff Orthopaedic Surgeon
　Methodist Hospital
Memphis, Tennessee

DIANE MOYNE SCHWAB, MS, PT

Champion Rehabilitation
San Diego, California

SUSAN W. STRALKA, PT

Director of Physical Therapy
　Campbell Clinic
Memphis, Tennessee

WILLIAM C. WARNER, Jr, MD

Assistant Professor
　University of Tennessee–Campbell Clinic
　Department of Orthopaedic Surgery;
Staff Orthopaedic Surgeon
　Campbell Clinic
Memphis, Tennessee

ARTHUR H. WHITE, MD

Medical Director
　SpineCare Medical Group;
Medical Director
　San Francisco Spine Institute;
Past President, North American Spine Society
San Francisco, California

KEVIN E. WILK, PT

National Director, Research and Clinical Education
　HealthSouth Rehabilitation Corporation;
Associate Clinical Director
　HealthSouth Rehabilitation Center;
Director of Rehabilitative Research
　American Sports Medicine Institute
Birmingham;
Adjunct Assistant Professor
　Marquette University
　Programs in Physician Therapy
Milwaukee, Wisconsin

To my loving wife Cynthia,
whose patience and understanding throughout the long process
has provided inspiration and encouragement,
and to my parents,
whose love and sacrifice over the years
have given me countless opportunities.

Preface

Although the literature describing orthopaedic surgical techniques and acute fracture care is sound and comprehensive, there is relatively little easily referenced information concerning postoperative or post-fracture rehabilitation. This void persisted despite the fact that rehabilitation therapy may have as much or more effect on long-term results than the initial treatment of an injury or condition. A technically superb surgical result may be compromised by improper postoperative rehabiliation techniques that allow scar formation, stiffness, rupture of incompletely healed tissue, or loss of function.

This textbook is designed to give the reader well-established rehabilitation protocols used by leading orthopaedic surgeons and therapists in specific specialty areas. Each protocol is preceded by background information and by the rehabilitation rationale needed for decision making during the rehabilitation process. These protocols are *not* intended to be used with a cookbook approach; they do not fit every possible situation or patient, but they are designed to give the reader a framework on which individualized programs can be built.

Many existing rehabilitation protocols are empirically based; they have been shaped by years of trial and error in large numbers of patients. Changes in rehabilitation approaches may be indicated in the future by the results of clinical research and biomechanical studies. At present, however, the principles outlined in this text are those accepted by most orthopaedic surgeons and therapists.

It is hoped that this text will provide physicians and therapists with a concise, easy-to-use guide for formulating rehabilitation protocols that will best serve their patients.

Acknowledgements

I would like to acknowledge the valuable contributions of a number of people who made this book possible. First, my thanks to all of the surgeons and therapists who were kind enough to invest the time and effort required to share their expertise. Thanks also to the Campbell Foundation crew: to Kay Daugherty for her editing skills, to Joan Crowson for her help in obtaining both obvious and obscure references, and to Linda Jones for her assistance in manuscript preparation. My special thanks to the staff of the Campbell Clinic for their generous and unfailing willingness to answer questions, give advice, and provide encouragement.

Of course, this text would not have been possible without the assistance and encouragement of all the staff at Mosby–Year Book. My thanks to all who believed the work was worthwhile and patiently guided a first-time author.

S. Brent Brotzman

Contents

Clinical Orthopaedic Rehabilitation

CHAPTER ONE

Rehabilitation of the Hand and Wrist

JAMES H. CALANDRUCCIO, MD

MARK T. JOBE, MD

KELLY AKIN, PT

Many of the rehabilitation protocols in this chapter are taken from *Diagnosis and Treatment Manual for Physicians and Therapists* by Nancy Cannon, OTR. These protocols are designated by an asterisk. We highly recommend this manual as a detailed reference text for hand therapy.

Flexor Tendon Injuries

REHABILITATION RATIONALE AND BASIC PRINCIPLES

Timing

The timing of flexor tendon repair influences the rehabilitation and outcome of flexor tendon injuries.

- *Primary repair* is performed within the first 12 to 24 hours after injury.
- *Delayed primary repair* is performed within the first 10 days after injury.

■ *If primary repair is not performed, delayed primary repair should be performed as soon as there is evidence of wound healing without infection.*

- *Secondary repair* is performed more than 10 to 14 days after injury.
- *Late secondary repair* is performed more than 4 weeks after injury.

After 4 weeks, it is extremely difficult to deliver the flexor tendon through the digital sheath, which usually becomes extensively scarred. However, clinical situations where tendon repair is of secondary importance often make late repair necessary, especially for patients with massive crush injuries, inadequate soft tissue coverage, grossly contaminated or infected wounds, multiple fractures, or untreated injuries. If the sheath is not scarred or destroyed, single-stage tendon grafting, direct repair, or tendon transfer may be performed. If extensive disturbance and scarring has occurred, two-stage tendon grafting with a Hunter rod technique should be used.

Before tendons may be secondarily repaired, the following certain requirements must be met:

- Joints must be supple and have useful passive range of motion (ROM) (Boyes' grade 1 or 2, see Table 1-1). Restoration of passive ROM is aggressively obtained with rehabilitation before secondary repair is performed.
- Skin coverage must be adequate.
- The surrounding tissue in which the tendon is expected to glide must be relatively free of scar tissue.
- Wound erythema and swelling must be minimal or absent.

Text and illustrations in this chapter marked with an asterisk (*) are modified or redrawn from Cannon NM: *Diagnosis and treatment manual for physicians and therapists,* ed 3, 1991, The Hand Rehabilitation Center of Indiana, PC.

TABLE 1-1 **Boyes' Preoperative Classification**

Grade	Preoperative condition
1	Good. Minimal scar with mobile joints and no trophic changes.
2	Cicatrix. Heavy skin scarring due to injury or prior surgery. Deep scarring due to failed primary repair or infection.
3	Joint damage. Injury to the joint with restricted range of motion.
4	Nerve damage. Injury to the digital nerves resulting in trophic changes in the finger.
5	Multiple damage. Involvement of multiple fingers with a combination of the above problems.

From Boyes JH: Flexor tendon grafts in the fingers and thumb: an evaluation of end results, *J Bone Joint Surg* 32A:489, 1950.

- Fractures must have been securely fixed or healed with adequate alignment.
- Sensation in the involved digit must be undamaged or restored, or it should be possible to repair damaged nerves at the time of tendon repair directly or with nerve grafts.
- The critical A2 and A4 pulleys must be present or have been reconstructed. Secondary repair is delayed until these are reconstructed. During reconstruction, Hunter rods (silicone) are useful to maintain the lumen of the tendon sheath while the grafted pulleys are healing.

Anatomy

The anatomic zone of injury of the flexor tendons influences the outcome and rehabilitation of these injuries. The hand is divided into five distinct flexor zones.

- Zone 1—from the insertion of the profundus tendon at the distal phalanx to just distal to the insertion of the sublimis.
- Zone 2—Bunnell's "no-man's land"—the critical area of pulleys between the insertion of the sublimis and the distal palmar crease.
- Zone 3—"area of lumbrical origin"—from the beginning of the pulleys (A1) to the distal margin of the transverse carpal ligament.
- Zone 4—area covered by the transverse carpal ligament.
- Zone 5—area proximal to the transverse carpal ligament.

■ *As a rule, repairs to tendons injured outside the flexor sheath have much better results than repairs to tendons injured inside the sheath (zone 2).*

It is essential that the A2 and A4 pulleys be preserved to prevent bow-stringing. In the thumb, the A1

and oblique pulleys are the most important. The thumb lacks vinculum for blood supply.

Tendon Healing

The exact mechanism of tendon healing is still unknown. Healing probably occurs through a combination of extrinsic and intrinsic processes. *Extrinsic* healing depends on the formation of adhesions between the tendon and the surrounding tissue, providing a blood supply and fibroblasts, but unfortunately it also prevents the tendon from gliding. *Intrinsic* healing relies on synovial fluid for nutrition and occurs only between the tendon ends.

Flexor tendons in the distal sheath have a dual source of nutrition via the vincular system and synovial diffusion. Diffusion appears to be more important than perfusion in the digital sheath (Green).

Several factors have been reported to affect tendon healing:

- Age—the number of vincula (blood supply) decreases with age.
- General health—cigarettes, caffeine, and poor general health delay healing. Patients should refrain from caffeine and cigarettes during the first 4 to 6 weeks after repair.
- Scar formation—the remodeling phase is not as effective in patients who produce heavy keloid or scar.
- Motivation and compliance—motivation and ability to follow the postoperative rehabilitation regimen are critical factors in outcome.
- Level of injury—zone 2 injuries are more apt to form limiting adhesions from the tendon to the surrounding tissue. In zone 4, where the flexor tendons lie in close proximity to each other, injuries tend to form tendon-to-tendon adhesions, limiting differential glide.
- Trauma and extent of injury—crushing or blunt injuries promote more scar formation and cause more vascular trauma, impairing function and healing. Infection also impedes the healing process.
- Pulley integrity—pulley repair is important in restoring mechanical advantage (especially A2 and A4) and maintaining tendon nutrition through synovial diffusion.
- Surgical technique—improper handling of tissues (such as forceps marks on the tendon) and excessive postoperative hematoma formation trigger adhesion formation.

■ *The two most frequent causes for failure of primary tendon repairs are formation of adhesions and rupture of the repaired tendon, respectively.*

Through experimental and clinical observation, Duran and Houser determined that 3 to 5 mm of tendon glide is sufficient to prevent motion-limiting tendon adhesions. Exercises are thus designed to achieve this motion.

Partial laceration involving less than 25% of the tendon substance may be treated by beveling the cut edges. Lacerations between 25% and 50% may be repaired with a 6-0 running nylon suture in the epitenon. Lacerations involving more than 50% should be considered complete and should be repaired with a core suture (such as a modified Kessler) and epitenon suture.

FDP lacerations should be repaired directly or advanced and reinserted into the distal phalanx with a pull-out wire, but should not be advanced more than 1 cm to avoid the quadriga effect (complication of a single digit with limited motion causing limitation of excursion, and thus motion of the uninvolved digits).

Rehabilitation

The rehabilitation protocol chosen for a patient depends on the *timing* of the repair (delayed primary or secondary), the *location* of the injury (zones 1 through 5), and the *compliance* of the patient (early mobilization for compliant patients or delayed mobilization for noncompliant patients and children younger than 7 years of age).

REHABILITATION PROTOCOL

Immediate (or Delayed Primary) Repair of Injury in Zone 1, 2, or 3 Modified Duran Protocol*

Prerequisites: compliant patient
clean or healed wound
repair within 14 days of injury

1 to 3 days
• Remove bulky compressive dressing and apply light compressive dressing.
• Digital level fingersocks or coban are utilized for edema control.
• Fit dorsal blocking splint (DBS) to wrist and digits for continual wear with following positions:
Wrist—20 degrees of flexion.
Metacarpophalangeal (MCP) joints—50 degrees of flexion.
Distal interphalangeal (DIP) and proximal interphalangeal (PIP) joints—full extension.
• Initiate controlled passive mobilization exercises, including passive flexion/extension exercises to DIP and PIP joints individually.

• Composite passive flexion/extension exercises to MCP, PIP, DIP joints of digits (modified Duran program). Active extension should be within the restraints of DBS. If full passive flexion is not obtained, the patient may begin prolonged flexion stretching with Coban or taping.
• 8 repetitions each of isolated passive flexion/extension exercises of the MCP, PIP, and DIP within the DBS (Figs. 1-1, 1-2, 1-3).

4.5 weeks
• Continue the exercises and begin active ROM for fingers and wrist flexion, allowing active wrist extension to neutral or 0 degrees of extension only.
• Patients should perform hourly exercises with the splint removed, including composite fist, wrist flexion and extension to neutral, composite finger flexion with the wrist immobilized (Fig. 1-4).

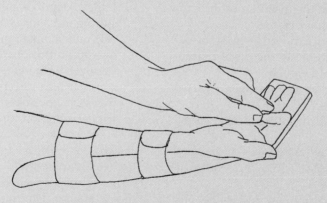

Figure 1-1 Passive flexion and extension exercises of the PIP joint in DBS.*

REHABILITATION PROTOCOL—cont'd

4.5 weeks —cont'd

- Have patient perform fist to hook fist (intrinsic minus position) exercise to extended fingers (Fig. 1-5).
- Watch for PIP flexion contractures. If an extension lag is present, add protected passive extension of PIP joint with MCP held in flexion—this should be performed only by reliable patients or therapists. The PIP joint should be blocked to 30 degrees of flexion for 3 weeks if a concomitant distal nerve repair is performed.
- Patients may reach a plateau in ROM 2 months after surgery; however, maximal motion is usually achieved by 3 months after surgery.

5 weeks

- FES (functional electrical stimulation) may be used to improve tendon excursion. Consider the patient's quality of primary repair, the nature of the injury, and the medical history before initiating FES.

5.5 weeks

- Add blocking exercises for PIP and DIP joints to previous home program.
- Discontinue DBS.
- Focus should be on gaining full passive ROM for flexion. Do not begin passive extension stretching at this time. A restraining extension splint may be used and positioned in available range if tightness is noted.

6 weeks

- Begin passive extension exercises of wrist and digits.
- Fit extension resting pan splint in maximum extension if extrinsic flexor tendon tightness is significant; frequently the patient may need only an extension gutter splint for night wear.

8 weeks

- Begin resistive exercises with sponges or a Nerf ball and progress to putty and a hand-helper. Allow use of the hand in light work activities but no lifting or heavy use of the hand.

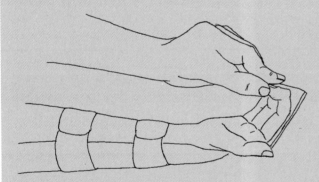

Figure 1-2 Passive flexion and extension exercises of the DIP joint in DBS.*

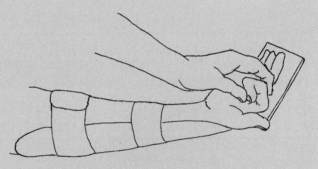

Figure 1-3 Combined passive flexion and extension exercises of the MCP, PIP, and DIP joints.*

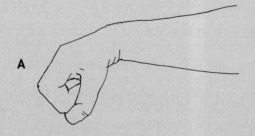

A

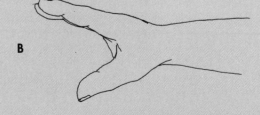

B

Figure 1-4 Bend the wrist in flexion. **A,** with a composite fist, then extend the wrist and fingers, **(B).***

Continued

REHABILITATION PROTOCOL—cont'd

Immediate (or Delayed Primary) Repair of Injury in Zone 1, 2, or 3 Modified Duran Protocol

10 to 12 weeks
- Allow full use of the hand in all daily activities.
- Use work simulator or strengthening program to improve hand strength.

The greatest achievement in total motion is seen between 12 to 14 weeks after surgery. It is not uncommon to see the patient begin to plateau in ROM between 6 to 8 weeks.

In patients with associated digital nerve repair with some degree of tension at the nerve site, the patient should be fitted with a separate digital dorsal blocking splint in 30 degrees of PIP joint flexion. This splint is worn for 6 weeks and is progressively adjusted into increased extension during that time frame (see the section on digital nerve repair).

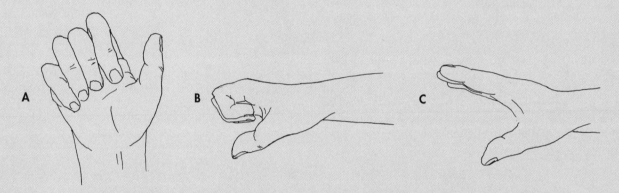

Figure 1-5 Patient makes a fist **(A)**, then straightens the MCP joints "back knuckles" **(B).** Then the fingers are straightened **(C)** with the wrist in neutral.*

REHABILITATION PROTOCOL

Early Mobilization of Immediate (or Delayed Primary) Repair of Zones 4 and 5 Modified Duran Protocol*

Prerequisites: compliant patient
clean or healed wound
repair within 14 days of injury

7 to 14 days
- Remove bulky compressive dressing and apply light compressive dressing. Use digital-level finger socks or Coban.
- Fit DBS to wrist and digits for continual wear in the following position:
    Wrist—30 degrees of palmar flexion.
    MCP joints—50 degrees of flexion.
    PIP and DIP joints—full extension.
- Begin hourly passive ROM exercises in flexion and extension within restraints of DBS. (See Figs. 1-1, 1-2, and 1-3.)

3 weeks
- Begin active ROM exercises (including blocking) 10 to 15 minutes each hour; exercises may be performed within restraints of DBS.

- FES or electrical muscle stimulation (EMS) may be initiated to improve tendon excursion within 2 days of initiation of active ROM.
- Begin scar massage, scar retraction, and scar remodeling techniques to remodel scar tissue and minimize subcutaneous adhesions.

4.5 weeks
- Begin active ROM exercises of wrist and digits outside of DBS. If nerve repair has been done at wrist level, ROM exercises are performed within the splint to alleviate additional stress at nerve repair site. (See the section on nerve repairs, p. 44.)

6 weeks
- Discontinue DBS.
- Begin passive ROM exercises of wrist and digits.

REHABILITATION PROTOCOL—cont'd

6 weeks —cont'd

- A full-extension resting pan splint or a long dorsal outrigger with a lumbrical bar may be used if extrinsic flexor tightness is present. Generally, this type of splinting is necessary with this level of repair.
- Do not allow lifting or heavy use of the hand.
- May begin gentle strengthening with a Nerf ball or putty.

7 weeks

- May upgrade progressive strengthening to include use of a hand-helper.

10 to 12 weeks

- Allow full use of the injured hand.

Once active ROM exercise is begun at 3 weeks, it is important to emphasize blocking exercises along with the composite active ROM exercises. If the patient is having difficulty recapturing active flexion, it is important to monitor progress carefully and request frequent patient visits to maximize flexion. *The first 3 to 7 weeks after surgery are critical for restoring tendon excursion.*

REHABILITATION PROTOCOL

Immediate (or Delayed Primary) Repair of Injuries in Zone 1, 2, or 3 Modified Early Motion Program

Prerequisites: compliant, motivated patient
good repair, wound healing

1 to 3 days

- Remove bulky compressive dressing and apply light compressive dressing.
- Use digital-level finger socks or Coban for edema at digital level.
- Fit DBS to wrist and digits for continual wear in the following position:
  Wrist—20 degrees of palmar flexion.
  MCP joints—50 degrees of flexion.
  DIP and PIP joints—full extension.
- Begin hourly passive ROM exercises in flexion and extension within restraints of DBS. (Refer to modified Duran protocol on p. 4.)

3 weeks

- Begin active ROM exercises in flexion and extension within restraints of DBS 4 to 6 times a day, in addition to modified Duran protocol. (See p. 4.)

4.5 weeks

- Begin hourly active ROM exercises of wrist and digits outside splint.
- Patient should wear DBS between exercise sessions and at night.

5.5 weeks

- Begin blocking exercises of DIP and PIP joint, as outlined in modified Duran protocol. (See Figs. 1-1 and 1-2.)

6 weeks

- Discontinue DBS.
- Begin passive ROM exercises in extension of wrist and digits as needed.
- Begin extension splinting if extrinsic flexor tendon tightness or PIP joint contracture is present.

8 weeks

- Begin progressive strengthening.
- Do not allow lifting or heavy use of the hand.

10 to 12 weeks

- Allow full use of hand, including sports.

This protocol differs from the modified Duran protocol because the patient may begin active ROM exercises within the restraints of the DBS at 3 weeks instead of exercising out of the splint at 4.5 weeks.

Noncompliant Patient With Injury in Zones 1 Through 5 Delayed Mobilization*

Indications:	crush injury younger than 11 years of age poor compliance and/or intelligence soft tissue loss, wound management problems
3 weeks	• Remove bulky dressing and apply light compressive dressing. • Fit DBS to wrist and digits for continual wear in the following position: Wrist—30 degrees of palmar flexion MCP joints—50 degrees of flexion PIP and DIP joints—full extension • Begin hourly active and passive ROM exercises within restraints of DBS; blocking exercises of PIP and DIP joints may be included. • Active ROM is begun earlier than in other protocols because of longer (3 weeks) immobilization in DBS.
4.5 weeks	• Begin active ROM exercises of digits and wrist outside of DBS; continue passive ROM exercises within restraints of splint. • May use FES or EMS to improve tendon excursion. • If an associated nerve repair is under any degree of tension, continue exercises
4.5 weeks —cont'd	within DBS that are appropriate for the level of nerve repair.6 weeks
6 weeks	• Discontinue DBS. • Begin passive ROM exercises in extension of wrist and digits. • May use extension resting pan splint for extrinsic flexor tendon tightness or joint stiffness. • Do not allow lifting or heavy use of hand.
8 weeks	• Begin progressive strengthening with putty and hand-helper.
10 to 12 weeks	• Allow full use of hand.

This delayed mobilization program for digital-level to forearm-level flexor tendon repairs is reserved primarily for significant crush injuries, which may include severe edema or wound problems. This program is best used for patients whose primary repair may be somewhat "ragged" because of the crushing or bursting nature of the wound. It also is indicated for young children who cannot comply with an early motion protocol, such as the modified Duran program. *It is not indicated for patients who have a simple primary repair.*

Repair of Flexor Pollicis Longus (FPL) of Thumb Early Mobilization*

Prerequisites:	compliant patient clean or healed wound
1 to 3 days	• Remove bulky compressive dressing and apply light compressive dressing; use finger socks or coban on thumb for edema control. • Fit DBS to wrist and thumb for continual wear in the following position: Wrist—20 degrees of palmar flexion Thumb MCP and interphalangeal (IP) joints—15 degrees of flexion at each joint Thumb carpometacarpal (CMC) joint—palmar abduction

■ *It is important to ensure that the thumb IP joint is in 15 degrees of flexion and is not extended. When the IP joint is left in a neutral position, restoration of IP flexion can be difficult.*

• Begin hourly controlled passive mobilization program within restraints of DBS:
8 repetitions passive flexion and extension of MCP joint (Fig. 1-6).
8 repetitions passive flexion and extension of IP joint (Fig. 1-7).
8 repetitions passive flexion and extension in composite manner of MCP and IP joints (Fig. 1-8).

REHABILITATION PROTOCOL—cont'd

4.5 weeks
- Remove DBS each hour to allow performance of the following exercises:
  10 repetitions active flexion and extension of wrist (Fig. 1-9).
  10 repetitions active flexion and extension of thumb (Fig. 1-10).
- Continue passive ROM exercises.
- Patient should wear DBS between exercise sessions and at night.

5 weeks
- May use FES or EMS within restraints of DBS to improve tendon excursion.

5.5 weeks
- Discontinue DBS.
- Begin hourly active ROM exercises:
  12 repetitions blocking of thumb IP joint (Fig. 1-11).
  12 repetitions composite active flexion and extension of thumb.
- Continue passive ROM exercises as necessary.

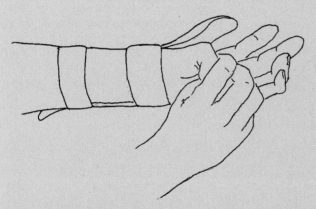

Figure 1-6 Passive flexion and extension of the MCP joint of the thumb.*

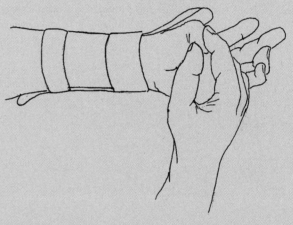

Figure 1-7 Passive flexion and extension of the IP joint of the thumb.*

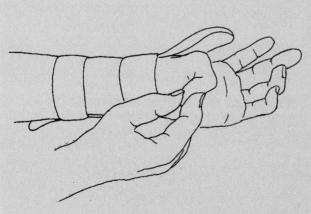

Figure 1-8 Passive flexion and extension of the MCP and IP joints in a composite manner.*

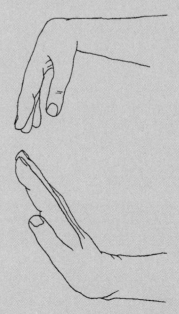

Figure 1-9 Active flexion and extension of the wrist.*

Continued

REHABILITATION PROTOCOL—cont'd

Repair of Flexor Pollicis Longus (FPL) of Thumb
Early Mobilization

6 weeks
- Begin passive ROM exercises in extension of wrist and thumb.
- If needed for extrinsic flexor tendon tightness in the FPL, a wrist and thumb static splint can be used to hold the wrist and thumb in extension. Often, a simple extension gutter splint in full extension can be used for night wear.

8 weeks
- Begin progressive strengthening with a Nerf ball and progress to a hand-helper.
- Do not allow lifting or heavy use of hand.

10 to
12 weeks
- Allow full use of the hand for most activities, including sports.
- ROM generally begins to plateau at approximately 7 to 8 weeks after surgery.
- If an associated digital nerve repair is under tension, position the thumb in 30 degrees of flexion at the MCP and IP joints.
- If passive flexion is limited, taping or dynamic flexion splinting may be used.
- Scar management, including scar retraction, scar massage, and the use of Otoform or Elastomer, may be used at 2 weeks after surgery.

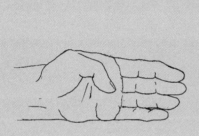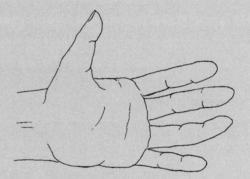

Figure 1-10 Active flexion and extension of the thumb.*

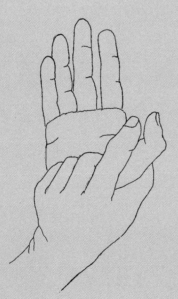

Figure 1-11 Blocking exercises of the thumb IP joint.*

REHABILITATION PROTOCOL

Repair of Flexor Pollicis Longus (FPL) of Thumb Delayed Mobilization*

Indications: crush injury
patient younger than 7 years of age
poor compliance and/or intelligence
soft tissue loss, wound management problems

3 weeks
• Remove bulky compressive dressing and apply light compressive dressing; use finger sock or Coban as needed for edema control.
• Fit DBS to wrist and thumb for continual wear in the following position:
Wrist—30 degrees of palmar flexion
Thumb CMC joint—palmar abduction
Thumb MCP and IP joints—15 degrees of flexion at each joint
• Begin hourly active and passive ROM exercises within restraints of DBS, including blocking exercises.
• If passive flexion of thumb is limited, taping or dynamic flexion splinting may be used.
• Begin scar massage and scar management techniques.

4.5 weeks
• Begin hourly active ROM exercises of wrist and thumb outside splint.
• May use FES or EMS to improve tendon excursion of FPL.

6 weeks
• Discontinue DBS.
• Begin passive ROM exercises in extension of wrist and thumb.
• If extrinsic flexor tendon tightness of FPL is present, a wrist and thumb static splint may be used as needed; the patient should wear the splint between exercise sessions and at night.
• Do not allow lifting or heavy use of the hand.

8 weeks
• Begin progressive strengthening with a Nerf ball or putty.

10 to 12 weeks
• Allow full use of hand for most activities.
• If associated digital nerve repair is under tension, position thumb MCP and IP joints in 30 degrees of flexion to minimize tension at repair site.
• Composite active flexion of the thumb tends to reach a plateau between 9 and 10 weeks after surgery.

The delayed mobilization program for FPL repairs is best reserved for patients with crush injuries, soft tissue loss, wound management problems, and patients in whom end-to-end repair was difficult.

REHABILITATION PROTOCOL

Two-Stage Reconstruction for Delayed Tendon Repair*

Stage 1 (Hunter rod)
BEFORE SURGERY
• Maximize passive ROM of digit with manual passive exercises, digital level taping, or dynamic splinting.
• Use scar management techniques to improve suppleness of soft tissues, including scar massage, scar retraction, and use of Otoform or Elastomer silicone molds.
• Begin strengthening exercises of future donor tendon to improve postoperative strength after stage 2 procedure.
• If needed for protection or assistance with ROM, use buddy taping of the involved digit.

AFTER SURGERY
5 to 7 days
• Remove bulky dressing and apply light compressive dressing; use digital-level finger socks or coban.
• Begin active and passive ROM exercises of hand for approximately 10 minutes, 6 times each day.
• Fit an extension gutter splint that holds the digit in full extension to wear between exercise sessions and at night.
• If pulleys have been reconstructed during stage 1, use taping for about 8 weeks during the postoperative phase.

Continued

Two-Stage Reconstruction for Delayed Tendon Repair

3 to 6 weeks • Gradually wean patient from extension gutter splint; continue buddy taping for protection.

■ *The major goal during stage 1 is to maintain passive ROM and obtain supple soft tissues before tendon grafting.*

Stage 2 (free tendon graft)
AFTER SURGERY
• Follow instructions for early motion program for zones 1 through 3 (modified Duran protocol) on p. 4 or the delayed mobilization program for zones 1 through 5 on p. 8.
• For most patients, the modified Duran program is preferable to the delayed mobilization program because it encourages greater excursion of the graft and helps maintain passive ROM through the early mobilization exercises.
• Do not use FES before 5 to 5.5 weeks after surgery because of the initial avascularity of the tendon graft. Also consider the reasons for failure of the primary repair.

TRIGGER FINGER AND THUMB

Trigger finger (stenosing flexor tenosynovitis) is a painful snapping or triggering of the digit during active motion. The smooth gliding of the flexor tendon below the first annular pulley (A1) is disrupted, causing snapping. Trigger finger usually can be treated with modification of activities that require repetitive grasping or power gripping. A conservative approach should be chosen for patients with mild symptoms or for those who have responded favorably to previous conservative measures. Even patients with locked thumbs or fingers who have had symptoms for a long time may respond to injection of the tendon sheath (not the tendon) with cortisone and splinting (see box). Some authors recommend an MCP block splint with the MCP joint immobilized at neutral for several weeks.

The length of the conservative program depends on the patient's avocational and vocational tolerance to the disability. Patients who have continued triggering or pain, especially involving more than one finger, and patients who have had symptoms for longer than 4 months are less likely to improve with conservative treatment and should be considered candidates for surgery.

Management of Trigger Finger and Thumb

Symptoms of Less than 3 Weeks Duration
• A thumb spica splint or dorsal MCP splint is used to block the MCP joint to 60 degrees of flexion.
• Nonsteroidal antiinflammatory medication
• Alleviation of inciting factors such as scissoring or gripping activities

Symptoms of More than 3 Weeks Duration
• Steroid injection
• Splinting
• Nonsteroidal antiinflammatory agent
• Alleviation of inciting factors

Trigger Digit Release

0 to 2 days • Remove soft postoperative dressing 24 to 48 hours after surgery. Encourage full active thumb and digital motion before and after removal of the dressing.
• Apply a light dressing 2 or 3 days after surgery. Initiate edema control with a compressive dressing or elastic stockinette.

1 week • Begin active and passive ROM exercises for 10 minutes each hour.
• Avoid splinting if possible.

2 to 4 weeks • Remove the sutures.
• Begin scar massage with lotion and/or the use of Otoform or Elastomer within 24 hours of suture removal.
• Gradually increase resistive exercises.

REHABILITATION PROTOCOL—cont'd

4 to 6 weeks	• Continue progressive strengthening as needed. Have patient avoid continuous and repetitive grasping and releasing of the hand for long periods. • Scar tenderness in the palm and the base of the thumb may persist for 6 weeks or longer and may require desensitization techniques.	• Tight-grip or full-grip strength activity may require protective padding over the surgery site for extended periods. • For patients with rheumatoid arthritis and those whose triggering results from a blunt or penetrating trauma, consider alternative sites of triggering, such as rheumatoid nodules more distally in the finger or irregularities from partial tendon ruptures or lacerations.

FLEXOR CARPI RADIALIS TUNNEL SYNDROME

Tenderness along the flexor carpi radialis (FCR) tendon with resisted wrist flexion is a relatively rare, disabling disorder. Pain relief with a Xylocaine injection into the FCR tendon sheath helps to make this diagnosis.

Conservative Management
• Avoidance of resisted wrist flexion activities
• Nightly splint wear for 6 weeks
• Daily splint wear for pain relief
• Nonsteroidal antiinflammatory medication
• Steroid injection into FCR tendon sheath

Nonoperative measures may be prolonged as long as the patient's vocational activities allows.

Surgical Management
Surgical management for FCR tunnel syndrome primarily consists of decompression of the FCR tendon and lysis of abnormal adhesions within the FCR tunnel.

REHABILITATION PROTOCOL

Decompression of Flexor Carpi Radialis Tunnel Syndrome

0 to 7 days	• Begin active wrist extension and flexion exercises in the soft surgical dressing.	2 to 4 weeks	• Begin gradual resisted flexion and extension exercises; continue full motion and desensitization techniques as necessary.
7 days	• Remove the surgical dressing and encourage free wrist flexion and extension exercises with interval splinting.	4 to 6 weeks	• Allow full activities with night splinting for comfort • Discontinue the splint at 6 weeks and allow full activity.
2 weeks	• Remove sutures and begin desensitization techniques.		

Extensor Tendon Injuries

REHABILITATION RATIONALE AND BASIC PRINCIPLES

Anatomy
Extensor mechanism injuries are conveniently grouped into eight anatomic zones according to Kleinert and Verdan. Odd-number zones overlie the joint levels so that zones 1, 3, 5, and 7 correspond to the DIP, PIP, MCP, and wrist joint regions, respectively (Figs. 1-12, 1-13, and Table 1-2). Normal extensor mechanism activity relies on concerted function between the intrinsic muscles of the hand and the extrinsic extensor tendons. Fig. 1-14 shows the normal relationships between these two systems and some fundamental relationships necessary to understanding digital extension.

Even though PIP and DIP joint extension is normally controlled by the intrinsic muscles of the hand (interossei and lumbricals), the extrinsic tendons may provide satisfactory digital extension when MCP joint hyperextension is prevented. Moreover, an injury at one zone typically produces compensatory imbalance in neighboring zones; for example, a closed mallet finger deformity may be accompanied by a more striking secondary swan-neck deformity at the PIP joint.

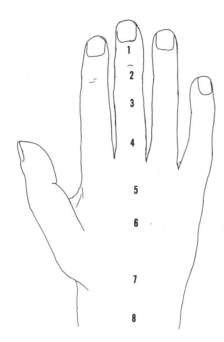

Figure 1-12 Zones of the extensor tendons.

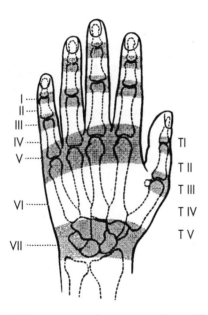

Figure 1-13 Extensor tendon zones. (From Kleinert HE, Schepel S, Gill T: Flexor tendon injuries, *Surg Clin North Am* 61:267, 1981.)

Disruption of the terminal slip tendon allows the extensor mechanism to migrate proximally and exert a hyperextension force to the PIP joint by the central slip attachment. Thus, extensor tendon injuries cannot be considered simply static disorders.

Treatment: Zones 1 and 2 Extensor Tendon Injuries

Pediatric

Injuries in children should be considered Salter-Harris type I or III physeal injuries (Fig. 1-15). Splint-

	Extensor	
Zone	**Finger**	**Thumb**
1	DIP joint	IP joint
2	Middle phalanx	Proximal phalanx
3	Apex PIP joint	MCP joint
4	Proximal phalanx	Metacarpal
5	Apex MCP joint	
6	Dorsal hand	
7	Dorsal retinaculum	Dorsal retinaculum
8	Distal forearm	Distal forearm

TABLE 1-2 Zones of Injury

From Kleinert HE, Verdan C: Report of the committee on tendon injuries, *J Hand Surg* 8:794, 1983.

ing of extremely small digits is difficult and fixing the joint in full extension for 4 weeks produces satisfactory results. Open injuries are especially difficult to splint and the DIP joint may be transfixed with a 22-gauge needle.

Adult

Closed mallet injuries in adults are managed with 6 weeks of splinting with a mallet-finger splint that holds the DIP joint in extension. When external splinting is not possible or when a mallet deformity results from an acute open injury, pinning for 6 weeks with a 0.045 Kirschner wire may be preferred. The wire is removed at 6 weeks and the remainder of the closed extensor program is followed.

Bony mallet deformities may be managed closed, unless the fragment is 50% or more of the articular surface. This may result in joint subluxation, and pin fixation and open reduction may be required. In any event, 6 weeks of immobilization precedes initiation of DIP exercises with interval splinting.

Mallet injuries that do not respond to a splinting program and those of 3 to 6 months duration are classified as *chronic*. Further splinting may be attempted, with full extension splinting for 8 weeks initially, or, if the deformity is unacceptable, surgical correction may be indicated. Motion-preserving procedures are reserved for nonarthritic DIP joints with a minimum passive ROM of 50 degrees. Fixed deformities and painful degenerative joints are best managed by arthrodesis.

Rehabilitation

Extensor tendon treatment protocol selection depends on the mechanism of injury and the time elapsed since the injury. The following protocols apply to isolated zonal extensor tendon disruptions.

Clearly, modifications of these programs will be dictated by other concomitant injuries.

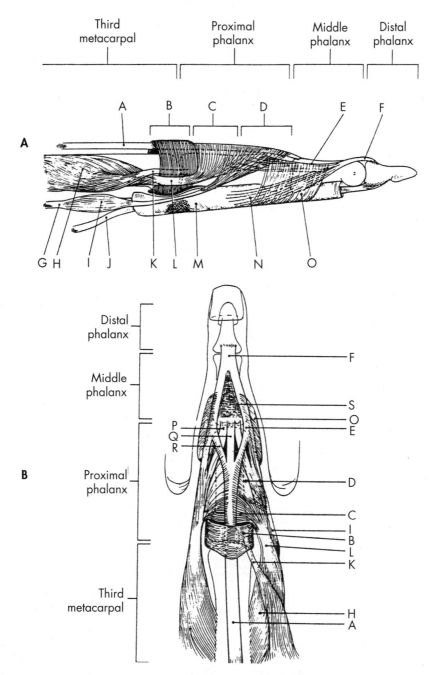

Figure 1-14 Diagrammatic representation of dorsal apparatus of finger. **A,** Radial side of left middle finger. **B,** Dorsum of left middle finger. *A,* Extensor digitorum communis tendon; *B,* sagittal bands; *C,* transverse fibers of intrinsic muscle apparatus; *D,* oblique fibers of intrinsic apparatus; *E,* conjoined lateral band; *F,* terminal tendon; *G,* flexor digitorum profundus tendon; *H,* second dorsal interosseous muscle; *I,* lumbrical muscle; *J,* flexor digitorum superficialis tendon; *K,* medial tendon of superficial belly of interosseous; *L,* lateral tendon of deep belly of interosseous; *M,* flexor pulley mechanism; *N,* oblique retinacular ligament; *O,* transverse retinacular ligament; *P,* medial band of oblique fibers of intrinsic expansion; *Q,* central slip; *R,* lateral slips; *S,* triangular ligament. (From Smith RJ: Balance and kinetics of the fingers under normal and pathological conditions, *Clin Orthop* 104:95, 1974.)

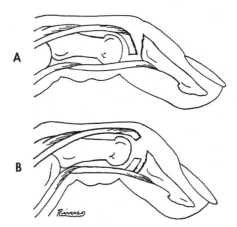

Figure 1-15 Two types of mallet equivalent epiphyseal fractures in child. **A,** Salter-Harris type I fracture. **B,** Salter-Harris type III fracture. (Redrawn from Wood VE: *Orthop Clin North Am* 7:527, 1976.)

REHABILITATION PROTOCOL

Acute Extensor Tendon Injuries in Zones 1 and 2

0 to 6 weeks	• Treat closed mallet injuries of adults with a mallet finger splint with the DIP joint in 0 to 15 degrees of of hyperextension. • Apply the mallet splint volar or dorsal to allow sensory input to the palmar surface of the finger. • Permit splint removal for hygienic purposes while the ipsilateral thumb maintains the splinted posture of the DIP joint. • Encourage full MCP and PIP joint motion during splinting.	6 to 9 weeks	• Begin weaning from the splint if no extensor lag is present after splint removal. Begin active DIP flexion with interval splinting between hourly exercises. Continue night splinting until the eighth week. • Should a DIP joint extensor lag exceed 10 degrees after the initial 6-week splinting period, reinstitute night splinting for 2 more weeks or until a satisfactory result is obtained.

REHABILITATION PROTOCOL

Chronic Extensor Injuries in Zones 1 and 2

Tenodermodesis

Tenodermodesis is a simple procedure used in relatively young patients who are unable to accept the mallet finger disability. With the use of a local anesthetic, the DIP joint is fully extended and the redundant pseudotendon is excised so that the edges of the tendon coapt (Fig. 1-16). A temporary Kirschner wire may be used to fix the DIP joint in full extension.

Central Slip Tenotomy (Fowler)

With the use of a local anesthetic, section the insertion of the central slip where it blends with the PIP joint dorsal capsule. The combined lateral band and the extrinsic contribution should be left undisturbed. Proximal migration of the dorsal apparatus improves the extensor force at the DIP joint. A 10- to 15-degree extensor lag at the PIP joint may occur.

Oblique Retinacular Ligament Reconstruction

Reconstruction of the oblique retinacular ligament is used for correction of a chronic mallet finger deformity and secondary swanneck deformity. A free tendon graft, such as the palmaris longus tendon, is passed from the dorsal base of the distal phalanx and volar to the axis of the PIP joint. The graft is anchored to the contralateral side of the proximal phalanx at the fibroosseous rim (Fig. 1-17). Kirschner wires temporarily fix the DIP in full extension and the PIP joint in 10 to 15 degrees of flexion.

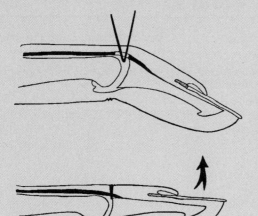

Figure 1-16 Technical principle: excision of skin and tendon callus. (From Iselin F, Levame J, Godoy J: A simplified technique for treatment of mallet fingers: tenodermodesis, *J Hand Surg* 2(2):118, 1977.)

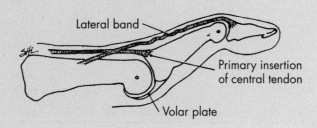

Lateral band

Primary insertion of central tendon

Volar plate

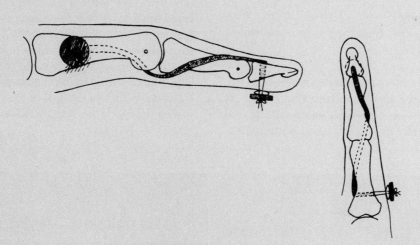

Figure 1-17 Palmaris longus tenodesis for oblique retinacular ligament reconstruction for swan-neck deformity, called the spiral oblique retinacular ligament. The pathology of the swan-neck deformity involves hyperextension of the PIP joint with extensor lag at the distal joint, combined with a laxity of the volar plate. The palmaris longus can be used to provide a tenodesis to correct the imbalance at both joints. This procedure uses the palmaris longus tendon as a graft rather than the oblique retinacular ligament, thus making a simpler dissection. It is also easier to adjust the tension of this tenodesis. (Redrawn from Thompson JS, Littler JW, Upton J: The spiral oblique retinacular ligament: SORL, *J Hand Surg* 3:482, 1978.)

Continued

REHABILITATION PROTOCOL—cont'd

Chronic Extensor Injuries in Zones 1 and 2

Tenodermodesis—cont'd		Central Slip Tenotomy (Fowler)—cont'd		Oblique Retinacular Ligament Reconstruction—cont'd	
3 to 5 days	• Remove the postoperative splint and fit the DIP joint with an extension splint. A pin protection splint may be necessary if the pin is left exposed; however, some patients have their pins buried to allow unsplinted use of the finger. PIP joint exercises are begun to maintain full PIP motion.	0 to 2 weeks	• The postsurgical dressing maintains the PIP joint at 45 degrees of flexion and the DIP joint at 0 degrees.	3 weeks	• Remove the bulky postoperative dressing and sutures. Withdraw the PIP joint pin and begin PIP joint active flexion and extension exercises.
		2 to 4 weeks	• Allow active DIP extension and flexion. Allow full extension of PIP joint from 45 degrees of flexion.	4 to 5 weeks	• Withdraw the DIP joint pin and begin full active and passive PIP and DIP joint exercises.
5 weeks	• Remove the Kirschner wire and begin active DIP motion with interval splinting. • Continue the nightly splinting for an additional 3 weeks.	4 weeks	• Begin full finger motion exercises.		• Supplement home exercises with a supervised program over the next 2 to 3 weeks to achieve full motion. • Continue the interval splinting of the DIP joint in full extension until 6 weeks after the operation.

EXTENSOR TENDON INJURIES IN ZONE 3

Boutonnière Deformity

■ *Rupture of the central slip is the cardinal anatomic disruption leading to boutonnière deformity.*

Anatomy

This injury results in an inability to extend the PIP joint from a 90-degree flexed posture (Fig. 1-18). As the triangular fibers become attenuated, the lateral bands migrate laterally and volarly and become flexors of the PIP joint. This volar subluxation of the lateral bands increases the force of the terminal slip, resulting in DIP joint hyperextension. Persistent deformity allows the lateral bands to become fixed volarly by the contracted transverse retinacular ligaments. The oblique retinacular ligaments also become contracted, so that extension of the PIP joint limits flexion of the DIP joint (Fig. 1-19).

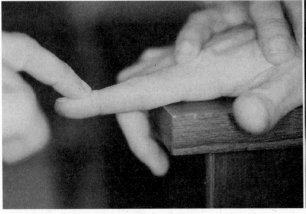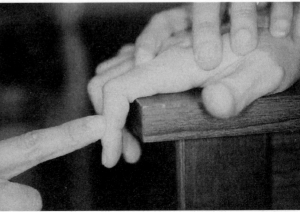

Figure 1-18 Slide Elson test.

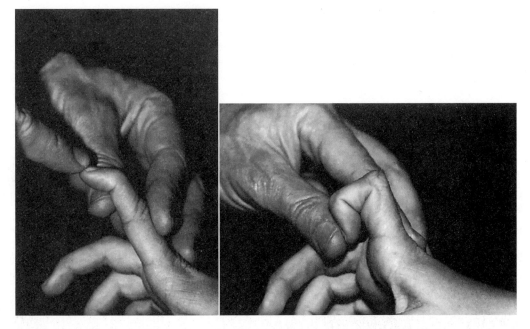

Figure 1-19 The oblique retinacular ligament tightness test. The DIP joint is passively flexed with the PIP joint held in extension. The DIP joint is then passively flexed with the PIP joint flexed. If there is greater motion when the PIP joint is flexed than when it is extended, there is a contracture of the ligament. Equal loss of DIP joint motion regardless of PIP joint position indicates a joint contracture. (From Hunter JM et al: *Rehabilitation of the hand*, ed 4, St. Louis, 1995, Mosby.)

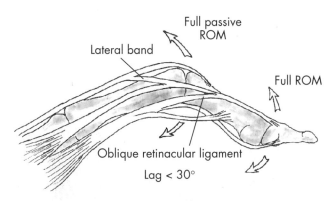

Figure 1-20 Range of motion in boutonnière deformity. (From Kiefhaber TR: *Boutonnière and swan-neck deformity*. Presented at the 45th annual instructional course symposium: *The extensor mechanism anatomy, injury, & reconstruction*, Toronto, Sept, 1990.)

	TABLE 1-3 **Stages of Boutonnière Deformity**		
Stage	**PIP extension lag**		**DIP changes**
1	<30 degrees active, full passive		Full flexion
2	>30 degrees, full passive		Full flexion
3	>30 degrees, full passive		Limited flexion
4	Fixed deformity		Fixed hyperextension
5	Arthritic joint		Fixed hyperextension

Classification

Central slip disruptions result in a predictable pattern of chronologic changes that has prompted a variety of staging systems for boutonnière deformities. These systems are designed to assist with outcome studies and to aid in treatment selection. Anatomic features of the deformities can be inferred from this grouping. These features will have some bearing on the treatment method chosen (Table 1-3).

Nonoperative treatment

Stage 1 (acute) deformity results from disruption of the central slip and translation of the lateral bands volar to the axis of the PIP joint flexion (Fig. 1-20). The patient can resist extension when the PIP joint is in full extension but is unable to extend this joint from a flexed posture. Fractures of the base of the middle phalanx are rare, and surgical intervention is indicated only when the fragment is large or the fragments are significantly displaced. Small fragments may be excised and the protocol for the open deformity followed.

In *stage 2 deformities,* more volar advancement of the lateral bands results in a greater flexed posture of the PIP joint than in stage 1 deformities. Because complete passive correction of the PIP and DIP joints is still possible in this stage, treatment is analogous to that of closed stage 1 deformity.

In *stage 3 deformities*, the PIP flexion deformity is passively correctable, although the oblique retinacular ligaments become contracted because of the relatively chronic boutonnière posture. *Emphasis on DIP joint flexion exercises is most important while maintaining full PIP joint extension splinting.* These deformities rarely require surgical intervention, but long-term splinting may be required. If a stage 3 deformity is not corrected after several months of splinting (PIP joint extensor lag greater than 20 degrees and DIP joint resting in hyperextension and active flexion less than 20 to 30 degrees), surgical intervention may be indicated.

REHABILITATION PROTOCOL
Stage 1, 2, or 3 Boutonnière Deformity

0 to 4 weeks (PIP immobilization phase)
- Hold the PIP joint in full extension with the DIP joint free.
- Begin active and passive flexion exercises to the DIP joint 5 minutes per hour daily (Fig. 1-21). This helps maintain or relocate the lateral bands dorsally, prevents contracture of the oblique retinacular ligaments, and maintains DIP joint motion.
- Allow removal of the splint for hygienic purposes while the PIP joint is maintained in full extension. The patient should perform gentle scar massage over the PIP joint twice daily to help prevent adhesions.

4 to 6 weeks (early PIP mobilization phase)
- Continue the splint at night, removing it hourly throughout the day; begin active PIP flexion exercises.
- At the fifth week from injury, begin active-assisted PIP joint exercises.

6 to 8 weeks (late PIP mobilization phase)
- Discontinue the splint during the day and begin gentle passive PIP flexion exercises.
- An extensor lag of more than 10 degrees during this period requires an additional 2 weeks of interval splinting.
- Continue night splinting.

8 to 10 weeks (aggressive PIP mobilization phase)
- Begin gentle passive flexion and resistive PIP joint extension. PIP joint flexion may be assisted by dynamic flexion or taping modalities (Fig. 1-22).
- Discontinue night splinting at the end of the tenth week only if an extensor lag does not develop.
- An extensor lag that develops during this period requires continued night splinting and a dynamic PIP extension splint during the day until elimination of the extensor lag.

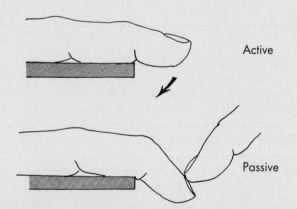

Figure 1-21 Active and passive DIP exercises for mallet deformity.

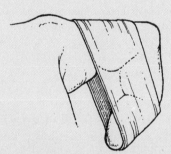

Figure 1-22 Taping for mallet finger. (From Fess EE, Gettle KS, Strickland JW: *Hand splinting principles and methods*, St. Louis, 1981, Mosby.)

Operative Treatment

Open boutonnière injuries require thorough PIP joint exploration and debridement before pinning the PIP joint in full extension. Tendon repair or reconstruction is performed once the PIP joint is fixed. Insufficient or severely damaged tendons, as may result from abrasion injuries, require rearrangement of local tissues for appropriate central and terminal slip reconstruction. The Snow technique uses a proximally based central section of the central tendon, and Aiche, Barsky, and Weiner use portions of the lateral bands to bridge the defect in the central tendon (Fig. 1-23).

In 1965, Dolphin described a technique in which the terminal slip is transected distal to the triangular ligament (Fig. 1-24). This procedure should be reserved for passively correctable (stage 2 or 3) deformities. At approximately 10 days after surgery, the postoperative dressing is removed and full use is resumed.

Fixed PIP flexion and DIP extension contractures signify *stage 4 deformities.* Besides contracture of the oblique retinacular ligaments, the lateral bands become fixed volarly by contracted transverse retinacular ligaments. The resultant recalcitrant PIP joint flexion contracture is often accompanied by collateral ligament, volar plate, and flexor tendon sheath contractures. These deformities almost always require operative correction.

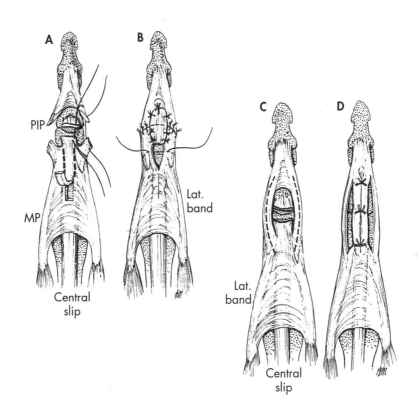

Figure 1-23 Acute boutonnière deformities associated with loss of substance of the extensor mechanism at the PIP joint are difficult to treat. In an attempt to solve this problem, a retrograde flap is taken from the central slip of the extensor **(A)** and applied as a reinforcing batten over the central slip repair. The retrograde flap is carefully sutured into place over the repair site to act as a reinforcement in the area of repair. The defect in the central slip is then closed with interrupted sutures **(B).** Cases of acute disruption of the extensor tendon over the PIP joint with shredded tendon and loss of tendon substance have been described. In those cases, primary reconstruction of the central slip is performed by identifying and dissecting free the two lateral bands from the oblique and transverse retinacular ligaments. These bands are then split longitudinally for about 2 cm **(C)** and their middle segments reapproximated in the midline over the base of the middle phalanx with 5-0 nonabsorbable suture **(D).** The lateral segments are left in position and represent the lumbrical insertions and retinacular ligaments, to aid in prevention of the boutonnière deformity. (From Doyle JR: *Extensor tendons—acute injuries.* In Green D, editor: *Operative hand surgery,* ed 3, 1993, Churchill Livingstone.)

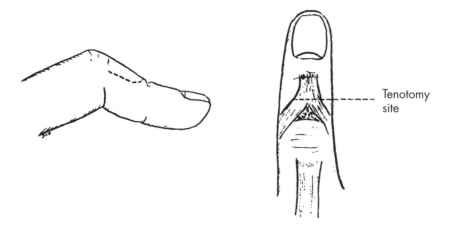

Figure 1-24 Extensor tenotomy. (Redrawn from Dolphin JA: Extensor tenotomy for chronic boutonnière deformity of the finger: report of two cases, *J Bone Joint Surg* 47A:161, 1965.)

Tenotomy site

Curtis, Reid, and Provost technique

The use of a local anesthetic allows the identification of the degree of deformity, which is corrected by a series of standardized steps.

Step 1 • Free the transverse retinacular ligaments with a blunt probe and perform an extensor tenolysis (Fig. 1-25). If full active PIP joint extension is not achieved, perform step 2.

Step 2 • Section the transverse retinacular ligaments along their length volar to the lateral bands, allowing the extensor mechanism to migrate proximally and the lateral bands dorsally. Full active PIP joint extension after these steps indicates the need for the following rehabilitation program:

0 to 7 days • Splint the PIP and DIP joints in full extension and the MCP joint in 70 degrees of flexion.

1 to 3 weeks • With a dorsal plaster splint, block the MCP joint to 70 degrees of flexion and apply a dynamic extension outrigger to the PIP joint.
• Allow active PIP and DIP joint flexion and extension.
• Discontinue splinting at 3 weeks.

The absence of full active extension indicates that the central slip has healed with laxity and requires a different approach.

Step 3 • Treat a PIP joint extensor lag of less than 20 degrees by step-cutting the lateral bands over the middle phalanx. The extensor mechanism will advance proximally and decrease the laxity of the central slip (Fig. 1-26). If there is full extension of the PIP joint after this step, use the following rehabilitation protocol.

0 to 4 weeks • Apply a mallet finger splint and leave the PIP joint free for full active motion.

4 to 6 weeks • Apply a mallet finger splint intermittently during the day and at night. Discontinue night splinting at the sixth week if an extensor lag does not develop.
• Advance DIP exercises as necessary during this period to achieve full motion.

Step 4 • A PIP joint extensor lag of more than 20 degrees requires shortening of the central slip (Fig. 1-27). A 4- to 6-mm section of the tendon is removed, overlapped, and sutured into a drill hole in the base of the middle phalanx. Alternatively, any of the anatomic central slip reconstruction procedures may be used in this step.

Anatomic Central Slip Reconstruction

The attenuated central slip and its resultant pseudotendon significantly decrease PIP joint extensor force. Procedures designed for direct correction of the central slip laxity are considered anatomic reconstructions. Adequate soft tissue over the PIP joints is a prerequisite for these procedures.

Elliott Procedure. A transverse portion of the lengthened central slip is removed and the tendon ends are repaired by sutures. An extensor tenolysis over the proximal and middle phalanges precedes dorsal relo-

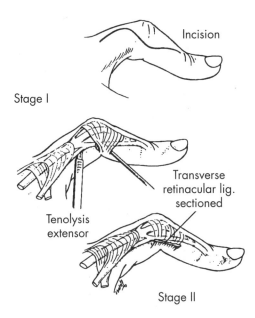

Figure 1-25 Stage 1, tenolysis of extensor tendon: freeing of transverse retinacular ligament, and stage 2, tenolysis of extensor tendon: sectioning of transverse retinacular ligament. (Redrawn from Curtis RM, Reid RL, Provost JM: A staged technique for the repair of traumatic boutonnière deformity, *J Hand Surg* 8(2):168, 1983.)

cation of the lateral bands and suture of the triangular ligament (Fig. 1-28).

Grundberg Procedure. This technique is similar to the Elliott procedure except that the lateral bands are not translocated dorsally. The undersurface of the proximal portion of the central slip exposes a 3-mm, yellowish, abnormal section of the tendon, which is excised. The lateral bands are not sutured to the central slip. The PIP joint is pinned in full extension and the tendon ends are sutured end to end with 5-0 merselene suture.

Urbaniak Procedure. A distally based capsular flap is combined with a proximally based tendon flap. The distally based flap is brought through an aperture in the proximally based triangular flap (Fig. 1-29). The PIP joint is pinned in full extension and the proximal flap is oversewn onto the distal flap.

Kilgore and Graham Procedure. A V-shaped segment of the central slip tissue is removed to allow a longer suture line and a more secure repair. If too large a segment of the central slip is excised, proper length can be restored with a V-Y suture technique.

Lateral Band Transfer

Matev Procedure. The lateral bands are used to compensate for deficient central slip tissue. The two lateral bands are sectioned, one proximally at the base of the middle phalanx and one distally at the inser-

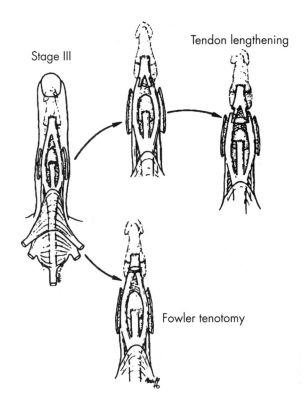

Figure 1-26 Stage 3, lengthening of lateral bands over middle phalanx or tenotomy of extensor tendon. (Redrawn from Curtis RM, Reid RL, Provost JM: A staged technique for the repair of traumatic boutonnière deformity, *J Hand Surg* 8(2):168, 1983.)

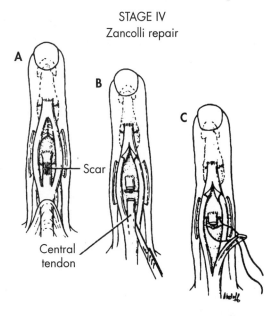

Figure 1-27 Stage 4, repair of central extensor tendon. (Redrawn from Curtis RM, Reid RL, Provost JM: A staged technique for the repair of traumatic boutonnière deformity, *J Hand Surg* 8(2):168, 1983.)

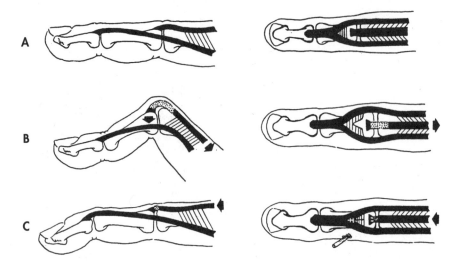

Figure 1-28 Correction of the established mobile boutonnière deformity. **A,** Normal anatomic relations. **B,** Deformity with retracted central tendon and scar bridge, tear in triangular ligament area, and displacement of lateral bands below axis of middle joint. **C,** Anatomic repair with fixation of middle joint in full extension. (From Elliott RA Jr: Injuries to the extensor mechanism of the hand, *Orthop Clin North Am* 1:335, 1970.)

tion to the distal phalanx (Fig. 1-30). The proximal segment is sutured into tissue at the base of the middle phalanx to reconstruct the central slip. The terminal slip is reconstructed by suturing the long proximal segment of one lateral band to the long distal segment of the contralateral lateral band.

Littler Procedure. Both lateral band segments are used to form the central slip. The remaining distal portions of the lateral bands are sutured to the reconstructed central slip. The lumbrical insertion to the terminal slip and the oblique retinacular ligaments are left undisturbed.

REHABILITATION PROTOCOL

Boutonnière Deformity (Open Injury or Surgically Treated)

0 to 2 weeks (immediate postoperative phase)
- Have patient perform DIP flexion exercises hourly from the time of surgery until the first follow-up office visit.
- Remove the sutures and initiate pin site and wound care management.
- Use nonsterile cotton swabs with hydrogen peroxide to remove crusted material from the pin-skin interface and allow free egress of fluid from the pin sites.
- Do not permit soaking of the hand, although showering over the exposed pin is allowed.
- Fashion a protective splint for night use.

2 to 4 weeks (PIP immobilization phase)
- Continue active and passive DIP motion exercises and scar massage to break up the postsurgical adhesions; this facilitates tendon glide during the period of PIP mobilization.
- Fit a PIP extension splint to be removed for hygienic purposes only.

4 to 6 weeks (early PIP mobilization phase)
- The remainder of the open protocol follows the plan for closed boutonnière deformities (see p. 20).

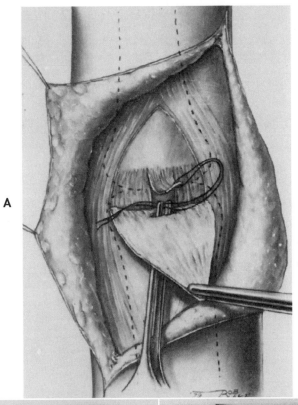

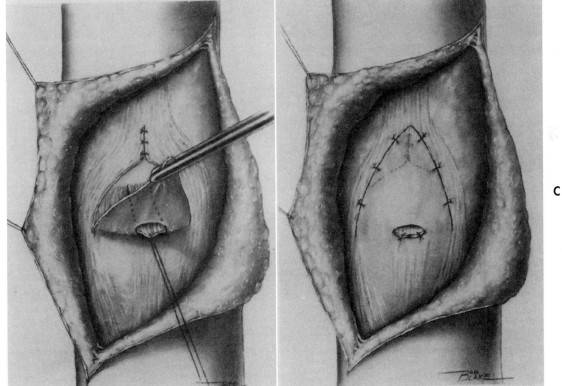

Figure 1-29 A, Dorsal view at PIP joint shows distally based capsular flap being pulled through transverse slit in proximally based flap to reconstruct central slip. **B,** Lateral bands are carefully approximated with two or three interrupted sutures after tongue of capsule is pulled through proximally based flap of extensor tendon. **C,** Final position of two triangular flaps. Proximally based flap is sutured over two distally approximated lateral bands. (From Urbaniak JR, Hayes MG: Chronic boutonnière deformity: an anatomic reconstruction. *J Hand Surg* 6(4):379, 1981.)

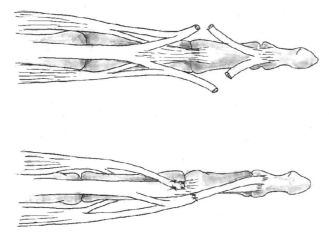

Figure 1-30 Matev procedure: Tenolysis of the extensor apparatus (Matev). Section one lateral band at the middle of P2 and the other at its insertion. Use the short proximal lateral band to reconstruct the central tendon. Transpose the longer proximal lateral band to the longest stump of the tendon. This lengthens the terminal tendon and allows DIP flexion. (From Matev, I: Transposition of the lateral slips of the aponeurosis in treatment of long-standing boutonnière deformity of the fingers, *Brit J Plas Surg* 17:281, 1964.)

REHABILITATION PROTOCOL
Stage 4 Boutonnière Deformity

0 to 4 weeks (PIP extension phase)
- Reestablishing full PIP joint extension requires dynamic splinting with aggressive PIP joint passive extension exercises. Serial casting may be beneficial in alleviating the flexion contracture.
- After full PIP joint extension is achieved, the DIP flexion phase can be initiated. Splint the PIP joint in full extension for 6 weeks once full extension is achieved.
- Failure to gain full PIP joint extension requires a surgical release of the PIP flexion contracture release by capsulotomy before a boutonnière reconstruction.

■ *Repeated recurrence of PIP joint contracture after nonoperative correction is an indication for early boutonnière reconstruction.*

6 to 10 weeks (DIP flexion phase)
- Address the DIP extension contracture by active, active-assisted, and passive DIP flexion exercises.

- The patient should spend 5 to 10 minutes each hour regaining DIP joint flexion.
- If 40 to 50 degrees of DIP flexion cannot be achieved, surgical intervention may be necessary.

10 to 14 weeks
- Splint the PIP joint in full extension for 6 weeks after full DIP flexion is achieved.
- Continue DIP joint flexion exercises 5 minutes hourly.

14 to 16 weeks
- Continue interval daily splinting between PIP joint flexion exercises and night splinting for 2 more weeks.
- A PIP joint extension lag greater than 10 to 15 degrees requires night and daily interval splinting until satisfactory results are obtained.
- If there is no PIP joint extensor lag at this point, the passive ROM and dynamic splinting may be used to gain motion.

Boutonnière Deformity in Patients With Rheumatoid Arthritis

Synovitis and subsequent capsular and central slip laxity at the PIP joint result in the rheumatoid boutonnière triad, which includes the following: PIP joint flexion, DIP joint hyperextension, and MCP joint hyperextension.

Rheumatoid boutonnière deformities are classified into 3 stages (Table 1-4), with treatment dependant on severity of the deformity (Table 1-5).

Rehabilitation

The rehabilitation of the surgically managed rheumatoid boutonnière deformity is the same as that for the nonrheumatoid boutonnière deformity (p. 20), unless arthroplasty or fusion is performed.

SWAN-NECK DEFORMITY (ZONE 3 EXTENSOR TENDON DISORDER)

Hyperextension at the PIP joint and flexion at the DIP joint may be caused by a variety of pathologic condi-

TABLE 1-4 **Classification of Rheumatoid Boutonnière Deformity**

Stage	MCP joint	PIP joint	DIP joint
1 (mild)	Normal	Slight extension lag (10 to 15 degrees)	With or without hyperextension; limited flexion
2 (moderate)	Hyperextension	Extensor lag of 30 to 40 degrees	Hyperextension
3 (severe)	Hyperextension	Fixed flexion	Fixed hyperextension

TABLE 1-5 **Treatment Options for Rheumatoid Boutonnière Deformity**

Stage	Treatment options
1	• Observation • Steroid injection • PIP synovectomy • Extensor tenotomy (Dolphin procedure) to improve PIP flexion
2	• Dolphin procedure and central slip reconstruction with local tissues
3	• PIP fusion arthroplasty • Soft tissue reconstruction (rare)

tions. Joint force imbalance may be associated with a pathologic condition at the PIP joint or may be secondary to tendon imbalance distally (as from a mallet finger deformity) or proximally (as with intrinsic muscle contracture). The treatment chosen should correct the original pathologic condition and the changes resulting from the chronicity of the pathologic process.

Classification

The staging system of swan-neck deformities developed by Nalebuff, Feldon, and Millender is based on intrinsic tightness and the passive mobility of the PIP and DIP joints (Table 1-6).

Treatment

■ *The primary goal of operative correction of swan-neck deformity is to limit PIP hyperextension; the early phase of the rehabilitation emphasizes this. These deformities almost always require surgical correction.*

Type I Deformities—Swan-Neck

Swan-neck deformities secondary to DIP joint pathology are related mainly to mallet finger disorders (see p. 14). Swan-neck deformities secondary to relative lengthening of the terminal slip can occur after middle phalanx shortening from bone loss or malunions. Treatment depends on the surgeon's preference; the appropriate rehabilitation protocol follows each procedure.

Beckenbaugh Procedure. Dorsal fracture-dislocations of the PIP joint, sublimis tendon lacerations, ruptures or transfers, and rheumatoid synovitis are some of the common problems that result in loss of volar soft tissue restraints. The Beckenbaugh procedure corrects PIP joint hyperextension by using the sublimis tendon(s) to recreate a competent volar soft-tissue sling. The sublimis tendon is anchored to the A2 pulley and serves as a static restraint to PIP joint hyperextension (Fig. 1-31). If DIP joint flexion persists at the end of the procedure, the DIP joint is pinned in full extension.

REHABILITATION PROTOCOL

Beckenbaugh Procedure for Swan-Neck Deformity

3 days	• Remove the postoperative dressing and begin motion exercises. • Fit a night extension splint to keep the MCP joints in full extension and the PIP joints in 20 degrees of flexion.	2 weeks	• Remove sutures and begin scar massage. Continue night splinting.
		3 weeks	• Pull the DIP pin and continue night splinting until 6 weeks after surgery.

Type II Deformities—Swan Neck

Causes of intrinsic contractures include trauma, rheumatoid arthritis, stroke, cerebral palsy, and closed head injury. Intrinsic tightness is present when MCP joint extension limits active and passive PIP joint flexion. One side of the intrinsics may be the primary deforming force, causing the involved finger to deviate toward the pathologic side with passive MCP joint extension. In this situation, selective intrinsic releases may be performed.

TABLE 1-6 **Classification of Swan-Neck Deformities**

Type	Tightness	PIP motion	Adhesions
I	No	Supple in any MCP position	None
II	Yes	Limited with MCP extended; full passive motion	None
III	Yes	Limited in any MCP position	Tendon adhesions, capsular contractures
IV	Yes	Fixed in hyperextension	Tendon adhesions, capsular contractures, joint destruction

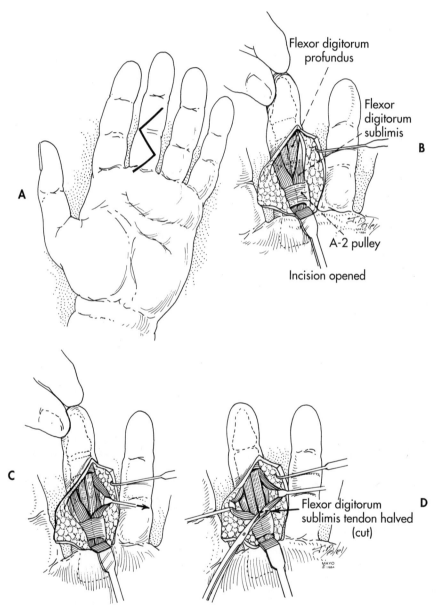

Figure 1-31 A-H, Beckenbaugh technique for correcting hyperextension deformity of the PIP joint. (From Phillip E, Wright PE II: *Arthritic hand.* In Crenshaw AH, editor: *Campbell's operative orthopaedics,* vol 5, ed 8, St. Louis, Mosby–Year Book, 1992.)

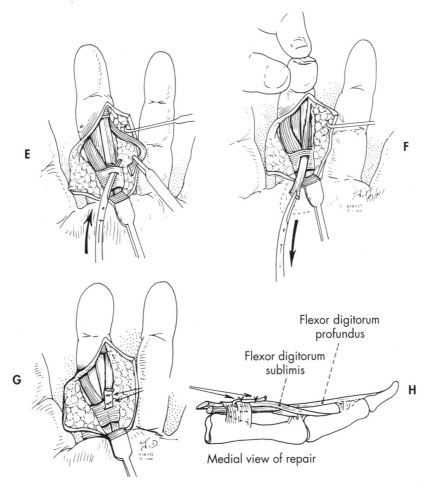

Figure 1-31 For legend see opposite page.

Littler intrinsic rerouting. The distal portion of the intrinsic tendon may be rerouted volar to Cleland's ligament to correct any remaining PIP hyperextension. The tendon is anchored volar to the axis of PIP motion into the flexor tendon sheath creating an oblique retinacular ligament. The PIP joint may be pinned in 20 degrees of flexion; if the DIP tends to fall into flexion, it is pinned in full extension.

Zancolli procedure. The lateral band is dissected from

the central slip and terminal slip and is routed volar to the axis of the PIP joint (Fig. 1-32). A dynamic sling is formed as the rerouted lateral band is held beneath the accessory collateral ligament. Sutures are placed at each end of the dissection. Tension may be altered by changing the suture positions. PIP joint pinning is performed as necessary.

Spiral oblique retinacular ligament (SORL) reconstruction. (See Fig. 1-17, p. 17.)

REHABILITATION PROTOCOL

Type II Swan-Neck Deformity After Reconstruction

0 to 2 weeks	• Mobilize the MCP joint for active MCP flexion and extension exercises.	4 weeks	• Remove the DIP pin and perform progressive active, active-assisted, and gentle passive flexion exercises to the PIP and DIP joints hourly.
2 to 4 weeks	• Remove sutures and PIP joint pin (if used) 2 weeks after surgery. Fit a splint to block the PIP joint in 20 degrees of flexion and begin active PIP flexion exercises.		• Have the patient wear a PIP splint between exercises and at night until 8 weeks after surgery.
			• If the PIP joint appears to be lax, continue the PIP joint dorsal blocking splint until satisfactory stabilization has been obtained.

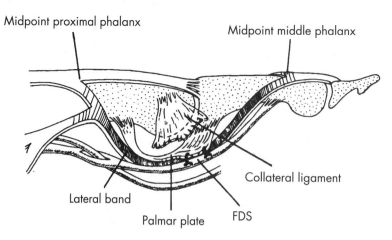

Figure 1-32 Zancolli procedure: Separation of the radial lateral band from the midpoint of the proximal phalanx to the midpoint of the middle phalanx. Release of accessory collateral ligament. Suture of palmar plate to FDS tendon to create retaining sling. (Redrawn from Tonkin et al: *J Hand Surg* 17A(2):262, 1992.)

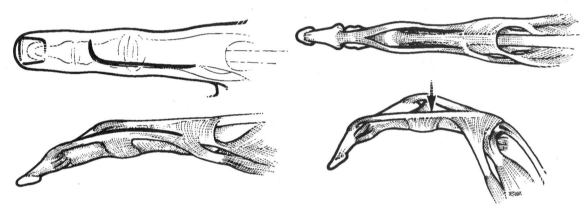

Figure 1-33 Nalebuff and Millender technique for correction of swan-neck deformity. Skin incision is shown curved to permit release of contracted skin. Incision should not be completely sutured. Lateral tendons are then mobilized by two longitudinal releasing incisions, and joint is flexed. (From Phillip E, Wright PE II: *Arthritic hand.* In Crenshaw AH, editor: *Campbell's operative orthopaedics*, vol 5, 1992.)

Nalebuff and Millender procedure. The lateral bands are released from their dorsal position by dissecting them from the central tendon. Flexion of the PIP joint allows the lateral bands to translate volarly (Fig. 1-33). The PIP joint is transfixed at 30 degrees of flexion with a Kirschner wire, and the MCP joints are protected with a dorsal blocking splint.

REHABILITATION PROTOCOL

Type II Swan-Neck Deformity After Nalebuff-Millender Procedure

2 weeks	• Remove the postoperative DBS and sutures. • Fit a protective removable splint and begin MCP joint active extension and flexion exercises.
3 weeks	• Remove the transfixing wire and fit the patient with a hand-based splint blocking the PIP joint at 30 degrees of flexion.

• The patient should wear splint nightly and between hourly active, active-assisted, and gentle passive flexion exercises.

6 weeks
• Discontinue the splint during the day but continue nightly wear for the next 4 weeks.
• If the PIP begins to extend within 10 degrees of full extension, continue the splint intermittently during the day as well.

■ *The goal of the surgery is a slight PIP flexion contracture of 10 to 15 degrees.*

Type III Swan-Neck Deformities

Extensor tenolyses and PIP capsulotomies are necessary adjuncts for these deformities. After full passive PIP flexion is achieved, any of the procedures outlined earlier in this section may be used to correct the deformity.

Type IV Swan-Neck Deformities

For joint destruction and fixed contractures, arthrodesis and arthroplasty are the only realistic options.

If MCP arthroplasties are present or planned, arthrodeses should be performed.

EXTENSOR TENDON INJURIES IN ZONES 4, 5, AND 6

Normal function usually is possible after unilateral injuries to the dorsal apparatus, and splinting and immobilization are not recommended. Complete disruptions of the dorsal expansion or central slip lacerations are repaired.

REHABILITATION PROTOCOL

Extensor Tendon Injury in Zone 4, 5, or 6, After Surgical Repair

0 to 2 weeks	• Allow active and passive PIP exercises; keep the MCP joint in full extension and the wrist in 40 degrees of extension.	4 to 6 weeks	• Begin MCP and wrist joint active flexion exercises with interval and night splinting with the wrist in neutral position. • Over the next 2 weeks, begin active-assisted and gentle passive flexion exercises.
2 weeks	• Remove the sutures and fit the patient with a removable splint • Keep the MCP joints in full extension and the wrist in neutral position. • Continue PIP exercises and remove the splint for scar massage and hygienic purposes only.	6 weeks	• Discontinue splinting unless an extensor lag develops at the MCP joint. • Use passive wrist flexion exercises as necessary.

Zone 5 Extensor Tendon Subluxations

Zone 5 extensor tendon subluxations rarely respond to a splinting program. The affected MCP joint may be splinted in full extension and radial deviation for 4 weeks with the understanding that surgical intervention probably will be required. Painful popping and swelling, in addition to a problematic extensor lag with radial deviation of the involved digit, usually require prompt reconstruction.

Acute injuries can be repaired directly and chronic injuries can be reconstructed with local tissue. Most reconstructive procedures, such as those described by Campbell, McCoy and Winsky, Wheeldon, and Kettlekamp, et al, use portions of the juncturae tendinum or extensor tendon slips anchored to the deep transverse metacarpal ligament or looped around the lumbrical tendon (Fig. 1-34).

REHABILITATION PROTOCOL

Zone 5 Extensor Tendon Subluxation

2 weeks	• Remove the postoperative dressing and sutures. • Keep the MCP joints in full extension. • Fashion a removable volar short-arm splint to maintain the operated finger MCP joint in full extension and radial deviation. • Allow periodic splint removal for hygienic purposes and scar massage. • Allow full PIP and DIP motion.	4 weeks	• Begin MCP active and active-assisted exercises hourly with interval daily and full-time night splinting. • At week 5, begin gentle passive MCP motion if necessary to gain full MCP joint flexion.
		6 weeks	• Discontinue the splint during the day and allow full activity.

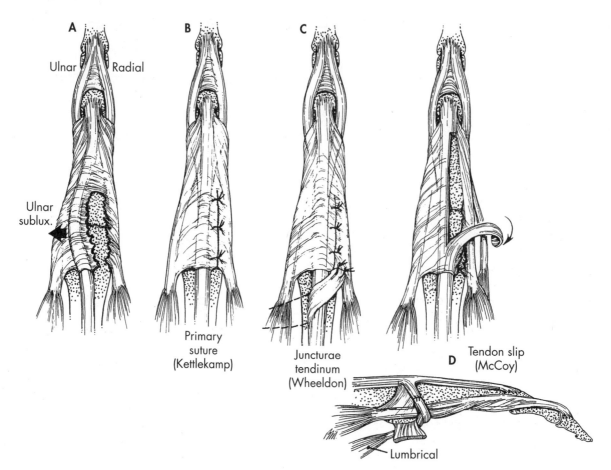

Figure 1-34 Subluxation or dislocation of the extensor tendon at the MCP joint may occur following laceration of the hood or following forceful flexion or extension of the finger. The lesion is secondary to a tear of the radial portion of the sagittal band **(A)**, which allows ulnar subluxation of the extensor tendon. Acute or fresh injuries are satisfactorily treated by primary suture of the defect in the hood and sagittal band **(B).** Late cases may require additional reconstruction. Wheeldon has described a method using a portion of the juncturae tendinum to stabilize the tendon over the dorsum of the joint **(C).** The junctura is lapped over the extensor tendon and sutured to the joint capsule on the radial side. McCoy and Winsky have also devised a technique **(D)** for stabilizing the extensor by removing a portion of the extensor tendon on the radial side of the finger, passing it around the lumbrical tendon, and suturing it back to itself. (From Doyle Jr: *Extensor tendons—acute injuries.* In Green D, editor: *Operative hand surgery,* ed 3, 1993, Churchill Livingstone.)

EXTENSOR TENDON INJURIES IN ZONES 7 AND 8

Extensor tendon injuries in zones 7 and 8 usually are from lacerations, but attritional ruptures secondary to remote distal radial fractures and rheumatoid synovitis may occur at the wrist level. These may require tendon transfers, free tendon grafts, or side-by-side transfers rather than direct repair. The splinting program for these, however, is identical to that for penetrating trauma.

REHABILITATION PROTOCOL

Zones 7 and 8 Extensor Tendon Injuries

0 to 2 week	• Maintain the wrist in 30 to 40 degrees of extension with a postoperative splint.
	• Encourage hand elevation and full PIP and DIP motion to reduce swelling and edema.
	• Treat any significant swelling by loosening the dressing and elevating the extremity.
2 to 4 weeks	• At 2 weeks, remove the postoperative dressing and sutures.
	• Fashion a volar splint to keep the wrist in 20 degrees of extension and the MCP joints of the affected finger(s) in full extension.
	• Continue full PIP and DIP motion exercises and initiate scar massage to improve skin-tendon glide during the next 2 weeks.

4 to 6 weeks	• Begin hourly wrist and MCP joint exercises, with interval and nightly splinting over the next 2 weeks.
	• From the fourth to the fifth week, hold the wrist in extension during the MCP flexion exercises and extend the MCP joints during the wrist flexion exercises.
	• Composite wrist and finger flexion from the fifth week onward. An MCP joint extension lag of more than 10 to 20 degrees requires interval daily splinting.
	• May discontinue the splinting program at 6 weeks.
6 to 7 weeks	• Begin gentle passive ROM.
	• Begin resistive extension exercises.

REHABILITATION PROTOCOL

Extensor Pollicis Longus Laceration

After repair of thumb extensor tendon lacerations, regardless of the zone of injury, apply a thumb spica splint with the wrist in 30 degrees of extension and the thumb in 40 degrees of radial abduction with full retroposition.

0 to 2 weeks	• Allow activity as comfortable in the postoperative splint.
	• Edema control measures include elevation and motion exercises to uninvolved digits.
2 to 4 weeks	• At 2 weeks after repair, remove the splint and sutures. Refit a thumb spica splint with the wrist and thumb positioned to minimize tension at the repair site as before.
	• Fit a removable splint for reliable patients and permit scar massage.
	• The vocational interests of some patients are best suited with a thumb spica cast. Continue edema control measures.
4 to 6 weeks	• Fit a removable thumb spica splint for night use and interval daily splinting between exercises.
	• During the next 2 weeks, the splint is removed for hourly wrist and thumb exercises. Between weeks 4 and 5 the patient should perform the thumb IP, MCP, and CMC flexion and extension exercises with the wrist held in extension.

	• Alternately, wrist flexion and extension motion is regained with the thumb extension.
	• After the fifth week, perform composite wrist and thumb exercises concomitantly.
6 weeks	• Discontinue the splinting program unless extensor lags develop.
	• Treat an extensor lag at the IP joint of more than 10 degrees with intermittent IP extension splinting in addition to nightly thumb spica splinting.
	• Problematic MCP and CMC extension lags require intermittent thumb spica splinting during the day and night for an additional 2 weeks or until acceptable results are obtained.
	• It may be necessary to continue edema control measures to 8 weeks or longer after surgery.
	• May use taping to gain full composite thumb flexion.
	• May use electrical stimulation for lack of extensor pull through.

Repairs performed 3 weeks or longer after the injury may weaken the extensor pollicis longus (EPL) muscle sufficiently for electrical stimulation to become necessary for tendon glide. The EPL is selectively strengthened by thumb retropulsion exercises performed against resistance with the palm held on a flat surface.

EXTENSOR TENOLYSES

Surgical intervention for extension contractures frequently follows an extensive period of presurgical therapy. Patients who have been active in their rehabilitation are more apt to appreciate that an early and aggressive postsurgical program is vital to their final outcome. Presurgical patient counseling should always be attempted to delineate the immediate postsurgical tenolysis program. The quality of the extensor tendon, bone, and joint encountered at surgery may alter the intended program, and the surgeon relays this information to the therapist and patient. Ideally, the surgical procedures are performed with the patient under local anesthesia or awakened from general anesthesia near the end of the procedure. The patient can then see the gains achieved and the surgeon can assess active motion, tendon glide, and the need for additional releases. Unusual circumstances may be well served by having the therapist observe the operative procedure.

Frequently, MCP and PIP capsular and ligament releases are necessary to achieve the desired joint motion. Complete collateral ligament resection may be required, and special attention may be necessary in the early postsurgical period for resultant instability.

Extensive tenolyses may require analgesic dosing before and during therapy sessions. Indwelling catheters also may be needed for the instillation of local anesthetics for this purpose.

REHABILITATION PROTOCOL

Extensor Tenolysis

0 to 24 hours	• Apply a light compressive postoperative dressing to allow as much digital motion as possible. Anticipate bleeding through the dressing and implement exercises hourly in 10-minute sessions to achieve as much of the motion noted intraoperatively as possible.
1 day to 4 weeks	• Remove the surgical dressings and drains at the first therapy visit. Apply light compressive sterile dressings. Edema control measures are critical at this stage. • Continue active and passive ROM exercises hourly for 10- to 15-minute sessions. Poor IP joint flexion during the first session is an indication for flexor FES. Extensor FES should be used initially with the wrist, MCP, PIP, and DIP joints passively extended to promote maximum proximal tendon excursion. After several stimulations in this position, place the wrist, MCP, and PIP joints into more flexion and continue the FES. • Remove the sutures at 2 weeks; dynamic flexion splints and taping may be required.

• Use splints to keep the joint in question in full extension between exercises and at night for the first 4 weeks. Extensor lags of 5 to 10 degrees are acceptable and are not indications to continue splint wear after this period.

4 to 6 weeks	• Continue hourly exercise sessions during the day for 10-minute sessions. Emphasis is on achieving MCP and IP joint flexion. Continue passive motion with greater emphasis during this period, especially for the MCP and PIP joints. • Continue extension night splinting until the sixth week.
6 weeks	• Encourage the patient to resume normal activity. Edema control measures may be required. Intermittent coban wrapping of the digits may be useful in conjunction with an oral antiinflammatory agent. Banana splints (foam cylindric digital sheaths) also appear to be quite effective for edema reduction.

REHABILITATION PROTOCOL—cont'd

The therapist must have acquired some critical information regarding the patient's tenolysis. Specific therapeutic programs and anticipated outcomes depend on the following:

- The quality of the tendon(s) undergoing tenolysis.
- The condition of the joint about which the tendon acts.
- The stability of the joint about which the tendon acts.

- The joint motions achieved during the surgical procedure. Passive motions are easily obtained; however, active motions in both extension and flexion are even more beneficial to guiding patient therapy goals.

■ *Achieving maximal MCP and PIP flexion during the first 3 weeks is essential. Significant gains after this period are uncommon.*

INTERSECTION SYNDROME

Approximately 4 cm proximal to the radial styloid, the abductus pollicis longus (APL) and extensor pollicis brevis (EPB) cross over the radial wrist extensors extensor carpi radialis longus (ECRL) and extensor carpi radialis brevis (ECRB). Pain, swelling, and tenderness in this region are the results of tendinitis at this crossover region, which is termed "intersection syndrome" (Grundberg and Reagan).

Conservative Management

Activity modification—discontinue repetitive wrist extension and flexion exercises.

Splint—fit a splint on the wrist in 15 degrees of extension; remove only for hygienic purposes for the first 2 weeks. The thumb may be incorporated, depending on the contribution of symptoms from thumb motion. Allow weaning from the splint during the day as symptoms warrant and pursue the resumption of activities in a graduated fashion.

Antiinflammatory agent—prescribe a systemic nonsteroidal antiinflammatory drug for 6 to 8 weeks.

Steroid injection—patients with moderate to severe symptoms who do not respond to the aforementioned modalities may benefit from a corticosteroid injection in the intersection region.

Persistent or worsening symptoms may require surgical decompression of the outcroppers and radial wrist extensors.

REHABILITATION PROTOCOL

Surgical Decompression of Intersection Syndrome

0 to 14 days	• Keep the wrist in neutral position within the surgical plaster splint. Encourage digital, thumb, and elbow motion as comfort allows. Remove the sutures at 10 to 14 days after surgery.
2 to 4 weeks	• Maintain the presurgical splint until the patient can perform the activities of daily living with little pain. Active and active-assisted wrist extension and flexion exercises should attain full preoperative values by 4 weeks after surgery.

4 to 6 weeks	• Advance the strengthening program. Anticipate full activities at the end of the sixth week after surgery. Use the splint as needed. • Scar desensitization techniques may be necessary, including the use of a transcutaneous electric nerve stimulation (TENS) unit if the scar region is still tender 6 weeks after surgery.

DEQUERVAIN'S TENOSYNOVITIS

Stenosing tenosynovitis of the abductor pollicis longus (APL) and extensor pollicis brevis (EPB) tendons usually causes discomfort localized to the region of the radial styloid (Fig. 1-35, *A*). Tenderness and swelling over the first dorsal compartment are usually accompanied by a positive Finkelstein's test (Fig. 1-35, *B*); however, resisted thumb MCP extension may be the only sign in more subtle cases.

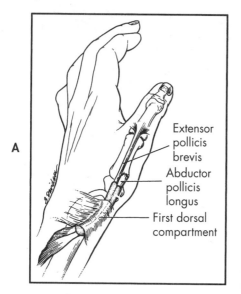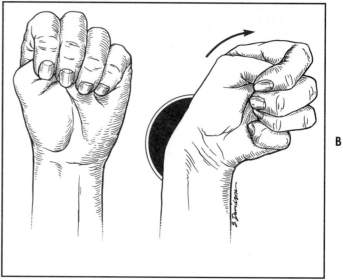

Figure 1-35 A, the anatomic arrangement of the first dorsal extensor compartment. The tunnel contains the extensor pollicis brevis tendon and one or more slips of the abductor pollicis longus tendon. **B,** Finkelstein's test. Flexion and ulnar deviation of the wrist with the fingers flexed over the thumb. Pain over the first compartment strongly suggests de-Quervain's stenosing tenosynovitis. (From Strickland JW, Idler RS, Creighton JC: Hand clinic: deQuervain's stenosing tenosynovitis, *Indiana Med* 83(5):340, 1990.)

Conservative Management

Thumb spica splint—immobilize the first dorsal compartment tendons with the use of a commercially available splint or, depending on the the patient's comfort, a custom-molded orthoplast device. The splint maintains the wrist in 15 to 20 degrees of extension and the thumb in 30 degrees of radial and palmar abduction. The IP joint is left free, and motion at this joint is encouraged. The patient wears the splint during the day for the first 2 weeks and at night until the next office visit, generally at 6 to 8 weeks. Splinting may continue longer, depending on the response to this form of treatment. Discontinue the splint during the day if symptoms permit and if daily activities are gradually resumed. Tailor workplace advancement accordingly.

Corticosteroid injection—offer a steroid injection to patients with moderate to marked pain or with symptoms lasting more than 3 weeks. The injection should distend individually the APL and EPB sheaths. Postinjection discomfort is variable, and a 2- to 3-day supply of mild analgesic is recommended.

Antiinflammatory agent—a systemic nonsteroidal antiinflammatory agent is commonly prescribed for the initial 6 to 8 weeks of treatment.

Activity modification—restrict thumb use so that the first dorsal compartment tendons are at relative rest.

Avoid activities that require prolonged thumb IP joint flexion, pinch, or repetitive motions.

Therapeutic modalities—edema control may be attempted through distal-to-proximal thumb coban wrapping, retrograde lotion or ice massage over the radial styloid, and phonophoresis with 10% hydrocortisone. Perform gentle active and passive thumb and wrist motion 5 minutes hourly to prevent joint contracture and tendon adhesions.

Often symptoms are temporarily relieved and the patient elects to repeat the management outlined above. Unsatisfactory symptom reduction or symptom persistence requires surgical decompression.

Anticipate separate compartments for the APL (which typically has 2 to 4 slips) and the EPB. Extreme caution in the approach will spare sensory branches of the lateral antebrachial cutaneous nerve and dorsal sensory branches of the radial nerve. Before decompression, fully expose the encasing circular retinacular fibers that arc across the radial styloid.

The floor of this compartment is the tendinous insertion of the brachioradialis tendon, which sends limbs to the volar and dorsal margins of the compartment. The APL and EPB tendons may be difficult to differentiate, especially in the absence of septation. When this "Y" tendinous floor is appreciated, it may serve as a landmark to indicate decompression of the first dorsal compartment.

Decompression for deQuervain's Tenosynovitis

0 to 2 days	• Leave the IP joint free and encourage motion as allowed by the soft compressive surgical dressing. • 2 days after surgery, remove the dressing. • Begin gentle active motion of the wrist and thumb.
2 to 14 days	• The presurgical splint is worn for comfort and motion exercises are continued. • At the tenth to fourteenth day, remove the sutures.
	• Commonly, patients complain of some hypersensitivity and of numbness at and distal to the incision site. Desensitization may be necessary. Digital massage of the area is usually sufficient, since the disturbance nearly always resolves.
2 to 6 weeks	• Advance the strengthening program and continue desensitization as necessary. • Anticipate the patient's release to unrestricted activity no earlier than about 6 weeks after surgery.

Nerve Compression Syndromes

CARPAL TUNNEL SYNDROME

Heightened awareness of carpal tunnel syndrome has increased the focus on conservative management because there are more patients with less intense symptoms of shorter duration. Objective neurologic loss (diminished two-point discrimination and thenar weakness) is uncommon in patients with recent onset of median nerve compression at the wrist.

Treatment

Regardless of the severity of this compression neuropathy, the first line of managment is to decrease the inciting and aggravating factors. Patients should avoid repetitive gripping and squeezing, and palmar impaction forces should be minimized. Patients should be educated about ergonomics and changes that may be required at work.

For *mild to moderate symptoms*, a forearm-based wrist splint, with the wrist in neutral position, is worn 24 hours a day for 2 weeks or until symptoms subside. Night splinting is continued for 6 weeks or longer. Although splinting appears to be the most effective treatment for nocturnal paresthesias, nonsteroidal antiinflammatory medications may be prescribed in addition to vitamin B_6. Activity modifications also may be helpful.

Patients with *severe symptoms* may benefit from steroid injection into the carpal tunnel; injections can be repeated several times, depending on the patient's response. Conservative treatment usually is not beneficial for patients with symptoms of more than 6 months duration, with objective neurologic loss, with recurrent carpal tunnel syndrome, or with symptoms that followed blunt trauma to the wrist.

Carpal Tunnel Syndrome, Open Release

0 to 7 days	• Encourage wrist extension and flexion exercises and full finger flexion and extension exercises immediately after surgery in the postsurgical dressing.
7 days	• Remove the dressing. Prohibit the patient from submerging the hand in liquids but permit showering. Discontinue the wrist splint if the patient is comfortable.
7 to 14 days	• Permit the patient to use the hand in activities of daily living as pain allows.
2 weeks	• Remove the sutures and begin ROM and gradual strengthening exercises. Achieve initial scar remodeling by using Elastomer or silicon gel-sheet scar pad at night and
	deep scar massage. If scar tenderness is intense, use desensitization techniques such as applying various textures to the area using light pressure and progressing to deep pressure. Textures include cotton, velour, wool, and Velcro. • Control pain and edema with the use of Isotoner gloves or electrical stimulation.
2 to 4 weeks	• Advance the patient to more rigorous activities; allow the patient to return to work if pain permits. The patient can use a padded glove for tasks that require pressure to be applied over the tender palmar scars. Begin pinch/grip strengthening with Baltimore Therapeutic Equipment work-simulator activities.

REHABILITATION PROTOCOL
Carpal Tunnel Syndrome, Endoscopic Release

0 to 1 day	• Encourage wrist extension and flexion exercises in the soft postsurgical dressing.	2 weeks	• Remove the sutures and advance activities to pain tolerance. Pillar tenderness (pain over the divided radial and ulnar portions of the transverse carpal ligament) may continue as a source of considerable discomfort and delay return to heavy work activities for 6 to 10 weeks after surgery.
2 days	• Remove the dressing. Protect wounds from immersion in liquids. Encourage activities as palmar tenderness allows.		

PRONATOR SYNDROME

A less common cause of median nerve entrapment occurs in the proximal forearm where the median nerve is compressed by either the pronator teres, the flexor superficialis arch, or the lacertus fibrosus in a condition referred to as pronator syndrome (Fig. 1-36). In addition to dysesthesias in the thumb and in the index, middle, and ring fingers, there may be a sensory disturbance of the volar base of the thenar eminence because of involvement of the palmar cutaneous branch of the median nerve.

Physical findings include marked proximal forearm tenderness; a proximal median nerve compression test will reproduce the symptoms. The most common

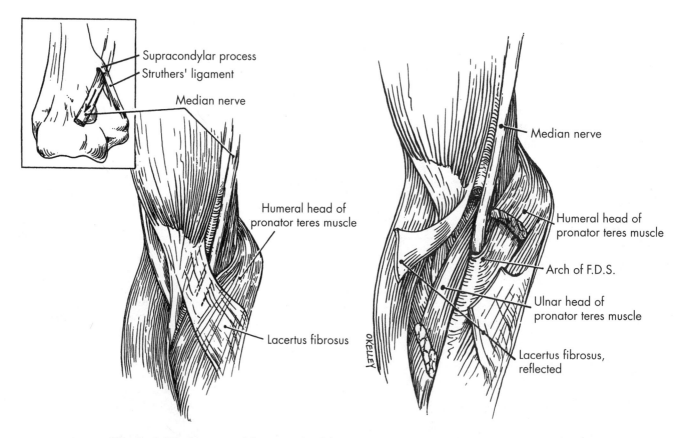

Figure 1-36 Anatomy of the antecubital fossa and structures overlying the course of the median nerve. The inset demonstrates the occasionally present supracondylar process. (From Idler RS, Strickland JW, Creighton JJ Jr: Hand clinic: pronator syndrome, *Indiana Med* 84(2):124, 1991.)

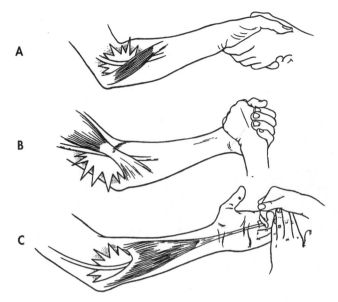

Figure 1-37 Provocative tests for pronator syndrome. **A,** Pronator teres: resisted forearm pronation with elbow relatively extended. **B,** Lacertus fibrosus: resisted elbow flexion with forearm supinated. **C,** FDS: resisted middle finger extension. (From Idler RS, Strickland JW, Creighton JJ Jr: Hand clinic: pronator syndrome, *Indiana Med* 84(2):124, 1991.)

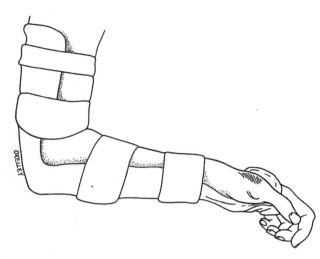

Figure 1-38 Immobilization splint for the conservative or postoperative management of pronator syndrome. (From Idler RS, Strickland JW, Creighton JJ Jr: Hand clinic: pronator syndrome *Indiana Med* 84(2):124, 1991.)

cause of this disorder is entrapment of the median nerve by the fascia of the pronator teres proximally, which can be tested by resisted pronation with gradual extension of the elbow (Fig. 1-37). A resisted middle finger flexion test may suggest median nerve entrapment by the flexor digitorum superficialis arch, and resisted supination with the elbow flexed may suggest entrapment by the lacertus fibrosus, a fascial extension of the biceps tendon.

Treatment

Nonoperative management of this disorder includes minimizing resisted pronation activities and repetitive gripping and squeezing. Long-arm splinting with the elbow at 90 degrees and the forearm in neutral rotation (Fig. 1-38), in addition to antiinflammatory medications and vitamin B_6, may be beneficial. Conservative management of this disorder often is ineffective, and surgery usually is required.

REHABILITATION PROTOCOL
Pronator Teres Syndrome, Surgical Decompression

0 to 7 days	• Keep a soft light compressive dressing in place to allow full elbow, forearm, and wrist motion.	4 weeks	• Permit moderate to heavy work.
		6 weeks	• Allow full, unprotected activity of the arm.
7 days	• Remove the dressing and encourage activities as tolerated, including light manual labor. Begin ROM to the wrist and elbow, including gripping in extension with putty.	Discomfort after surgical decompression of the median nerve in the proximal forearm is less than after decompression of the median nerve at the wrist level, and desensitization techniques rarely are necessary.	
2 weeks	• Remove the sutures and encourage progressive strengthening and use of the upper extremity.		

ULNAR TUNNEL SYNDROME

Compression of the ulnar nerve at the wrist level may result from a pathologic condition within Guyon's canal, such as an ulnar artery aneurysm, thrombosis, ganglia, anomalous muscle bellies, or anomalous ligaments. External compression of the nerve may be caused by idiopathic fascial thickening, repetitive trauma, palmaris brevis hypertrophy, and other muscle anomalies or hypertrophies. Conservative management for this disorder is similar to that of carpal tunnel syndrome, although injections should be performed with caution because of the proximity to the ulnar artery.

REHABILITATION PROTOCOL

Ulnar Tunnel Syndrome, Surgical Decompression

0 to 7 days	• Fit the patient with a a soft splint and encourage wrist flexion and extension exercises.		• Begin resistive exercises (hand-helper, clothes-pin pinch, forearm and wrist curls).
7 days	• Remove the splint and increase wrist extension and flexion exercises to full motion.	4 to 6 weeks	• Encourage normal activity. • Allow the patient to begin work-related activities.
7 to 14 days	• Emphasize light grip activities and finger motion (marble hunt in corn or rice or soft putty exercises). • Remove sutures at 2 weeks.		• Desensitization techniques may be necessary for palmar scar tenderness, and a padded glove may allow the patient an early return to moderate to heavy work activities.
2 to 4 weeks	• Treat the scar with deep friction massage and a silicone-based scar pad.		

CUBITAL TUNNEL SYNDROME

Few patients with cubital tunnel syndrome respond to nonsurgical measures, but modification of workplace activities, including a decrease in forceful grip use of the hand and prolonged elbow flexion, may be beneficial. Long-arm night splints with the elbow in 40 degrees of flexion, antiinflammatory medication, and vitamin B_6 are prescribed. Elbow pads to decrease impaction on the cubital tunnel also are worthwhile, especially if the cubital tunnel syndrome is accompanied by medial epicondylitis. Nonsurgical management for this disorder may be used as long as the patient desires, but 3 to 6 months seems reasonable.

Sites of ulnar nerve compression include the medial intramuscular septum, the arcade of Struthers, the ligament of Struthers, the ligament of Osborne (proximal fascial margins of the flexor carpi ulnaris muscle), and the deeper muscular fascia within the flexor carpi ulnaris muscle.

Postsurgical therapy for cubital tunnel syndrome depends on the surgical technique used.

REHABILITATION PROTOCOL

Cubital Tunnel Syndrome, In Situ Decompression

0 to 7 days	• Fit the patient with a long-arm splint with the elbow at 90 degrees of flexion and the forearm in neutral position. • Emphasize shoulder and digital motion.	7 days	• Remove the splint and apply a light compressive dressing to the elbow. Begin elbow, forearm, and wrist active and active-assisted exercises. • Control edema with high-voltage galvanic stimulator (HVGS).

REHABILITATION PROTOCOL—cont'd

7 days —cont'd	• Instruct the patient to avoid repetitive activities.	4 weeks	• Begin resistive strengthening exercises for forearm pronation and supination, wrist curls, and grip/pinch exercises.
2 weeks	• Remove the sutures and begin an active ROM program. Emphasize full elbow extension, flexion, and forearm pronation and supination. Continue edema control, scar management, and desensitization as necessary.	6 weeks	• Allow full activity.

REHABILITATION PROTOCOL

Medial Epicondylectomy and Anterior Transposition Procedure

0 to 2 weeks	• Fit the patient with a long-arm splint that keeps the elbow in 90 degrees of flexion, the forearm in 40 degrees pronation, and the wrist in 40 degrees of flexion. Encourage thumb and finger ROM. • Remove the sutures at 2 weeks.	4 weeks	• Discontinue the splint. Advance from active and active-assisted elbow exercises to passive to regain full motion. Full concomitant forearm and wrist motion should be present at 4 weeks.
2 to 4 weeks	• Fashion a removable long-arm splint to keep the elbow at 90 degrees of flexion and the forearm and wrist in neutral. The splint is removed hourly for 10-minute sessions of gentle active elbow, forearm, and wrist motion. Begin edema control with compression sleeve (tubi-grip), retrograde massage, and HVGS. • Begin scar management.	5 weeks	• Begin strengthening exercises: wrist curls and forearm rotation Velcro board activities for wrist flexion, extension, pronation/supination, and pinch; hand-helper for grip.
		6 weeks	• Allow activity as comfort permits. Begin gradual repetitive activities.
		8 weeks	• Allow full unrestricted activity.

RADIAL TUNNEL SYNDROME/POSTERIOR INTEROSSEOUS SYNDROME

Entrapment of the posterior interosseous nerve may be associated with pain and tenderness in the proximal forearm without weakness (radial tunnel syndrome) or with motor loss (posterior interosseous nerve syndrome). Sites of compression include fibrous bands over the radiocapitellar joint, synovitis of the radiocapitellar joint (as in rheumatoid arthritis), the vascular leash of Henry, the proximal fascial edge of the extensor carpi radialis brevis muscle, the arcade of Frohse (proximal edge of superficial head of supinator muscle), and the distal edge of the supinator. Although often associated with tennis elbow, this syndrome may exist as an isolated compression neuropathy.

Treatment
Conservative management of entrapment of the posterior interosseous nerve includes long-arm splinting with the elbow at 90 degrees and the forearm in neutral, refraining from resisted supination and wrist extension types of activities. Antiinflammatory medications and vitamin B_6 may be prescribed.

Rehabilitation after posterior interosseous nerve decompression may vary, depending on the surgical approach. The interval between the brachioradialis and the extensor carpi radialis longus gives excellent exposure of the posterior interosseous nerve from the radiocapitellar articulation through the proximal half of the supinator. Rehabilitation may be easier because the muscle fibers of the brachioradialis are not violated.

REHABILITATION PROTOCOL

Radial Tunnel/Posterior Interosseous Syndrome, Surgical Decompression

0 to 7 days	• Remove light compressive surgical dressing at 3 to 5 days. • Initiate full active forearm and elbow flexion and extension exercises.		• Continue edema control with compressive sleeve and HVGS.
7 to 14 days	• Remove the dressing at 7 days. • Begin active and active-assisted wrist, forearm, and elbow exercises.	2 to 4 weeks 6 weeks	• Begin resistive exercises for wrist and forearm supination. • Allow unrestricted activity.

THORACIC OUTLET SYNDROME

Suggested causes of thoracic outlet syndrome include congenital anomalous cervical ribs and elongated cervical transverse processes, trauma, fibromuscular bands, hypertrophic scalene musculature, hypotonia with subsequent postural shoulder changes, and narrowing of the costoclavicular interval with shoulder bracing.

Clinical Signs and Symptoms

Brachial plexus compression occurs in for 94% to 97% of patients, whose symptoms may be divided into less common upper plexus and more common lower plexus symptoms (Fig. 1-39). Lower plexus compression results in subjective pain in the medial arm, forearm, and ulnar one and one-half digits. Upper plexus compression may produce symptoms referable to the eye, face, anterior neck, chest, and shoulder.

Compression of the subclavian artery or vein in addition to the brachial plexus may result in varied manifestations of this disorder. Cyanosis and edema progress to venous thrombosis in 2% to 3% of patients with subclavian vein compression. Symptoms of arterial insufficiency, such as pain, pallor, and coolness, may be associated with Raynaud's phenomenon in patients with subclavian artery compression.

Unfortunately, there are no definitive tests for this syndrome. The diagnosis relies heavily on physician acumen, and the history and physical examination are most important. The Roos test (repetitive gripping with the arms in external rotation, shoulders and elbows at 90 degrees for 3 minutes) is considered the most reliable test for this condition. The reproduction of symptoms, sensations of heaviness and fatigue, or sudden inability to main-

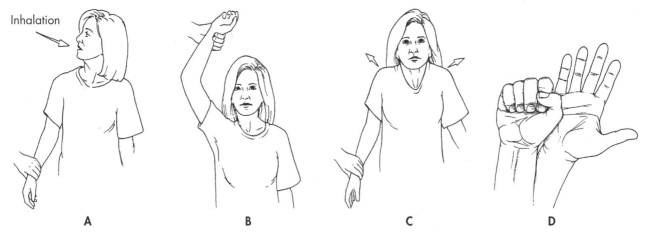

Figure 1-39 Provocative maneuvers used in evaluation of patients with suspected thoracic outlet syndrome (TOS). Symptoms must be reproduced for tests to be considered positive. **A,** Adson's maneuver. **B,** Wright's maneuver. **C,** Costoclavicular, or military brace, maneuver. **D,** overhead exercise test. (From Leffert RD: Thoracic outlet syndrome, *JAAOS* 2(6):317, 1994.

tain the provocative test position is considered positive. However, the same findings can be present in patients with carpal tunnel and other peripheral nerve compression syndromes of the upper extremity.

Treatment

Conservative treatment is successful in approximately two thirds of patients with thoracic outlet syndrome and should include the following:

- Activity modification.
- Extremity resting.
- Postural changes and breast support.
- Shoulder girdle musculature strengthening.
- Antiinflammatory agents.
- Transcutaneous nerve stimulation.
- Biofeedback.
- Ultrasound.

Surgery is indicated when conservative treatment does not relieve symptoms. Cervical rib resection, thoracic rib resection, scalenectomy, scalenotomy, and fibromuscular band excision may be used individually or in combinations.

Nerve Injuries

Nerve injuries are most commonly caused by direct trauma, laceration, traction or stretching, entrapment, or compression. Obtaining optimal hand function after nerve injury depends on preservation of passive range of motion of the hand and prevention of secondary damage from attenuation or stretching of involved structures due to poor positioning or substitution patterns. Combined with the appropriate exercise regimens, splinting techniques can be effective for attaining these goals.

Median nerve lesions result in a loss of coordination, decreased strength, and a decrease in or loss of sensory input from the thumb, index, long, and ring fingers. Distal lesions primarily impair opposition and adduction, and splinting is aimed primarily at preventing first web contracture and maintaining passive motion of the thumb CMC joint.

Ulnar nerve lesions compromise coordination, pinch and grip strength, and thumb stability and frequently cause "clawing" of the ring and small fingers. Splinting is aimed at prevention of this clawing, while allowing full digital flexion and IP extension.

Radial nerve lesions result in loss of active extension of the wrist, thumb and fingers, weakness of thumb abduction, decreased grip strength, and diminished coordination. The emphasis of splinting is on providing wrist stability and maintaining thumb position.

SPLINTING FOR NERVE PALSIES*

Median Nerve

Splint recommendation: web spacer

Purpose	• The web spacer splint maintains the width of the first web space, preventing a first web contracture.
	• This is necessary because of the paralysis of the thenar musculature.
Warning/ Precautions	• When fabricating the splint, avoid hyperextension of the thumb MCP joint or stress to the ulnar collateral ligament (UCL) of the MCP joint.
Wearing Time	• Night only.
	• If any first web space contracture is noted, periodic daywear is added.

Ulnar Nerve

Splint recommendation: single Wynn-Parry splint or static MCP extension block.

Purpose	• These splints are used to prevent clawing of the ring and small fingers, yet allow full digital flexion and IP extension.
	• The splint is required because of paralysis of the ulnar innervated intrinsics.
Warning/ Precautions	• Monitor carefully to prevent pressure sores in patients who do not have sensory return.
Wearing Time	• Continuous wear until the MCP volar plates tighten so that hyperextension is no longer present, the intrinsics return, or tendon transfers are performed to replace the function of the intrinsics.

Radial Nerve

Splint recommendation: wrist immobilization splint or possibly a long dorsal outrigger.

Purpose	• Positioning the wrist in approximately 15 to 20 degrees of dorsiflexion allows improved functional use of the hand and prevents wrist drop.
	• Incorporation of the outrigger component of the splint allows assistance with extension at the MCP level of the digits.

Wearing Time • The patient wears the splint until there is return of the radial nerve innervated muscles or tendon transfers are performed to improve wrist and/or finger extension.

DIGITAL NERVE REPAIR

Most lacerations of digital nerves should be repaired as soon as possible (within 5 to 7 days of injury) if the wound is clean and sharp. The condition of the patient, the presence of other injuries that may take precedence over nerve repair, skin conditions such as extensive soft-tissue loss, wound contamination, and the availability of personnel and equipment also must be considered in the timing of digital nerve repair.

REHABILITATION PROTOCOL
Repair of Digital Nerve*

2 weeks	• Remove bulky dressing and initiate edema control with coban or finger socks. • Fit DBS in 30 degrees of flexion at the PIP joint for continual wear, assuming the repair is near the PIP level or slightly distal to this point. The DBS may be fitted in more flexion at the MCP or PIP level if the digital nerve repair is under more tension. **Note:** If nerve repair is near the MCP joint, the DBS should include the MCP joint only, with approximately 30 degrees of flexion of the MCP joint. • Begin active and passive ROM exercises 6 times a day within the restraints of the dorsal blocking gutter. • Begin scar massage with lotion and/or the use of Otoform or Elastomer within 24 hours after suture removal.	3 to 6 weeks	• Adjust the dorsal blocking gutter splint into extension 10 degrees each week until neutral is reached at 6 weeks.
		6 weeks	• Discontinue DBS. • Initiate passive extension at the MCP joint. • May begin extension splinting if passive extension is limited, but generally patients regain extension and extension splints are not necessary. • Begin progressive strengthening.
		8 to 10 weeks	• Begin sensory reeducation when some sign of sensory return (protective sensation) is present.

Wrist Disorders

DORSAL AND VOLAR CARPAL GANGLION CYSTS

Dorsal carpal ganglion cysts rarely originate from sites other than near the scapholunate interval. These cysts may decompress into the EPL or common extensor tendon sheaths and may appear to arise from sites remote from their origin.

A dorsal transverse incision in a Langer's line over the scapholunate interval clearly exposes the pathology through a window bounded by the second and third dorsal compartments radially, the fourth compartment ulnarly, the dorsal intercarpal ligament distally, and the dorsal radiocarpal ligament proximally.

Volar carpal ganglion cysts originate from the flexor carpal radialis tendon sheath or from the articulations between the radius and scaphoid, the scaphoid and trapezium, or the scaphoid and lunate. Excision of these cysts, as with dorsal carpal ganglion cysts, should include a generous capsulectomy at the site of the cyst origin.

REHABILITATION PROTOCOL

Excision of Wrist Ganglion Cyst

2 weeks	• Remove the short-arm splint and sutures. Initiate active and active-assisted wrist extension and flexion. Continue interval splint wear during the day between exercises and at night.	4 to 6 weeks	• Allow normal activities to tolerance.
2 to 4 weeks	• Advance ROM exercises to resistive and gradual strengthening exercises. • Discontinue the splint at 4 weeks.	6 weeks	• Allow full activity.

The time it takes to achieve full wrist extension and flexion depends on the the patient. Return of motion, however, is quite predictable, and only rarely is formal therapy necessary after 4 to 6 weeks.

WRIST LIGAMENT RECONSTRUCTION

Reconstruction of the intrinsic wrist ligaments is essentially confined to the scapholunate ligament. Methods of reconstruction are varied and include direct anatomic repair of the scapholunate ligament and reconstruction with tendon grafts or dorsal wrist capsule. Early intervention for reduction of intercarpal subluxations and dislocations is warranted because degenerative arthritis appears to follow a predictable pattern, especially in scapholunate injuries.

In the Blatt capsulodesis, rotatory subluxation of the scaphoid is reduced by a capsuloligamentous flap attached to the distal pole of the scaphoid (Fig. 1-40). A 0.045 in Kirschner wire is driven obliquely through the reduced scaphoid and the capitate into the base of the third metacarpal, and the capsular flap is secured to the distal pole of the scaphoid with a 4-0 stainless steel pull-out wire through a button on the volar tubercle of the scaphoid.

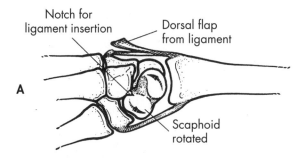

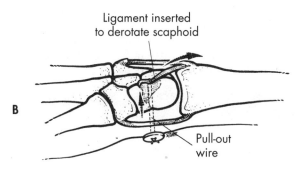

Figure 1-40 Dorsal capsulodesis (Blatt). **A,** Proximal-based ligamentous flap is developed from dorsal wrist capsule. Notch for ligament insertion is created in dorsal cortex of distal scaphoid pole. **B,** Scaphoid has been derotated and ligament has been inserted with pull-out wire suture. (Redrawn from Blatt G: Capsulodesis in reconstructive hand surgery: dorsal capsulodesis for the unstable scaphoid and volar capsulodesis following excision of the distal ulna, *Hand Clin* 3:81, 1987.)

REHABILITATION PROTOCOL
Wrist Ligament Repair (Blatt Capsulodesis)

2 weeks	• Remove postoperative dressing and sutures. • Shoulder ROM exercises
2 months	• Remove the pull-out wire. • Apply a removable splint. • Begin active wrist extension and flexion exercises.
3 months	• Remove the Kirschner wire, and allow intercarpal extension and flexion.
4 to 6 months	• Encourage motion and gradually increase resistive exercises.

SCAPHOLUNATE LIGAMENT REPAIR

Reconstruction of the scapholunate ligament by direct ligament repair augmented with capsulodesis is advocated by Lavernia, Cohen, and Taleisnik. This procedure includes repair of the dorsal scapholunate ligament into a roughened trough on the proximal pole of the scaphoid augmented with a Blatt capsulodesis.

REHABILITATION PROTOCOL
Direct Scapholunate Ligament Repair

0 to 8 weeks	• Place the forearm in slight pronation and the wrist in neutral angulation in a splint that limits forearm rotation. • Shoulder, finger, and elbow ROM exercises daily.
8 weeks	• Remove the pull-out sutures and Kirschner wires.
	• Begin ROM exercises. A removable splint is worn for 2 to 4 more weeks.
10 to 14 weeks	• Encourage normal activities. Do not allow palmar impaction and resisted wrist extension for at least 6 months after surgery.

RHEUMATOID ARTHRITIS

The radioulnar joint is a frequent site of proliferative synovitis in patients with rheumatoid arthritis. Initially, this synovitis may cause only slight swelling and tenderness over the ulnar head, but gradually forearm rotation, especially supination, becomes restricted and painful and the ligamentous structures of the wrist are stretched and disrupted. Progressive laxity of the distal radioulnar joint results in dorsal subluxation and sometimes dislocation of the ulnar head. Synovectomy of the distal radioulnar joint often is combined with resection of the ulnar head (Darrach procedure) for the treatment of these problems. The wrist should be carefully evaluated clinically and roentgenographically before surgery to determine if any instability is present at the radiocarpal joint; if so, arthroplasty or arthrodesis of the wrist usually is required in addition to ulnar head resection.

REHABILITATION PROTOCOL
Darrach Resection of the Distal Ulna*

0 to 3 weeks	• Apply a bulky compressive splint with the forearm supinated and the elbow flexed 90 degrees. • At 2 weeks, replace the bulky dressing with a long-arm splint.
3 weeks	• Fit a wrist immobilization splint with 15 degrees of dorsiflexion to wear between exercise sessions and at night (some authors prefer to use a long-arm splint until 6 weeks after surgery)

REHABILITATION PROTOCOL—cont'd

3 weeks —cont'd	• Begin hourly active and passive ROM exercises to the wrist and forearm. **Be sure to perform passive exercises proximal to the wrist and not distally by turning the hand.** • Discomfort along the distal ulna when attempting forearm rotation is typical for the first 6 weeks. ■ *If the Darrach procedure is performed in conjunction with multiple procedures for rheumatoid arthritis, active ROM exercises may begin 3 to 5 days after surgery at the discretion of the physician. If the Darrach surgical area is painful, exercises may need to be minimized in the initial 2 to 3 weeks.*		• Patients with dorsal subluxation of the distal ulna may derive comfort from a distal ulnar strap applied 2 inches proximally to the distal ulna to help hold the ulna in an anatomic position.
		6 weeks	• Discontinue wrist immobilization splint if the patient is experiencing no pain. • Initiate gentle strengthening exercises.

Dupuytren's Contracture

The manifestations of Dupuytren's disease are variable and may be confined to a single digit, but palmar and digital involvement of the ring and small fingers is more common. Diffuse involvement of the first web space and thumb in addition to the fingers is less common.

No exact criteria exist for surgical intervention in Dupuytren's disease. Some patients who have severe MCP and PIP contractures have surprisingly few complaints of functional disability, whereas some patients with pretendinous cords and nodules without contractures desire surgical intervention.

Guidelines for surgical intervention include the following:

• 30 degrees of MCP joint contracture.
• 15 degrees of PIP joint contracture.
• Inability to place the hand into a pocket, lay it flat on a table, or bring it together with the opposite hand (as in prayer).

Regardless of the criteria used for surgical intervention, the PIP joint contracture is the most difficult to correct and warrants early intervention.

Surgical procedures used in the treatment of Dupuytren's contracture include subcutaneous fasciotomy, partial selective fasciectomy, complete fasciectomy, fasciectomy with skin grafting, and amputation.

SUBCUTANEOUS FASCIOTOMY

In elderly patients with MCP joint contracture, subcutaneous fasciotomy is ideal, regardless of whether one or two digits are involved. This procedure may be done in the office with local anesthesia.

Technique of Subcutaneous Fasciotomy

With the palm anesthetized, a #15 blade is introduced across the palm between the skin and the pretendinous cord. The finger is extended and the knife blade is gently pressed onto the taut cord. An abrupt release of the MCP joint contracture follows when the cord transection is complete. Manipulation of the fingers may result in some tearing of the palmar skin; however, this usually is minor, and the wound can be left open and covered with a sterile dressing.

REHABILITATION PROTOCOL

Dupuytren's Contracture, Subcutaneous Fasciotomy

0 to 7 days	• Encourage the patient to work on stretching exercises immediately after the surgery. Maintain digital extension with a resting pan splint with Velcro straps.	• Have the patient wear the splint during the day between exercises and at night for the first week. • Continue night splints for 6 weeks after surgery.

Surgical procedures other than cordotomy for Dupuytren's disease require considerable dissection, and subsequent palmar and finger hematomas become more likely. Small suction drain systems may be incorporated to prevent these hematomas.

Replantation

Replantation of amputed parts and revascularization for salvaging mangled extremities require intense commitment from both the patient and the surgeon. Emotional and financial investments are enormous, and successful replantation and revascularization require long postsurgical rehabilitation programs that are frequently interrupted and prolonged by multiple reconstructive surgical procedures.

■ *Proper candidate selection is critical to the success of replantation and revascularization of amputated parts.*

CONTRAINDICATIONS

Absolute contraindications for replantation and revascularization include multiple-trauma victims with significant associated injuries in whom treatment of other organ systems takes precedence over extremity salvage. Digits have been refrigerated and replanted up to 3 days after injury. Extensive injury to the affected limb, chronic illness, previously nonfunctioning parts, and psychiatric illness also prohibit salvage procedures.

Relative contraindications include avulsion injuries, lengthy ischemia time, and patients older than 50 years. Major limbs are defined as those with significant skeletal muscle content. These may be salvaged if appropriately cooled 12 hours after the injury; up to 6 hours of warm ischemia time can be tolerated.

Only under unusual circumstances should single digits be replanted, especially those proximal to the flexor digitorum superficialis insertion.

INDICATIONS

The ideal candidate for replantation is a young patient with a narrow zone of injury. Power saws and punch presses often result in replantable parts. Indications for replantation include any upper or lower extremity in a child, as well as thumbs, multiple digits, hands, and wrist-level and some more proximal-level amputations in adults.

POSTSURGICAL CONSIDERATIONS

Postsurgical care typically begins in the operating room, where brachial plexus blocks are given before the patient leaves. A bulky, noncompressive dressing reinforced with plaster splints is applied in the operating room and usually is kept in place for 3 weeks. When the likelihood of thrombosis is increased, such as in wide zone injuries, heparin may be used. Postsurgical orders include keeping the patient NPO for 12 to 24 hours after surgery, because vascular compromise may necessitate emergency surgical intervention. The replanted part is kept warm either with a thermal blanket or by elevating the room temperature to 78° to 80° F. Caffeine-containing products, such as coffee, tea, cokes, and chocolate, are prohibited, as is smoking and the use of tobacco products by both the patient and visitors. Ice and iced drinks are not allowed, and visitation is limited to one to two visitors at a time to try to prevent emotional disturbance. The patient is restricted to bed rest for approximately 3 days, and the replanted part is kept at or slightly above heart level.

REHABILITATION PROTOCOL
Replantation and Revascularization in Adults

1 day	• Appropriate and liberal use of analgesics is recommended, although postoperative discomfort usually is minimal with replantations. Revascularization procedures typically require more postoperative pain management, especially when neural connections remain. • Low-molecular–weight dextran 40 in 500 cc of D_5-W is given over 6 to 24 hours. In patients with pulmonary problems, continuous intravenous infusion at a lower rate is recommended.

• Aspirin (325 mg, 1 by mouth 2 times a day).
• Thorazine (25 mg by mouth 3 times a day).
• Antibiotics—cefazolin or a similar antibiotic is used for 3 to 5 days.
• Administer low-molecular–weight dextran 40 and 500 cc of D_5-W at a rate of 10 ml/kg/day for 3 days to the pediatric patient.

REHABILITATION PROTOCOL—cont'd

1 day—cont'd

- Automated monitors with alarms provide continuous feedback, although hourly visual inspection for the first 12 hours provides important information, including color, capillary refill, turgor, and bleeding of the replanted part.

Management of Early Complications

- 5 to 10 days of hospitalization are necessary after replantation. After that time, replantation failure from vascular compromise occurs infrequently. Arterial insufficiency from thrombosis or vasoconstriction usually requires immediate return to the operating room. Give a plexus block, explore the arterial anastomosis, excise the damaged segment, and perform vein grafting if necessary. Administer heparin in salvage procedures of this sort and attempt to keep the partial thromboplastin time 1.5 to 2.0 times normal.
- Venous congestion indicates either insufficient venous outflow or venous thrombosis. At the first sign of venous congestion, loosen all postoperative dressings to eliminate external constriction. Digital replantations with venous congestion may benefit from a longitudinal laceration through the digital pulp or removal of the nail plate. Heparinized-saline drops applied to the nail bed and pulp may promote venous drainage. If the venous outflow from the nail bed or drainage site is inadequate but present, leech therapy may be indicated. Apply a medical leech to the finger or area of congestion with the remaining sites shielded by plastic sheathing. A leech cage may be fashioned from the plastic bag in which intravenous bags are stored. Tape the open end of the plastic bag around the bulky postoperative dressing, introduce a leech through a vertical slit in the bag, then tape the vertical slit. Adequate oxygenization occurs through the porous surgical dressing. Leeches have a long-lasting anticoagulant and vasodilating effect in addition to withdrawing approximately 5 cc of blood. However, arterial inflow must be present for the leech to attach. If the leech does not attach, the digit may have arterial as well as venous insufficiency and further salvage requires immediate surgical exploration of the artery and venous anastomoses.

5 to 10 days

- The patient may be discharged from the hospital if the appearance of the replanted part is acceptable.
- Dietary and environmental restrictions remain the same, and the patient receives aspirin (325 mg) twice daily for an additional 2 weeks.

3 weeks

- Remove the dressing and assess the wound. Replanted digits usually are markedly edematous with granulating wounds.
- Wound care management consists of hydrogen peroxide wound cleansing and silver nitrate cauterization of redundant granulation tissue.
- Apply soft, nonadherent dressings and fit the wrist with a splint in slight wrist flexion and MCP joint flexion to about 50 to 60 degrees.
- Begin passive wrist flexion and MCP joint flexion exercises, with emphasis on flexor tendon glide.

6 weeks

- Begin active and active-assisted ROM and flexion and extension with interval splinting.
- Continue edema control measures.

8 weeks

- Accelerate active and active-assisted flexion and extension exercises of all joints and use electrical stimulation if necessary.
- Remove temporary bony fixation.

4 months

- Perform soft tissue and bony reconstruction procedures.
- PIP joint injuries are commonly treated by fusion. Active digital extension and flexion are often inhibited by tendon adhesions.
- Motion is best achieved through a two-stage tenolysis program. Perform extensor tenolyses first, followed by a flexor tenolysis approximately 2 to 3 months after the initial procedure.

MAJOR LIMB REPLANTATION

Major limb replantation requires the wrist and hand to be splinted in a functional position. Full passive motion of each joint at the more proximal soft tissue and neurologic injury is allowed. Motion exercises are continued until proximal neuromuscular function returns. The results of replantation primarily depend on the outcome of the nerve repairs. The age of the patient, mechanism of injury, level of injury, and the quality of the replantation procedure, especially the extent of revascularization, also are important factors.

Arthroplasty

PROXIMAL INTERPHALANGEAL JOINT ARTHROPLASTY

PIP joint arthroplasty is primarily indicated for pa-
tients who are relatively free of disease at the MCP joints. This usually precludes patients with rheumatoid arthritis with significant MCP joint involvement. The best treatment option for these patients is MCP joint arthroplasty and either soft tissue procedures for correction of the soft tissue deformities or PIP joint fusion. Patients with osteoarthritis may benefit from isolated PIP joint arthroplasty, other than the index finger.

A volar approach for placement of the implant may be used when the extensor mechanism does not require repair or corrective surgery. Active flexion and extension exercises may be started immediately after surgery.

Rehabilitation after PIP joint arthroplasty depends on whether the arthroplasty is done for a stiff IP joint, for reconstruction with lateral deviation, or to correct a boutonnière deformity.

REHABILITATION PROTOCOL

Proximal Interphalangeal Joint Arthroplasty for Joint Stiffness

0 to 3 weeks	• Begin active flexion and extension exercises at 3 to 5 days after surgery. • Have the patient use a padded aluminum splint between hourly exercises to maintain full PIP joint extension.	6 weeks	• Begin resistive exercises. • Continue interval splinting to correct any angular deviation and extensor lag of more than 20 degrees. • Have the patient wear protective splint at night for 3 months after surgery.
3 to 6 weeks	• Continue interval PIP joint splinting during the day for 6 weeks.		

The ideal ranges of motion obtained are 0 to 70 degrees of flexion in the ring and small fingers, 60 degrees of flexion in the middle finger, and 45 degrees of flexion in the index finger.

REHABILITATION PROTOCOL

Proximal Interphalangeal Joint Arthroplasty for Lateral Deviation

The central slip and collateral ligaments are reconstructed in this deformity.

			• Have the patient wear splints for 6 to 8 weeks after surgery.
2 to 3 weeks	• Use an extension splint and gutter splints to correct residual angular deformities. • Perform active exercises 3 to 5 times a day with taping or radial outriggers.	6 to 8 weeks	• Continue night splinting for 3 to 6 months.

REHABILITATION PROTOCOL

Proximal Interphalangeal Joint Arthroplasty for Boutonnière Deformity

0 to 2 weeks	• Leave the DIP joint free for active and active-assisted flexion exercises.		• Continue interval splinting between exercises and at night.
2 to 3 weeks	• Begin active flexion and extension PIP joint exercises.	6 weeks	• Begin resistive exercises. • Continue night splinting for 3 to 6 months or until the PIP joint is stable.

REHABILITATION PROTOCOL

Eaton Volar Plate Arthroplasty

Acute and chronic fracture dislocations of the PIP joint may be treated by soft tissue arthroplasty with volar plate advancement. Eaton and Malerich recommend this procedure when more than 40% of the base of the middle phalanx is involved.		3 weeks	• Remove the pull-out wire.
		4 weeks	• Allow light work. Buddy tape the affected finger to the adjacent finger. (Moderate swelling may persist for 3 to 5 months and ROM will improve within 2 years.)
2 weeks	• Remove the Kirschner wire. Begin active guarded flexion exercises with a dorsal block splint.	5 weeks	• Use a dynamic extension splint to achieve complete extension.

METACARPOPHALANGEAL JOINT ARTHROPLASTY

MCP joint arthroplasty is indicated primarily for patients with rheumatoid arthritis, although unusual posttraumatic or osteoarthritic conditions may require implant arthroplasty. Correction of radial deviation of the metacarpals as well as intrinsic imbalance are necessary for acceptable results. The procedure increases the range of functional motion of the fingers, although grip and pinch strength do not improve significantly.

REHABILITATION PROTOCOL

Metacarpophalangeal Joint Arthroplasty

0 to 7 days	• Remove drains 2 days after surgery. • Use postoperative splint to maintain MCP joints in full extension and neutral to slight radial deviation.	4 weeks	• Allow light hand use and activities of daily living. • Continue night splinting for 4 months to help reduce extensor lag.
7 days	• Fashion dynamic extension outrigger splint and resting hand splints. • Begin active MCP joint exercises. • Apply a supinator tab to index finger.		Note: If MCP joint motion is not obtained in 2 weeks, the PIP joint should be splinted in full extension and flexion force concentrated at the MCP joint level. Careful follow-up is necessary during the first 3 weeks, when the desired motion should be achieved. At 3 weeks, the capsular structures are significantly tight, and no further ROM should be expected. Dynamic flexion may be necessary to regain early MCP joint flexion.
2 to 4 weeks	• Remove the sutures. Continue the night resting pan splint. • Continue dynamic extension outrigger splint for daily use.		

THUMB CARPOMETACARPAL JOINT ARTHROPLASTY

The arthritic basilar joint of the thumb offers another clear example that roentgenographic appearance has no correlation with the severity of clinical symptoms. Roentgenographic evidence of advanced arthritic change may be an incidental finding, whereas a roentgenographically normal thumb may have significant disability. Treatment regimens with steroid injection, splinting, and nonsteroidal antiinflammatory agents should be exhausted before surgical intervention.

Total joint arthroplasty, implant arthroplasty, interposition arthroplasty, suspension arthroplasties, and CMC joint fusion have been used to alleviate pain and restore function in the diseased basilar joint of the thumb.

Silastic Trapezial Arthroplasty

The low-demand rheumatoid thumb is most suitable for silicone implant arthroplasty, because this implant has a 25% failure rate. More than 80% satisfactory results are reported, despite 56% scaphoid cysts and 74% intramedullary metacarpal radiolucency and/or cysts at long-term follow-up.

REHABILITATION PROTOCOL
Silastic Trapezial Arthroplasty

2 weeks	• Remove the well-padded volar surgical splint and surgical dressing, as well as the temporary Kirschner wire. • Apply a short-arm thumb spica cast.	9 weeks	• Discontinue the splinting.
6 weeks	• Remove the cast and begin controlled CMC, MCP, and IP active ROM exercises with interval protective thumb spica splinting.	3 to 6 months	• Allow the patient to resume normal activities of daily living.

Interposition and Sling Suspension Arthroplasties

Trapezial excision techniques combined with soft tissue interposition or sling suspension arthroplasties have similar postsurgical protocols. Sling suspension arthroplasties are designed to prevent thumb osteoarticular column shortening and provide stability beyond that afforded by simple trapezial excision.

REHABILITATION PROTOCOL
Interposition and Sling Suspension Arthroplasties

2 weeks	• Remove the surgical thumb spica splint and sutures. Apply a short-arm thumb spica cast for an additional 2 weeks.	8 weeks	• Encourage light to moderate activity. • The wrist and thumb static splint may be discontinued in the presence of a painfree and stable joint.
4 weeks	• Begin active, active-assisted, and passive ROM exercises with interval splinting. • Ideally the splint or cast should include only CMC joint leaving the MP or IP free for ROM.	3 months	• Allow normal activity.
6 weeks	• Begin gentle strengthening exercises.		

Discomfort frequently lasts for 6 months after surgery. The function and strength of the thumb will improve over a 6- to 12-month period.

TOTAL WRIST ARTHROPLASTY

Numerous designs of total wrist implants have followed the Swanson flexible silicone implant introduced in 1967. In 1992 Jolly et al. and Lundkvist and Barfred reported silicone synovitis in 30% of patients and prosthetic fracture in 75%. Despite the various metal-on-plastic total wrist arthroplasty designs that have evolved, additional surgery has been required in 35% of patients with total wrist implants because of loosening, tendon imbalance, prosthetic dislocation, and malalignment. Therefore, total wrist arthroplasty appears to be indicated only for the low-demand upper extremity in patients older than 50 years of age with rheumatoid arthritis.

REHABILITATION PROTOCOL

Total Wrist Arthroplasty*

3 to 7 days	• Remove the bulky surgical dressing. • Fashion a contour splint with the wrist in 20 to 30 degrees of extension for night use and interval splinting. Note: The hand is splinted in slight radial deviation to counter ulnar deviation forces. • Dynamic splinting of the digits may be initiated if required.
10 to 12 days	• Begin active-assisted wrist motion. • Avoid ulnar deviation during wrist flexion and extension. • Perform selective strengthening of wrist extensors. • Maintain a dynamic splint for approximately 3 months postoperatively. • Use a resting splint at night.
6 weeks	• Initiate full passive ROM of wrist minimizing radial and ulnar deviation.
8 weeks	• Continue progressive strengthening of hand and wrist.
3 months	• Gradual resumption of normal activities. Note: The total wrist arthroplasty is a low-demand prosthesis, and patients are not to lift objects weighing more than 5 lbs. Problems with silicone synovitis, stability, and bone resorption have limited the use of this procedure.

Fractures and Dislocations

Fractures and dislocations involving the hand are classified as stable or unstable injuries to determine the appropriate treatment. Stable fractures are those that should not displace if some degree of early digital motion is allowed. Unstable fractures are those that displace to an unacceptable degree if early digital motion is allowed. Although some unstable fractures can be converted to stable fractures with closed reduction, it is very difficult to predict which of these will maintain their stability throughout the early treatment phase. For this reason most unstable fractures should undergo closed reduction and percutaneous pinning or open reduction and internal fixation to allow for early protected digital motion and thus prevent stiffness. Those fractures that often require surgical intervention include open fractures, comminuted displaced fractures, fractures associated with joint dislocation or subluxation, displaced spiral fractures, displaced intraarticular fractures particularly around the PIP joint, fractures in which there is loss of bone, and multiple fractures.

METACARPAL AND PHALANGEAL FRACTURES

Nondisplaced metacarpal fractures are stable injuries and are treated with the application of an anterior-posterior splint in the *position of function:* the wrist in 30 to 60 degrees of extension, the MCP joints in 70 degrees of flexion, and the IP joints in 0 to 10 degrees of flexion. In this position, the important ligaments of the wrist and hand are maintained in maximum tension to prevent contractures.

Allowing early PIP and DIP joint motion is essential. Motion prevents adhesions between the tendons and the underlying fracture and controls edema. The dorsal fiberglass splint should extend from below the elbow to the fingertips of all of the involved digits and one adjacent digit. The anterior splint should extend from below the elbow to the distal aspect of the proximal phalanx (Fig. 1-41, *A*), allowing the patient to resume PIP and DIP active flexion and extension exercises immediately (Fig. 1-41, *A*).

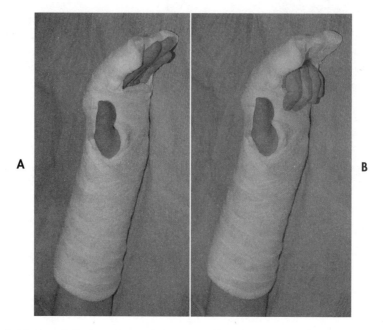

Figure 1-41 A and **B,** Anterior and posterior fiberglass splints typically used to treat metacarpal and proximal phalangeal fractures. PIP and DIP flexion and extension are allowed. The anterior splint should extend 2 cm distal to the level of the fracture.

REHABILITATION PROTOCOL

Nondisplaced Metacarpal Fracture

0 to 3 weeks	• Begin active PIP and DIP flexion and extension exercises. • Elevate hand for edema control.	• Begin gentle active and active-assisted ROM exercises. • Begin strengthening exercises with silicone putty.
3 weeks	• Discontinue splinting. • Protect fingers with buddy taping.	• Continue exercises until grip strength is restored.

Displaced transverse metacarpal fractures, after closed reduction, are treated similarly to nondisplaced fractures. Roentgenograms in the splint should be obtained at weekly intervals to be certain that acceptable skeletal alignment is maintained. Extension contractures of the MCP joints are common after metacarpal fractures and are caused by inadequate splinting in MCP flexion or excessive dorsal angulation of the metacarpal, resulting in intrinsic weakness and clawing. Extension contractures should be treated with aggressive, dynamic flexion splinting, such as a knuckle-bender splint.

Nondisplaced extraarticular phalangeal fractures are treated with similar anterior-posterior splints; however, the anterior splint must also extend out to the fingertips to support the fracture in the position of function. ROM exercises are begun at 3 weeks.

Unstable metacarpal and phalangeal fractures require closed reduction and percutaneous pinning or open reduction and internal fixation. Stable fracture fixation is imperative to allow early ROM.

REHABILITATION PROTOCOL
Postsurgical Metacarpal and Phalangeal Fractures

0 to 4 days	• Apply a bulky hand dressing with an anterior-posterior splint in the position of function.		• If fixation is tenuous but alignment is adequate, immobilize the hand in the position of function for a full 3 weeks.
4 days	• Remove the splint and apply an anterior-posterior splint or a well-molded orthoplast splint that allows PIP and DIP motion. The MCP joint may be immobilized in flexion during this period.	3 to 6 weeks	• Begin active motion before pin removal.

Comminuted phalangeal fractures, especially those that involve diaphyseal segments with thick cortices, may be slow to heal and may require fixation for up to 6 weeks (Fig. 1-42).

0-4 weeks	• Before pin removal, begin active ROM exercises while the therapist supports the fracture site.
4-6 weeks	• Active and active-assisted intrinsic stretching exercises (i.e., simultaneous MCP extension and IP flexion) are recommended.
	• Prevent PIP joint flexion contractures by ensuring that the initial splint immobilizes the PIP joint in an almost neutral position.
	• When the fracture is considered solid on roentgenogram, a dynamic splinting program can be started. The LMB dynamic extension splint and the Capner splint are quite useful. They should be worn for 2-hour increments, 6 to 12 hours a day (Fig. 1-43), and alternated with dynamic flexion strapping (Fig. 1-44).
	• Therapy may be prolonged for up to 3 to 6 months after injury.

Volar PIP joint dislocations are less common than dorsal dislocations and often are difficult to reduce by closed techniques because of entrapment of the lateral bands around the flare of the proximal phalangeal head. If not treated properly, these injuries may result in a boutonnière deformity (combined PIP flexion and DIP extension contracture). Usually the joint is stable after closed or open reduction; however, static PIP extension splinting is recommended for 6 weeks to allow healing of the central slip.

Avulsion fractures involving the dorsal margin of the

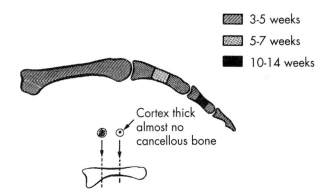

▨ 3-5 weeks
▨ 5-7 weeks
■ 10-14 weeks

Cortex thick
almost no
cancellous bone

Figure 1-42 Time required for fracture healing varies, depending on ratio of cortical to cancellous bone at the fracture site. Healing is the slowest where ratio of cortical to cancellous bone is the highest. (Redrawn from Wilson RE, Carter MS: *Management of Hand Fractures.* In Hunter JM et al, editors: *Rehabilitation of the hand,* St. Louis, 1990, Mosby.)

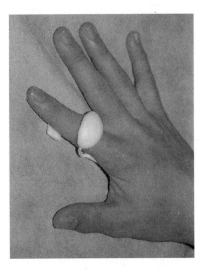

Figure 1-43 Dynamic PIP extension splint (LMB).

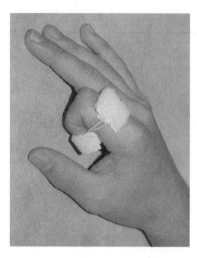

Figure 1-44 Flexion strap used to help regain PIP and DIP flexion.

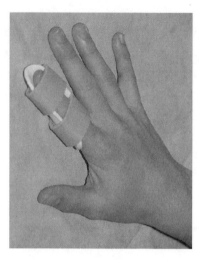

Figure 1-45 Static PIP and DIP extension gutter splint. May be shortened to allow DIP motion.

middle phalanx occur at the insertion of the central slip. These fractures may be treated by closed technique; however, if the fragment is displaced more than 2 mm proximally with the finger splinted in extension, open reduction and internal fixation of the fragment are indicated.

- After closed reduction, fit an extension gutter splint with the PIP joint in neutral position for continuous wear (Fig. 1-45).
- The patient should perform active and passive ROM exercises of the MCP and DIP joints approximately 6 times a day.
- Do not allow PIP joint motion for 6 weeks.
- Begin active ROM exercises at 6 weeks in combination with intermittent daytime splinting and continuous night splinting for an additional 2 weeks.
- After open reduction and internal fixation of a dorsal marginal fracture, remove the transarticular pin between 2 and 4 weeks after the wound has healed, and ensure continuous splinting in an extension gutter splint for a total of 6 weeks. The remainder of the protocol is similar to that used after the closed technique.

■ *Continue extension splinting as long as an extensor lag is present, and avoid passive flexion exercises as long as an extension lag of 30 degrees or more is present.*

Dorsal fracture-dislocations of the PIP joint are much more common than volar dislocations. If less than 50% of the articular surface is involved, these injuries usually are stable after a closed reduction and protective splinting in flexion.

- If the injury is believed to be stable after closed reduction, apply a DBS with the PIP joint in 30 degrees of flexion. This allows for full flexion but prevents the terminal 30 degrees of extension (Fig. 1-46).

- After 3 weeks, adjust the DBS at weekly intervals to increase PIP extension by about 10 degrees each week.
- The splint should be in the neutral position by the sixth week and then discontinued.
- Begin an active ROM program and use dynamic extension splinting as needed.
- Begin progressive strengthening exercises at 8 weeks.

Dorsal fracture-dislocations involving more than 50% of the articular surface may be unstable, even with the digit in flexion, and may require surgical intervention. The Eaton volar plate advancement is probably the most common procedure used. The fracture fragments are excised, and the volar plate is advanced into the remaining portion of the middle phalanx. The PIP joint usually is pinned in 30 degrees of flexion.

- At 3 weeks after surgery, remove the pin from the PIP joint and fit a DBS with the PIP joint in 30 degrees of flexion for continuous wear.
- Begin active and active-assisted ROM exercises within the restraints of the DBS.
- At 5 weeks discontinue the DBS and continue active and passive extension exercises.
- At 6 weeks dynamic extension splinting may be necessary if full passive extension has not been regained.

Flexion contractures are not uncommon after this procedure. Agee described the use of an external fixator combined with rubber bands that allows early active ROM of the PIP joint in unstable fracture-dislocation while maintaining reduction. The bulky hand dressing is removed 3 to 5 days after surgery, and active ROM exercises are carried out for 10-minute sessions every 2 hours. Pins should be cleansed twice daily with the use of cotton swabs and

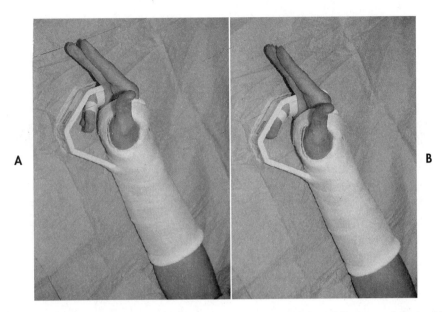

Figure 1-46 **A** and **B,** Extension block splint allowing full digital flexion and limited PIP extension.

hydrogen peroxide, protecting the base of the pin with gauze. The external fixator may be removed between 3 and 6 weeks. An unrestricted active and passive ROM exercise program is started.

Dorsal dislocations of the PIP joint without associated fractures usually are stable after closed reduction. Stability is tested after reduction under digital block and, if the joint is believed to be stable, buddy taping for 3 to 6 weeks, early active ROM exercises, and edema control are necessary. If instability is present with passive extension of the joint, a DBS, similar to that used in fracture-dislocations, should be used.

Intraarticular fractures involving the base of the thumb metacarpal are classified as either *Bennett fractures* (if a single volar ulnar fragment exists) or *Rolando fractures* (if there is a T-condylar fracture pattern). These fractures often displace because of the proximal pull of the APL on the base of the proximal thumb metacarpal.

Nondisplaced Bennett fractures are treated in a short-arm thumb spica cast, which can be removed at 6 weeks if the fracture has healed clinically. Active and gentle passive ROM exercises are begun. At that time the patient is also fitted with a removable thumb spica splint. This should be used between exercise sessions and at night for an additional 2 weeks. Strengthening exercises are then started using silicone putty. The patient generally returns to normal activity between 10 and 12 weeks. If there is persistent joint subluxation after application of a short-arm cast with the thumb positioned in palmar and radial abduction, closed reduction and percutaneous pinning are carried out. After pinning, the thumb is placed in a thumb spica splint and protected for 6 weeks. After the pin is re-

moved, therapy progresses as described for nondisplaced fractures.

Rolando fractures have poor prognoses. The choice of treatment usually depends on the severity of comminution and the degree of displacement. If large fragments are present with displacement, open reduction and internal fixation with Kirschner wires or a mini-fragment plate are performed. If severe comminution is present, manual molding in palmar abduction and immobilization in a thumb spica cast for 3 to 4 weeks are recommended. After stable internal fixation, motion may be started at 6 weeks in a manner similar to that for Bennett fractures.

INJURIES TO THE ULNAR COLLATERAL LIGAMENT OF THE THUMB METACARPOPHALANGEAL JOINT (GAMEKEEPER'S THUMB)

Injuries to the ulnar collateral ligament of the thumb MCP joint are common. They may be partial or complete ruptures of the ligament. Complete ruptures are called gamekeeper's thumb or skier's thumb and can be differentiated from partial tears by obtaining anterior-posterior (AP) stress views of the thumb MCP joint. If the thumb MCP joint angulates more than 30 degrees with radial directed stress compared with the uninjured side, the injury is considered a complete tear, and surgical intervention is indicated.

Partial injuries are treated with a thumb spica cast for 4 weeks. The cast is then removed, and the patient is placed in a removable thumb spica splint, beginning gentle silicone putty strengthening exercises. The thumb is protected during activity for an additional 6 weeks.

After repair of the thumb ulnar collateral ligament (UCL), the MCP joint is pinned in the reduced position, allowing placement of the thumb ray in palmar

and radial abduction without stressing the joint in the splint. The pin is removed between 4 and 6 weeks after surgery, and the thumb is protected during activity for an additional 6 weeks while putty strengthening exercises are instituted.

REHABILITATION PROTOCOL

Ulnar Collateral Ligament (UCL) Strain of Thumb Metacarpophalangeal Joint

Mechanism:	Typically, a ski pole or gamekeeper's thumb type of mechanism, but *not an unstable injury* (only a strain), that can be treated nonoperatively.
0 to 3 weeks	• Fit opponens splint with thumb in palmar abduction; splint is worn continuously.
3 to 6 weeks	• Reevaluate stability and discomfort. • Begin active and gentle passive ROM exercises of thumb.

• If ROM is unstable or painful, have physician reevaluate.
• Patient should wear the splint for protection and comfort and remove it several times a day for exercise sessions.

8 weeks
• Patient should be asymptomatic.
• Discontinue splint except for sports, heavy lifting, or repetitive pinching.
• Use progressive strengthening exercises.

REHABILITATION PROTOCOL

Repair or Reconstruction of Ulnar Collateral Ligament of Thumb Metacarpophalangeal Joint*

Indications:	Typically after repair of gamekeeper's thumb.
3 weeks	• Remove bulky dressing. • Remove MCP pin if used for joint stabilization. • Fit with wrist and thumb static splint for continual wear.
6 weeks	• Begin active and gentle passive ROM exercises of thumb for 10 minutes each hour.

■ *Avoid any lateral stress to the MCP joint of the thumb.*

• Begin dynamic splinting if necessary to increase passive ROM of thumb.

8 weeks
• Discontinue splinting. Wrist and thumb static splint or short opponens splint may be useful during sports-related activities or heavy lifting.
• Begin progressive strengthening.

12 weeks
• Allow the patient to return to unrestricted activity.

SCAPHOID FRACTURES

Nondisplaced scaphoid fractures are treated initially in a long-arm thumb spica cast for 6 weeks, followed by a short-arm spica cast for an additional 6 weeks until roentgenographic union is evident. Fractures involving the proximal and central portions of the scaphoid often require longer periods of immobilization. Active ROM exercises to the forearm, wrist, and thumb should be carried out 6 to 8 times daily after prolonged immobilization. A wrist and thumb static splint often is fitted with the wrist in neutral to be worn between exercise sessions and at night.

Displaced fractures usually require open reduction and internal fixation using either multiple Kirschner wires, a small cancellous screw, or a Herbert screw. Usually, the fracture is treated in a short-arm thumb spica splint until roentgenographic union is achieved, usually in 8 to 12 weeks. Occasionally, if good screw fixation is achieved (as determined by the surgeon intraoperatively), an extremely compliant patient may be treated initially in a short-arm splint for 3 to 4 weeks, followed by application of a removable orthoplast thumb spica splint to be worn during activity until there is roentgenographic evidence of a union. The splint should be removed only 3 times a day for gentle ROM exercises and for bathing. At 4 months after surgery, dynamic wrist flexion and extension may be initiated to increase passive wrist motion. Usually the patient is able to resume normal use of the hand without restriction by 6 months after surgery, provided ROM has been regained and union is evident on roentgenogram.

COLLES' FRACTURES OF THE WRIST

Classification Systems

Frykman (Fig. 1-47)
- Even-numbered fractures (types II, IV, VI, and VIII) have an associated fracture of the distal ulna.
- Types III through VI are intraarticular fractures.
- Higher numbers in the classification have worse prognoses.
- Joint involvement

I, II	Extraarticular
III, IV	Radiocarpal joint
V, VI	Radioulnar joint
VII, VIII	Both radiocarpal and radioulnar joints

Melone (Fig. 1-48)
- The four basic components of intraarticular distal radial fractures:

  Shaft

  Radial styloid

  Dorsal medial facet

  Volar medial facet

  The major fragment of this four-part fracture is the medial facet (fragments 3 and 4).
- This classification recognizes the importance of the lunate facet.
- Types I through IV are different grades of a four-part fracture of the radius; type V is an extremely comminuted unstable fracture without any identifiable facet fragments.

GENERAL PRINCIPLES: WRIST FRACTURE

Because the radius carries 80% of the axial load of the forearm, changes in forearm length ratio (such as with a settled distal radial fracture) increase radial loading beyond physiologic limits.

Biomechanical studies with cadavers show significant increases in axial load transmitted to the ulnar shaft when the radius is shortened by small amounts (2.5 mm). This theoretically could lead to ulnar wrist pain and degenerative joint disease, as could the loss of volar tilt (Fig. 1-49).

Knirk and Jupiter found intraarticular distal radial fractures that healed with more than 1 mm of articular depression resulted in symptomatic posttraumatic arthritis in more than 90% of patients.

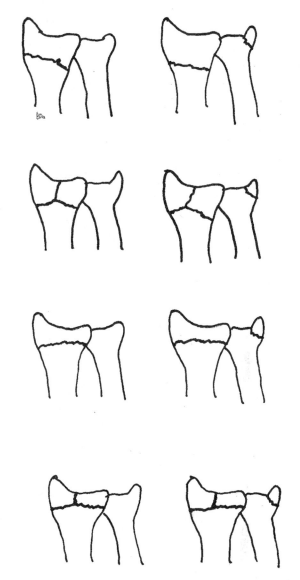

Figure 1-47 Frykman classification of distal radius fractures.

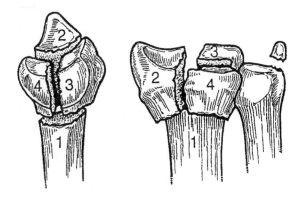

Figure 1-48 Melone classification of distal radius fracture. (From Palmer A: *Fractures of the distal radius.* In Green D, editor: *Operative hand surgery,* ed 3, 1993, Churchill Livingstone.)

Other biomechanical studies show that distal radial tilt dorsally decreases the contact area of the articular surface with the scaphoid and lunate, as well as shifting the contact area dorsally.

Kaukonen et al. noted that closed treatment of distal radial fractures resulted in malposition of the fracture in 85% of patients; the investigators concluded that casting was *not* adequate support for many unstable fractures.

Although maintaining normal ROM (Table 1-7) is desirable Ryu et al found that 40 normal subjects could perform "normal" activities with 60 degrees of extension, 45 degrees of flexion, 40 degrees of ulnar deviation, and 17 degrees of radial deviation.

Goals of Treatment
- Restoration of radial length (Fig. 1-49, *B*).
- Restoration of volar tilt (Fig. 1-49, *C*).

- Restoration of anatomic articular congruity.
- Avoidance of complications.
- Appropriate treatment with consideration of patient's physiologic age, functional demands, occupation, and handedness.
- Early motion of a stable construct.

TABLE 1-7 **Normal Range of Motion**	
Movement	**Degree**
Flexion and extension	120
Radial/ulnar deviation	50
Forearm rotation at distal radioulnar joint	150

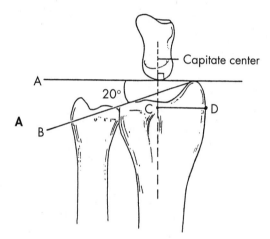

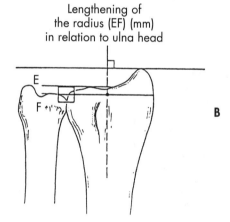

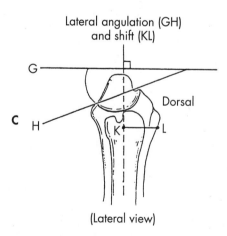

(Lateral view)

Figure 1-49 The location of lines to be drawn for measuring radial slope, radial length, and volar inclination of the distal radius are shown in **A**, **B**, and **C**, respectively. (From Putnam MD: *Fractures and dislocations of the carpus including the distal radius.* In Gustillo RB, Kyle RF, Templeman D, editors: *Fractures and dislocations*, St. Louis, 1993, Mosby–Year Book.)

Complications

- Stiff wrist and/or fingers
- Posttraumatic arthritis
- Residual deformity
- Reflex sympathetic dystrophy
- Malunion, nonunion, delayed union
- Transient or permanent neuropathy

Treatment Considerations

The algorithm described by Palmer bases treatment on physiologic age and demand, stability, displacement, articular congruity, shortening, and angulation (Table 1-8).

TABLE 1-8 Palmer Treatment Algorithm

Fracture type	Treatment protocol	
	Group 1 (physiologically young and/or active)	**Group 2** (physiologically old and/or inactive)
Nondisplaced fracture	STS-3 weeks SAC-3 weeks Splint (R)-3 weeks	STS-2 weeks SAC-2 weeks Splint (R)-3 weeks
Displaced fracture	Closed reduction X-ray findings	Closed reduction 1. STS-2 weeks 2. SAC-3 weeks Splint (R)-3 weeks 3. Late-distal ulna resection

Closed reduction X-ray findings branches into:

Acceptable Reduction → **Stable Fracture** and **Unstable Fracture**

Unacceptable Reduction
(>2 mm radial shortening)
(>2 mm displacement of articular fragment)
(>15° dorsiflexion radius)

Stable Fracture

STS-3 weeks
LAC-3 weeks
Splint (R)-3 weeks

Unstable Fracture

1. External fixation
   with supplemental
   percutaneous pins
   Ex fix-6 weeks
   Pins-8 weeks
   Splint (R)-3 weeks

2. ORIF (plate)
   SAS-10 days
   Splint (R)-5 weeks

3. Percutaneous pins

   STS-3 weeks
   SAC-3 weeks
   Pins-6 weeks
   Splint (R)-3 weeks

Unacceptable Reduction leads to:

1. External fixation with fragment
   elevation (pins optional) and
   iliac crest bone graft-5 weeks

2. ORIF (K-wire) with iliac crest bone graft
   Ex fix-6 weeks
   Pins-6 weeks
   SAS-6 weeks
   Splint (R)-4 weeks

STS = Sugar Tong Splint
SAC = Short-Arm Cast
LAC = Long-Arm Cast
SAS = Short-Arm Splint

From Palmar AK: *Fractures of the distal radius.* In Green D: *Operative hand surgery,* ed 3, New York, 1993, Churchill Livingstone. Our protocol for the treatment of nondisplaced and displaced distal radial fractures in the physiologically young and/or active (group I) and the physiologically old and/or inactive (group II). Nondisplaced fractures are easily treated with immobilization alone in both groups. Displaced fractures require reduction in both groups, but only in group I do we recommend further treatment. Based on the reduction and whether the fracture is stable or not, immobilization is recommended with or without operative treatment. Fractures where the reduction is unacceptable require reduction of the fragments with external fixation and/or internal fixation and bone grafting. *R,* removable; *STS,* sugar tong splint; *SAC,* short-arm cast; *LAC,* long-arm cast; *SAS,* short arm splint.

REHABILITATION PROTOCOL

Stable Colles' Fracture*

1 day
- Use a sugar tong splint.
- Ice for 72 hours.
- Elevate in cradle boot or on pillows for 2 to 3 days at home.
- Begin active and passive ROM exercises to thumb, digits, and shoulder to be performed 10 minutes each hour.
- Use dynamic splinting of the thumb and/or digits 4 to 6 times a day as needed.
- Begin edema control with coban or finger socks to the thumb and digits.

■ Watch for increased levels of edema and pain, which may result in reflex sympathetic dystrophy.

4 to 6 weeks
- Remove splint.
- Fit wrist immobilization splint for continual wear or between exercises and at night (depending on radiographic evidence of healing of fracture).

- Begin active ROM exercises to wrist and forearm for 10 minutes each hour (assuming the fracture is well healed).
- If necessary, begin FES to thumb, digits, wrist, and forearm.
- Continue edema control as needed.

6 to 8 weeks
- Begin passive ROM exercises to wrist and forearm, 10 minutes each hour: flexion, extension, supination, and pronation.
- If needed, begin dynamic splinting of wrist and/or forearm 4 to 6 times a day.
- Decrease or discontinue wrist immobilization splint as comfort permits.
- Begin progressive strengthening as needed.
- Joint mobilization may help to improve ROM of the wrist and forearm, but is indicated only if the fracture is well healed on radiograph.

REHABILITATION PROTOCOL

Colles' Fracture Treated With External Fixation*

(Fig. 1-50)

1 day
- Ice for 72 hours
- Elevate in cradle boot or pillows for 72 hours.
- Perform routine neurovascular checks.

3 days
- Remove bulky compressive dressing and apply light compressive dressing evenly and carefully around pins.
- Clean pin tracts twice a day with hydrogen peroxide and sterile cotton swab.
- Apply gauze at base of pins to absorb drainage and prevent infection.
- Begin active ROM and gentle passive ROM to fingers, elbow, shoulder, and thumb. Apply passive forearm rotation proximal to the fracture site only within the comfort level of the patient.
- It usually is necessary to concentrate on passive motion of the thumb and index finger because of the proximity of the fixator pins to the EPL and extensor indicis pollicis (EIP)/extensor digitorum communis (EDC).

6 to 8 weeks
- Remove fixator (dependent on healing).
- Begin active ROM exercises of wrist and forearm 10 minutes each hour.
- Continue wrist immobilization splint at night and between exercise sessions for protection.
- Begin strengthening with putty and/or hand exercise.

8 to 10 weeks
- Begin passive ROM exercises to wrist (if fracture is healed).
- Begin dynamic splinting of wrist as necessary.
- Begin gentle progressive resistive exercises of wrist.

Advantages of External Fixation Include the Following:
- Supplementation of internal fixation that is maintaining articular alignment.
- Maintenance of length of radius to avoid fracture settling.
- Alleviation of compressive load forces to the wrist.
- Early forearm ROM and unrestricted active and passive ROM of digits and thumb.

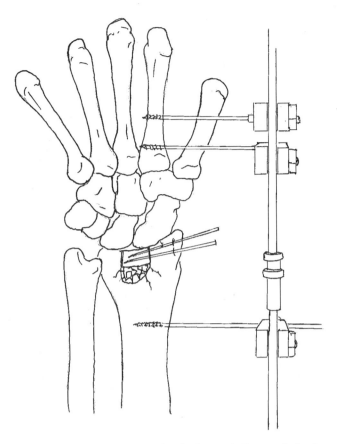

Figure 1-50 External fixator with elevated die punch fracture.

Bibliography
TENDON INJURIES

Trigger Digits

Boyes JH: Flexor tendon grafts in the fingers and thumb: an evaluation of end results, *J Bone Joint Surg* 32A:489, 1950.

Bunnell S: Surgery of the hand, 3rd ed, Philadelphia, JB Lippincott, 1956.

Cannon NM: Diagnosis and treatment manual for physicians and therapists, 3rd edition, The Hand Rehabilitation Center of Indiana, PC, 1991.

Creighton JJ, Idler RS, Strickland JW: Hand Clinic, Trigger finger and thumb, Indiana Medicine 83(4):260, 1990.

Dinham JM, Meggitt BF: Trigger thumbs in children: a review of the natural history and indications for treatment in 105 patients, *J Bone Joint Surg* 56B:153, 1974.

Duran RJ, Houser RG: Controlled passive motion following flexor tendon repair in zones 2 and 3. AAOS Symposium on Tendon Surgery in the Hand. St. Louis, Mosby–Year Book, 1975, pp: 105-114.

Fahey JJ, Bollinger JA: Trigger finger in adults and children, *J Bone Joint Surg* 36A:1200, 1954.

Green D: Operative hand surgery, 3rd edition, Churchill Livingston, 1993.

Hunter JH: Rehabilitation of the hand 3rd edition. Mosby, St. Louis, 1992.

Idler RS: Anatomy and biomechanics of the digital flexor tendons. *Hand Clin* 1:3, 1985.

Rhoades CE, Gelberman RH, Manjarris JF: Stenosing tenosynovitis of the fingers and thumbs, *Clin Orthop* 190:236, 1984.

Flexor Carpi Radialis Tendinitis

Bishop AT, Gabel G, Carmichael, SW: Flexor carpi radialis tendinitis, *J Bone Joint Surg* 76A:1009, 1994.

Gabel G, Bishop AT, Wood MB: Flexor carpi radialis tendinitis. I. Operative anatomy, *J Bone Joint Surg* 76A:1009, 1994.

Gabel G, Bishop AT, Wood, MB: Flexor carpi radialis tendinitis. II. Results of operative treatment. *J Bone Joint Surg* 76A:1015, 1994.

Kleinert HE, Schepel S, Gill T: Flexor tendon injuries, *Surg Clin North Am* 61:267, 1981.

Kleinert HE, Verdan C: Report of the Committee on Tendon Injuries, *J Hand Surg* 8:794, 1983.

Smith, RJ: Balance and kinetics of the fingers under normal and pathological conditions. *Clin Orthop* 104:92, 1974.

Smith RJ: Intrinsic muscles of the fingers: function, dysfunction, and surgical reconstruction, *AAOS Instructional Course Lectures* 24:200, 1975.

Tubiana R, Valentin P: The anatomy of the extensor apparatus of the fingers, *Surg Clin North Am* 44:897, 1964.

Mallet Finger

Bowers WH, Hurst LC: Chronic mallet finger: the use of Fowler's central slip release, *J Hand Surg* 3:373, 1978.

Fess EE, Gettle KS, Strickland JW: Hand splinting principles and methods. St. Louis, Mosby, 1981.

Hillman FE: New technique for treatment of mallet fingers and fractures of the distal phalanx, *JAMA* 161:1135, 1956.

Iselin F, Levame J, Godoy J: A simplified technique for treating mallet fingers: tenodermodesis, *J Hand Surg* 2:118, 1977.

Kleinman WB, Peterson DP: Oblique retinacular ligament reconstruction for chronic mallet finger deformity, *J Hand Surg* 9A:399, 1984.

Stark HH et al: Operative treatment of intraarticular fractures of the dorsal aspect of the distal phalanx of digits, *J Bone Joint Surg* 69A:892, 1987.

Stern PJ, Kastrup JJ: Complications and prognosis of treatment of mallet finger, *J Hand Surg* 13A:329, 1988.

Wehbe MA, Schneider LH: Mallet fractures, *J Bone Joint Surg* 66A:658, 1984.

Wood VE: Fractures of the hand in children. *Orthop Clin North Am* 7:527, 1976.

Boutonnière Deformity

Aiche A, Barsky AJ, Weiner DW: Prevention of boutonnière deformity. *Plast Reconstr Surg* 46:164, 1979.

Chabon SJ, Kuzma GR: Assessing common tendon injuries of the hand, *J Amer Acad Physician Assistants* 1:365, 1988.

Curtis RM, Reid RL, Provost JM: A staged technique for the repair of the traumatic boutonnière deformity, *J Hand Surg* 8:167, 1983.

Dolphin JA: Extensor tenotomy for chronic boutonnière deformity of the finger, *J Bone Joint Surg* 47A:161, 1965.

Doyle JR: Extensor tendons—acute injuries. In Green D, editor: *Operative hand surgery,* ed 3, New York, Churchill Livingston, 1993.

Elliott RA Jr: Injuries to the extensor mechanism of the hand, *Orthop Clin North Am* 1:335, 1970.

Elson RA: Rupture of the central slip of the extensor hood of the finger: a test for early diagnosis, *J Bone Joint Surg* 68B:229, 1986.

Fowler SB: The management of tendon injuries. *J Bone Joint Surg* 41A: 579, 1959.

Green D: *Operative hand surgery,* ed 3, New York, Churchill Livingston, 1993.

Grundberg AB: Anatomic repair of boutonnière deformity, *Clin Orthop* 153:226, 1980.

Hunter JM et al: *Rehabilitation of the hand,* ed 4, St. Louis, 1995, Mosby–Year Book.

Kettelkamp DB, Flatt AE, Moulds R: Traumatic dislocation of the long-finger extensor tendon: a clinical, anatomical, and biomechanical study. *J Bone Joint Surg* 53A:229, 1971.

Kiefhaber TR: Boutonnière & swan-neck deformity. Instructional course, Annual Meeting of the American Society for Surgery of the Hand, Toronto, Canada, Sept, 1990.

Kilgore ES, Graham WP: The hand: surgical and nonsurgical management, Philadelphia, Lea & Febiger, 1977.

Littler JW, Eaton RG: Redistribution of forces in the correction of the boutonnière deformity, *J Bone Joint Surg* 49:1267, 1967.

Matev I: Transposition of the lateral slips of the aponeurosis in treatment of long-standing "boutonnière deformity" of the fingers, *Brit J Plast Surg* 17:281, 1963.

McCoy FJ, Winsky AJ: Lumbrical loop operation for luxation of the extensor tendons of the hand, *Plast Reconstr Surg* 44:142, 1969.

Nalebuff EA, Millender LH: Surgical treatment of the boutonnière deformity in rheumatoid arthritis, *Orthop Clin North Am* 6:753, 1975.

Snow JW: Use of a retrograde tendon flap in repairing a severed extensor tendon in the PIP joint area. *Plast Reconstr Surg* 51:555, 1973.

Thompson JS, Littler JW, Upton J: The spiral oblique retinacular ligament: SORL, *J Hand Surg* 3:482, 1978.

Tonkin Hughes J, Smith KL: Lateral band translocation for Swan-Neck deformity. *J Hand Surg* 17A(2):260, 1992.

Urbaniak JR, Hayes MG: Chronic boutonnière deformity: an anatomic reconstruction, *J Hand Surg* 6:379, 1981.

Wheeldon FT: Recurrent dislocation of extensor tendons in the hand, *J Bone Joint Surg* 36B:612, 1954.

Wright PE II: Arthritic hand. In Crenshaw AH, editor: *Campbell's operative orthopaedics,* vol 5, St. Louis, Mosby, 1992.

deQuervain's Disease

Edwards EG: deQuervain's stenosing tendo-vaginitis at the radial styloid process, *The South Surg* 16:1081, 1950.

Jackson WT et al: Anatomical variations in the first extensor compartment of the wrist, *J Bone Joint Surg* 68A:923, 1986.

Minamikawa Y et al: deQuervain's syndrome: surgical and anatomical studies of the fibrosseous canal, *Orthopaedics* 14:545, 1991.

Strickland JW, Idler RS, Creighton JC: Hand Clinic deQuervain's stenosing tenovitis, *Indiana Medicine* 83(5):340, 1990.

Totten PA: Therapist's management of deQuervain's disease. In Hunter JM et al, editors *Rehabilitation of the hand, surgery and therapy,* St. Louis, 1990, Mosby.

Intersection Syndrome

Grundberg AB, Reagan DS: Pathologic anatomy of the forearm: intersection syndrome, *J Hand Surg* 10A:299, 1985.

NERVE COMPRESSION SYNDROMES

Pronator Syndrome

Gainor BJ: The pronator compression test revisited, *Orthop Rev* 19:888, 1990.

Hartz CR, et al: The pronator teres syndrome: compressive neuropathy of the median nerve, *J Bone Joint Surg* 63A:886, 1981.

Idler RS, Strickland JW, Creighton JJ: Pronator syndrome, Hand Clinic, Indiana Center for Surgery and Rehabilitation of the Hand and Upper Extremity, Indianapolis.

Ulnar Tunnel Syndrome

Amadio PC, Beckenbaugh RD: Entrapment of the ulnar nerve by the deep flexor-pronator aponeurosis, *J Hand Surg* 11:83, 1986.

Dupont C et al: Ulnar-tunnel syndrome at the wrist, *J Bone Joint Surg* 47A:757, 1965.

Johnson RK, Spinner M, Shrewsbury MM: Median nerve entrapment syndrome in the proximal forearm, *J Hand Surg* 4:48, 1979.

Kleinert HE, Hayes JE: The ulnar tunnel syndrome, *Plast Reconstr Surg* 47:21, 1971.

Kleinman WB: Anterior intramuscular transposition of the ulnar nerve, *J Hand Surg* 14A:972, 1989.

Kuschner SH, Gelberman RH, Jennings C: Ulnar nerve compression at the wrist, *J Hand Surg* 13A:577, 1988.

Leffert RD: Anterior submuscular transposition of the ulnar nerves by the Learmonth technique, *J Hand Surg* 7:147, 1982.

Magassy CL et al: Ulnar tunnel syndrome, *Orthop Rev* 11:21, 1973.

Roles NC, Maudsley RH: Radial tunnel syndrome: resistant tennis elbow as a nerve entrapment, *J Bone Joint Surg* 54B:499, 1972.

Shea JD, McClain EJ: Ulnar nerve compression syndromes at and below the wrist, *J Bone Joint Surg* 51A:1095, 1969.

Cubital Tunnel Syndrome

Craven PR, Green DP: Cubital tunnel syndrome, *J Hand Surg* 62A:986, 1980.

Radial Tunnel Syndrome

Lister GD, Belsole RB, Kleinert HE: The radial tunnel syndrome, *J Hand Surg* 4:52, 1979.

Spinner M: The arcade of Frohse and its relationship to posterior interosseous nerve paralysis, *J Bone Joint Surg* 50B:809, 1968.

Sponseller PD, Engber WD: Double-entrapment radial tunnel syndrome, *J Hand Surg* 8:420, 1983.

Thoracic Outlet Syndrome

Fechter JD, Kuschner SH: The thoracic outlet syndrome, *Orthopaedics* 16:1243, 1993.

Leffert RD: Thoracic outlet syndrome, *J Amer Acad Orthopaedic Surgeons*, 2(6):317, 1994.

WRIST AND DISTAL RADIOULNAR JOINT DISORDERS

Wrist Ligament Injury

Blatt G: Capsulodesis in reconstructive hand surgery, *Hand Clin* 3:81, 1987.

Lavernia CJ, Cohen MS, Taleisnik J: Treatment of scapholunate dissociation by ligamentous repair and capsulodesis, *J Hand Surg*, 17A:354, 1992.

Watson HK, Ballet FL: The SLAC wrist: scapholunate advanced collapse pattern of degenerative arthritis, *J Hand Surg* 9A:358, 1984.

REPLANTATION

Entin MA: Crushing and avulsing injuries of the hand, *Surg Clin North Am* 44:1009, 1964.

Kleinder HE, Kasdan ML: Salvage of devascularized upper extremities, including studies on small vessel anastomosis, *Clin Orthop* 29:29, 1963.

Moberg E: The treatment of mutilating injuries of the upper limb, *Surg Clin North Am* 44:1107, 1964.

ARTHROPLASTY

Finger Arthroplasty

Bieber EJ, Weiland AJ, Volenec-Dowling S: Silicone-rubber implant arthroplasty of the metacarpophalangeal joints for rheumatoid arthritis, *J Bone Joint Surg* 68A:206, 1986.

Blair WF, Shurr DG, Buckwalter JA: Metacarpophalangeal joint implant arthroplasty with a silastic spacer, *J Bone Joint Surg* 66A:365, 1984.

Cannon NM: Diagnosis and treatment manual for physicians and therapists, 3rd edition, The Hand Rehabilitation Center of Indiana, PC, 1991.

Eaton RG, Malerich MM: Volar plate arthroplasty of the proximal interphalangeal joint: a review of ten years' experience, *J Hand Surg* 5:260, 1980.

Swanson AB: Flexible implant arthroplasty for arthritic finger joints, *J Bone Joint Surg* 54A:435, 1972.

Swanson AB: Silastic HP 100 Swanson finger joint implant for metacarpophalangeal and proximal interphalangeal joint arthroplasty and Dow Corning Wright Swanson finger joint Grommet II for metacarpophalangeal implant arthroplasty, Down Corning Wright, 1988.

Swanson AB, Leonard JB, deGroot Swanson G: Implant resection arthroplasty of the finger joints, *Hand Clin* 2:107, 1986.

Swanson AB et al: Flexible implant arthroplasty in the proximal interphalangeal joint of the hand, *J Hand Surg* 10A:796, 1985.

Thumb Carpometacarpal Joint Arthroplasty

Burton RI, Pellegrini VD: Surgical management of basal joint arthritis of the thumb. II. Ligament reconstruction with tendon interposition arthroplasty, *J Hand Surg*, 11A:324, 1986.

Cannon NM: Diagnosis and treatment manual for physicians and therapists, 3rd edition, The Hand Rehabilitation Center of Indiana, PC, 1991.

Creigton JJ, Steichen JB, Strickland JW: Long-term evaluation of silastic trapezial arthroplasty in patients with osteoarthritis, *J Hand Surg* 16A:510, 1991.

Dell PC, Brushart TM, Smith RJ: Treatment of trapeziometacarpal arthritis: Results of resection arthroplasty, *J Hand Surg* 3:243, 1978.

Eaton RG, Littler JW: Ligament reconstruction for the painful thumb carpometacarpal joint, *J Bone Joint Surg* 55A:1655, 1973.

Kleinman WB, Eckenrode JF: Tendon suspension sling arthroplasty for thumb trapeziometacarpal arthritis, *J Hand Surg* 16A:983, 1991.

Hofammann DY, Ferlic DC, Clayton ML: Arthroplasty of the basal joint of the thumb using a silicone prosthesis, *J Bone Joint Surg* 69A:993, 1987.

Pellegrini VD, Burton RI: Surgical management of basal joint arthritis of the thumb. I. Long-term results of silicone implant arthroplasty, *J Hand Surg* 11A:309, 1986.

Wrist Arthroplasty

Beckenbaugh RD: Current status of total joint replacement in the upper extremity, *J Am Geriatr Soc* 25:68, 1977.

Beckenbaugh RD: Implant arthroplasty in the rheumatoid hand and wrist: current state of the art in the United States, *J Hand Surg* 8:675, 1983.

Beckenbaugh RD: New concepts in arthroplasty of the hand and wrist, *Arch Surg* 112:1094, 1977.

Beckenbaugh RD: Total joint arthroplasty: the wrist, *Mayo Clin Proc* 54:513, 1979.

Beckenbaugh RD, Linscheid RL: Total wrist arthroplasty: a preliminary report, *J Hand Surg* 2:337, 1977.

Cooney WP, Beckenbaugh RD, Linscheid RL: Total wrist arthroplasty: problems with implant failures, *Clin Orthop* 187:121, 1984.

Dennis DA, Ferlic DC, Clayton ML: Volz total wrist arthroplasty in rheumatoid arthritis: a long-term review, *J Hand Surg* 11:483, 1986.

Ferlic DC: Implant arthroplasty of the rheumatoid wrist, *Hand Clinics* 3:169, 1987.

Figgie HE et al: Preliminary results of total wrist arthroplasty in rheumatoid arthritis using the trispherical total wrist arthroplasty, *J Arthroplasty* 3:9, 1988.

Figgie MP et al: Trispherical total wrist arthroplasty in rheumatoid arthritis, *J Hand Surg* 15A:217, 1990.

Johnson BM, Flynn MJG, Beckenbaugh RD: A dynamic splint for use after total wrist arthroplasty, *Am J Occup Ther* 35:179, 1981.

Jolly SL et al: Swanson silicone arthroplasty of the wrist in rheumatoid arthritis: a long-term follow-up, *J Hand Surg* 17A:142, 1992.

Linscheid RL, Beckenbaugh RD: Total arthroplasty of the wrist to relieve pain and increase motion, *Geriatrics* 31:48, 1976.

Lundkvist L, Barfred T: Total wrist arthroplasty, *Scand J Plast Reconstr Hand Surg* 26:97, 1992.

Menon J: Total wrist replacement using the modified Volz prosthesis, *J Bone Joint Surg* 69A:998, 1987.

Siemionow M, Lister GD: Tendon ruptures and median nerve damage after Hamas total wrist arthroplasty, *J Hand Surg* 12:374, 1987.

FRACTURES AND DISLOCATIONS

Agee JM: Unstable fracture-dislocations of the proximal interphalangeal joint: treatment with the force couple splint. *Clin Orthop* 214:101, 1987.

Crenshaw AH: *Campbell's operative orthopaedics,* ed 8, St. Louis, 1992, Mosby.

Jobe MT: Fractures and dislocations of the hand. In Gustilo RB, Kyle RK, Templeman D, editors: *Fractures and dislocations,* St Louis, 1993, Mosby.

Greene D: *Operative hand surgery,* ed 3, New York, Churchill Livingston, 1993.

Hunter JM, et al: *Rehabilitation of the hand: surgery and therapy,* ed 3, St. Louis, 1990, Mosby.

Indiana hand rehabilitation manual, Indianapolis, 1993.

Kaukonen JP, Porras M, Karaharju E: Anatomical results after distal forearm fractures. *Ann Chir Gynaecol* 77:21, 1988.

Knirk JL, Jupiter JB: Intra-articular fractures of the distal end of the radius in young adults. *J Bone Joint Surg* 63-A: 647, 1986.

Moberg E: *Emergency surgery of the hand,* Edinburgh, 1968, Churchill Livingstone.

Putnam MD: Fractures and dislocations of the carpus including the distal radius. In Gustillo RB, Kyle RF, Templeman D, editors: *Fractures and dislocations,* St. Louis, 1993, Mosby.

Ryu J, Watson HK, Burgess RC: Rheumatoid wrist reconstruction utilizing a fibrous nonunion and radiocarpal arthrodesis, *J Hand Surg* 10A:830, 1985.

CHAPTER TWO

Elbow Rehabilitation

JAMES R. ANDREWS, MD
KEVIN E. WILK, PT
DAVID GROH, PT

Elbow Dislocation

REHABILITATION RATIONALE

Elbow dislocations most frequently occur as a result of hyperextension, in which the olecranon process is forced into the olecranon fossa with such impact that the trochlea is levered over the coronoid process (Fig. 2-1). Most elbow dislocations occur in a directly posterior or posterolateral direction. Anterior dislocations occur in only 1% to 2% of patients.

Classification

The traditional classification of elbow dislocations divides injuries into anterior and posterior dislocations. Posterior dislocations are further subdivided according to the final resting position of the olecranon in relation to the distal humerus: posterior, posterolateral (most common), posteromedial (least common), or pure lateral.

Morrey makes a clinical distinction between complete dislocation and "perched" dislocation (Fig. 2-2). Because perched dislocations have less ligament tearing, they have a more rapid recovery and more rapid rehabilitation. For a complete dislocation the anterior capsule must be disrupted. The brachialis must also be torn or significantly stretched.

Many elbow dislocations are accompanied by some type of ulnar collateral ligament (UCL) involvement. More specifically, the anterior oblique band of the UCL is affected. Tullos et al found that the anterior oblique band of the UCL was torn in 34 of 37 patients who had previously experienced a posterior elbow dislocation. Repair of this ligament is sometimes indicated in athletes if the injury occurs in the dominant arm. This optimizes the chance for full return to the athlete's previous level of competition.

Associated fractures occur in 25% to 50% of patients with elbow dislocations, most commonly a fracture of the radial head.

GENERAL REHABILITATION CONSIDERATIONS

■ *The most common sequela of elbow dislocations is the loss of motion, especially extension.*

At 10 weeks, a flexion contracture averaging 30 degrees is common, and at 2 years a 10-degree flexion contracture often is present. This condition does not improve with time.

Rehabilitation is focused on restoring early range of motion (ROM) within the limits of elbow stability. *Valgus stress* to the elbow is *avoided* during rehabilitation.

Stability after reduction of an elbow dislocation must be determined to ensure proper rehabilitation. The elbow is moved through a gentle passive ROM, avoiding any valgus stressing. Redislocation of the el-

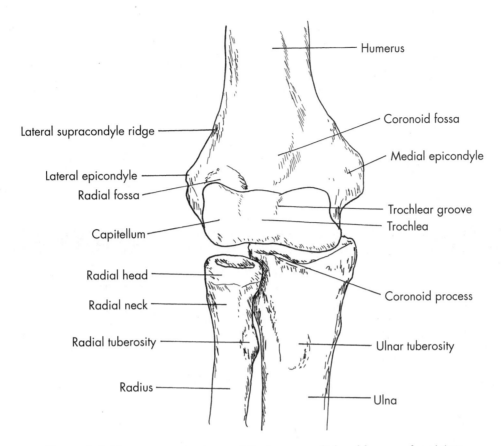

Figure 2-1 The osseous structures of the humeroradial and humeroulnar joints.

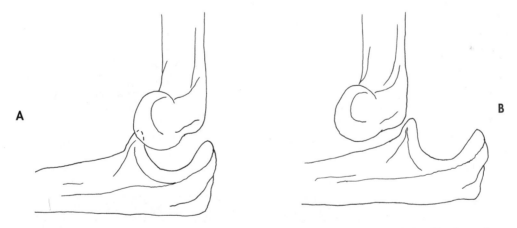

Figure 2-2 Simplified classification of elbow dislocation has prognostic implications. **A,** Perched (subluxed). **B,** Complete (dislocated). (From Morrey BF: Biomechanics of the elbow and forearm, *Orthop Sports Med* 17:840, 1994.)

bow with simple passive ROM implies severe valgus instability with rupture of the medial collateral ligaments and forearm flexors.

For dislocations that are *stable* after reduction, best results are obtained with early protected motion before 2 weeks. Prolonged immobilization (more than 2 weeks) is associated with more severe flexion contracture and more pain at follow-up, and it does not de-

crease symptoms of instability. Stable elbow dislocations are effectively treated with early ROM and general strengthening, as with other rehabilitation protocols for the elbow. Inherent osseous stability allows early extension and flexion if valgus stress is prevented after reduction.

Unstable dislocations require repair of the medial collateral ligament. Rehabilitation of unstable dislocations requires a longer protection phase. Starting at week 1, a ROM brace preset at 30 to 90 degrees is implemented. Each week, motion in this brace is increased by 5 degrees of extension and 10 degrees of flexion. This progression is controlled directly by the collagen synthesis and remodeling process that takes place within the involved tissues.

Recurrence of elbow dislocations is uncommon, occurring after only 1% to 2% of simple elbow dislocations. Recurrent instability is more likely if the initial dislocation involved a posterior fracture or if the first incident took place during childhood or adolescence.

A rehabilitation program that is too aggressive may cause recurrent subluxation, and one that is too conservative can lead to a flexion contracture; the occurrence of flexion contractures is a much greater probability. Full elbow extension is less critical for the nonathlete and thus may be sacrificed slightly to ensure that the joint structure and ligaments are given more time to heal and to decrease the risk of recurrent subluxation or dislocation.

REHABILITATION PROTOCOL

Stable Elbow Dislocation ANDREWS AND WILK

1 to 4 days	• Immobilize the elbow in a posterior splint for 3 to 4 days. • Begin light gripping exercises. • Begin active ROM in all planes. • Begin shoulder isometrics. Avoid valgus stress to the elbow. • Use pulsed ultrasound and high-voltage galvanic stimulation (HVGS) modalities as required.	10 to 14 days	• Discard the splint. • Continue active ROM exercises. • Initiate full elbow rehabilitation program, including passive ROM. • Begin progressive resistance exercises as tolerated for elbow; begin supination and pronation also. • Perform isotonic exercises; use caution with external rotation (ER) to avoid valgus stress to the elbow. • A hinged brace may be used and locked from 15 to 90 degrees for up to 4 weeks if borderline stability is a concern.
5 to 9 days	• The splint should be removed for exercises. • Begin gentle active ROM exercises of elbow out of the splint several times a day but no passive ROM. • Begin active ROM in elbow flexion/extension, supination/pronation, and slow Upper Body Ergonometer (UBE). • Begin isometrics in elbow flexion/extension at varying angles. • Begin shoulder strength progression with stabilization of elbow; begin wrist isotonics.	Return to sports	• Do not allow return to participation in sports until strength, power, and endurance is 85% to 90% of the uninvolved limb. • Brace is worn and locked on parameters to prevent elbow hyperextension and valgus stress once the athlete returns to competition.

REHABILITATION PROTOCOL

Unstable Elbow Dislocation ANDREWS AND WILK

Phase 1—Immediate Postreduction Phase			

0 to 3 weeks	• Goals:
	  Protect healing tissue.
	  Decrease pain/inflammation.
	  Retard muscular atrophy.
	• Set splint or brace ROM at 10 degrees less than active ROM elbow extension limit.
	• Perform elbow flexion to patient tolerance.
	• Perform wrist active ROM flexion/extension and supination/pronation exercises, 5
		0 to 3 weeks— cont'd	degrees of extension and 10 degrees of flexion per week (as long as there is no associated fracture).
			• *Avoid any varus/valgus stress on the elbow.*
			• Initiate further exercises:
			  Gripping exercises.
			  Wrist ROM.
			  Shoulder "straight plane isometrics" (no shoulder internal rotation [IR] or ER); biceps multiangle isometrics.

REHABILITATION PROTOCOL—cont'd

Phase 1—Immediate Postreduction Phase—cont'd

0 to 3 weeks—cont'd
- Use cryotherapy.
- Use pulsed ultrasound or HVGS.

Phase 2—Intermediate Phase

4 to 8 weeks
- Goals:
  Gradually increase elbow extension ROM (10 degrees per week).
  Promote healing of damaged tissue.
  Regain and improve muscle strength.

4 weeks
- Set functional brace at 10 degrees greater than it was in the previous week.
- Begin light resistance exercises for arm (1 lb).
  Wrist curls, extensions.
  Pronation/supination.
  Elbow flexion/extension.
- Progress shoulder program. Emphasize rotator cuff strengthening (avoid IR/ER until the sixth week).
- Begin gentle passive ROM for elbow flexion/extension.

6 weeks
- Progress elbow strengthening exercises.
- Initiate shoulder ER strengthening.
- Progress shoulder program.

Phase 3—Advanced Strengthening Phase

9 to 13 weeks
- Goals:
  Increase strength, power, endurance.
  Maintain full elbow ROM.
  Gradually initiate sports activities.

9 weeks
- Initiate eccentric elbow flexion/extension.
- Continue isotonic program for forearm and wrist.
- Continue shoulder program (Thrower's Ten Program, p. 82).
- Begin manual resistance diagonal patterns.
- Initiate plyometric exercise program.

11 weeks
- Continue all exercises.
- Patient may begin light sports activities (such as golf and swimming).

Ulnar Collateral Ligament Reconstruction

ANATOMY

The UCL originates at the medial epicondyle and is composed of three bands: the anterior oblique, which remains taut throughout full ROM; the posterior oblique, which is taut during flexion and lax during extension; and the transverse oblique, which remains taut throughout elbow ROM but plays only a minor role in providing medial stability (Fig. 2-3).

Among the soft tissue structures of the elbow, the UCL provides the primary resistive force to valgus stresses that occur during throwing activities (e.g., acceleration and follow-through phases of pitching). It is the structure usually torn as a result of a valgus force or injured as a result of the repetitive trauma of overhead throwing.

RECONSTRUCTION

Reconstruction of the UCL is one of the most commonly performed surgical procedures in throwing athletes. During the acceleration phase of throwing, tremendously high and repetitive stresses are applied to the medial elbow joint, frequently resulting in liga-

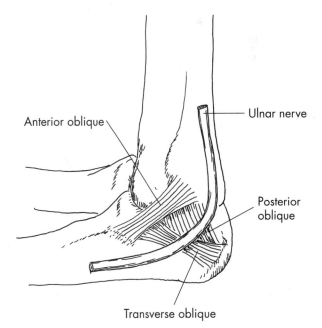

Figure 2-3 The ulnar collateral ligament complex of the elbow, consisting of three bundles: anterior, posterior, and transverse oblique. (From Wilk KE, Arrigo CA, Andrews JR: Rehabilitation of the elbow in the throwing athlete, *J Orthop Sports Phys Ther* 17:305, 1993.)

mentous failure, tendonitis, or osseous changes. These can vary in degree from an overuse flexor/pronator muscular strain to ligamentous sprains of the UCL. Besides throwing, sports activities that can stress the UCL include the forehand stroke in tennis, an improper golf swing, and arm wrestling. Because the UCL is the primary stabilizer to valgus stress at the elbow, reconstruction is vital to competitive throwing athletes who wish to return to their previous levels of performance.

Usually an autogenous graft, such as the palmaris longus extensor hallucis, is used to reconstruct the UCL. The graft then simulates the function of the UCL, particularly the anterior oblique portion, providing the primary restraint to valgus stress during throwing. During this surgical procedure, the ulnar nerve is transposed subcutaneously medially and is held in place with fascial slings.

Immediate postoperative precautions must be observed, especially in relation to the soft tissue of the fascial slings that stabilize the ulnar nerve. For this reason, the patient is placed in a 90-degree posterior splint for 1 week. This does not delay the entire rehabilitation process, however, because submaximal isometrics for the wrist musculature and elbow flexors and extensors at multiple angles may be initiated within the first week if all valgus stress is eliminated. In the second week the patient is placed into a ROM brace preset at 30 to 90 degrees. Each week the motion is increased by 5 degrees of extension and 10 degrees of flexion, with full motion restoration at 6 to 7 weeks.

REHABILITATION PROTOCOL

Reconstruction of the Ulnar Collateral Ligament
ANDREWS AND WILK

Phase 1—Immediate Postoperative Phase

0 to 3 weeks
- Goals:
  Protect healing tissue.
  Decrease pain/inflammation.
  Retard muscular atrophy.

1 week
- Set posterior splint at 90 degrees of elbow flexion.
- Begin wrist active ROM extension/flexion.
- Use elbow compression dressing (2 to 3 days).
- Begin exercises:
  Gripping exercises.
  Wrist ROM.
  Shoulder isometrics (except shoulder ER).
  Biceps isometrics.
- Use cryotherapy.

2 weeks
- Apply ROM brace settings from 30 to 100 degrees.
- Initiate wrist isometrics.
- Initiate elbow flexion/extension isometrics.
- Continue all exercises listed above.

3 weeks
- Advance brace 15 to 110 degrees (gradually increase ROM; 5 degrees of extension and 10 degrees of flexion per week).

Phase 2—Intermediate Phase

4 to 8 weeks
- Goals:
  Gradually increase ROM.
  Promote healing of repaired tissue.
  Regain and improve muscular strength.

4 weeks
- Set ROM brace (10 to 120 degrees).
- Begin light resistance exercises for arm (1 lb):
  Wrist curls, extensions.
  Pronation/supination.
  Elbow extension/flexion.
- Progress shoulder program; emphasize rotator cuff strengthening (avoid ER until the sixth week).
- Begin gentle passive ROM for elbow flexion/extension.

6 weeks
- Set ROM brace at 0 to 130 degrees; perform active ROM at 0 to 145 degrees (without brace).
- Progress elbow strengthening exercises.
- Initiate shoulder ER strengthening.
- Progress shoulder program.

Phase 3—Advanced Strengthening Phase

9 to 13 weeks
- Goals:
  Increase strength, power, endurance.
  Maintain full elbow ROM.
  Gradually initiate sporting activities.

9 weeks
- Initiate eccentric elbow flexion/extension.
- Continue isotonic program; continue forearm and wrist exercises.
- Continue shoulder program (Thrower's Ten Program, p. 82).
- Perform manual resistance diagonal patterns.
- Initiate plyometric exercise program. Include trunk rotation and plyoball with minitramp.

REHABILITATION PROTOCOL—cont'd

Phase 3—Advanced Strengthening Phase—cont'd
11 weeks
- Continue all exercises listed above.
- The patient may begin light sports activities (such as golf and swimming).

Phase 4—Return to Activity Phase
14 to 26 weeks
- Goals:
  Continue to increase strength, power, and endurance of upper extremity musculature.
  Gradual return to sports activities.

14 weeks
- Initiate interval throwing program (phase 1).
- Continue strengthening program.
- Emphasize elbow and wrist strengthening and flexibility exercises.

22 to 26 weeks
- Patient may return to competitive throwing (competitive athletes only).

REHABILITATION PROTOCOL

Reconstruction of Ulnar Collateral Ligament
JOBE, BREWSTER, AND SETO

This rehabilitation program is designed to return throwing athletes to their competitive levels at approximately 1 year after surgery. Jobe reports that it is critical to allow this complete period for tendon revascularization to occur and to promote its viability.

0 to 2 weeks
- Immobilize elbow.
- Begin gripping exercises.

2 to 4 weeks
- Remove splint.
- Begin passive ROM and active-assisted elbow ROM.
- Begin active shoulder ROM exercises (if necessary).

4 to 6 weeks
- Perform active elbow and shoulder ROM exercises.
- Begin strengthening exercises:
  Wrist flexion/extension.
  Forearm pronation/supination.

6 weeks to 3 months
- Continue shoulder and elbow ROM exercises.
- Continue wrist and forearm strengthening exercises.
- Add elbow strengthening exercises.
- Add resistive radial and ulnar deviation as required.

3 to 5 months
- Avoid valgus stress to elbow and ballistic movement in terminal elbow ranges.
- May begin shoulder strengthening exercises with light resistance, with emphasis on rotator cuff muscles.
- Start total body conditioning exercises.

- May begin easy tossing at 30 feet, progressing to 50 feet, no wind up, 2 to 3 times per week, 10 to 15 minutes per session.

5 to 5.5 months
- Continue upper extremity strengthening exercises.
- Continue easy tossing, 50 to 60 feet, no wind up, 2 to 3 times per week, 10 to 15 minutes per session.

5.5 to 6 months
- Add shoulder IR exercise in side-lying position.
- Continue strengthening exercises and total body conditioning program.
- Lob ball on alternate days, no more than 30 feet, 10 to 15 minutes per session.

6 to 6.5 months
- Lob with easy wind up, 40 to 50 feet, 15 to 20 minutes per session, 2 to 3 times per week.

6.5 to 7 months
- Lob with occasional straight throw at half speed, 60 feet, 20 minutes per session, 2 to 3 times per week.

7 to 7.5 months
- Increase throwing distance to 100 feet at half speed, 20 to 25 minutes per session, 2 to 3 times per week.

7.5 to 8 months
- Progress to long, easy throws from 150 feet, with ball back to home plate on 5 to 6 bounces, 20 to 25 minutes per session.
- Begin 12-day throwing cycle: throw 2 days, rest 1 day; repeat 4 times.

Continued

REHABILITATION PROTOCOL—cont'd

Reconstruction of Ulnar Collateral Ligament
JOBE, BREWSTER, AND SETO

8 to 8.5 months	• **OUTFIELDERS** Increase throwing distance to 200 to 250 feet, with ball reaching home plate on numerous bounces, 20 to 25 minutes per session. Use a 12-day throwing cycle. • **PITCHERS AND INFIELDERS** In-and-out drill: Begin throwing at half speed, gradually increasing the throwing distance up to 150 feet. Gradually decrease throwing distance until reaching normal throwing position distance. Perform this drill 30 to 35 minutes on the 12-day throwing cycle.
8.5 to 9 months	• **OUTFIELDERS** Increase throwing distance to 300 to 350 feet, with ball reaching home plate on 1 to 2 bounces at three-quarter speed to full speed, 30 to 35 minutes per session. Use a 12-day throwing cycle. • **PITCHERS AND INFIELDERS** In-and-out drill: Gradually reduce time throwing "in and out" and increase throwing time from normal playing position, three-quarter speed to full speed, 30 to 35 minutes per session. Use a 12-day throwing cycle.

9 to 9.5 months	• **OUTFIELDERS AND INFIELDERS** Begin short, crisp throws from 100 to 150 feet, three-quarter to full speed, 30 minutes per session. Use a 12-day throwing cycle. • **PITCHERS** Throw batting practice at three-quarter to full speed, 30 minutes per session. Use a 12-day throwing cycle.
9.5 to 10.5 months	• **ALL PLAYERS** Return to throwing from normal playing position, three-quarter to full speed, with emphasis on technique and accuracy; 25 to 30 minutes per session. Use a 12-day throwing cycle.
10.5 to 11 months	• **ALL PLAYERS** Continue throwing from normal playing position, seven-eighths to full speed, gradually increasing throwing time.
11 to 12 months	• **ALL PLAYERS** Simulate game day situation. • **PITCHERS** Warm-up with appropriate number of pitches and throw for an average number of innings, taking the usual rest breaks between innings. Repeat this simulation 2 to 4 times with a 3- to 4-day rest period in between.

OVERVIEW OF REHABILITATION PROTOCOL

Reconstruction of Ulnar Collateral Ligament
JOBE, BREWSTER, AND SETO

0 to 2 weeks	• Initiate gripping exercises with a soft ball while the patient is still immobilized in the postoperative splint.
2 to 4 weeks	• Remove the splint. • Begin gentle passive and active-assisted elbow ROM exercises. • Use gentle active shoulder exercises to maintain ROM; however, avoid IR and ER, because when the elbow is flexed and a force causing shoulder rotation is applied below the elbow, an inappropriate valgus force is placed on the elbow.

4 weeks	• Progress to elbow and wrist strengthening exercises at full range.
	    Elbow strengthening exercises:
	      Flexion and extension.
	      Pronation and supination.
	    Wrist strengthening exercises:
	      Flexion and extension.
	• Continue active shoulder exercises.
	• Continue resistive gripping exercises, provided no pain is produced at the elbow.

6 weeks	• Add radial and ulnar deviation as a strengthening exercise.

OVERVIEW OF REHABILITATION PROTOCOL—cont'd

6 weeks —cont'd	• Carefully monitor the amount of resistance for wrist flexion and forearm pronation and supination. Excessive weight may lead to soft tissue discomfort as a result of the flexor pronator mass having been split at the time of surgery.
3 to 4 months	• Patient should have full elbow ROM without pain or discomfort at the end of the range. • Start endurance activities (e.g., running, swimming, bicycling). • At 4 to 5 months, add light resistance to shoulder strengthening (emphasis on rotator cuff). • *Avoid* valgus forces to the elbow joint, shoulder internal rotation in the supine position with the arm in 90 degrees of abduction, and ER.
3 to 5 months	• **THROWING PROGRAM** • Patients perform throwing program on alternative days to minimize stress and fatigue placed on the graft.

• Apply heat to the shoulder and elbow for 10 to 15 minutes before each throwing session to increase circulation and promote tissue flexibility.
• Apply ice for 10 to 15 minutes after a session to minimize the inflammatory response.
• Do not progress the regimen if there is more than minor pain or pain of long duration (i.e., longer than 15 to 20 minutes after completion of throwing).
• The first step is easy tossing with no wind-up to minimize valgus forces.
• The initial throwing distance is 30 to 40 feet, with throwing 10 to 15 minutes per session. This is slowly progressed to 50 feet at 6 months.
• At 6 months the reconstructed ligament can tolerate valgus stresses and lobbing the ball with an easy wind-up may begin.
• At the 8-month mark the throwing program differs for outfielders, infielders, and pitchers (see outline, p. 74).

Lateral and Medial Epicondylitis

REHABILITATION RATIONALE

Classic lateral epicondylitis (tennis elbow) is caused by repetitive microtrauma that results in degeneration of the extensor carpi radialis brevis tendon. Repetitive eccentric muscle overload has been implicated in the development of lateral epicondylitis. A change in the patient's regular activity or an overuse syndrome should be sought in the history as a precipitating cause. Pain with resisted wrist extension and full elbow extension differentiates involvement of the extensor carpi radialis longus from that of the extensor carpi radialis brevis.

Mechanism

Lateral Epicondylitis. In tennis players, improper backhand stroke and wrist extension or flipping of the wrist may produce an overuse extensor tendonitis, especially of the extensor carpi radialis brevis muscle (Fig. 2-4). Serving with the racquet in pronation and snapping the wrist to impart spin also may cause lateral epicondylitis. Activities involving repetitive use of the extensor wad other than tennis may cause lateral epicondylitis.

Medial Epicondylitis. "Golfer's elbow" is produced in the right elbow in a right-handed golf swing by

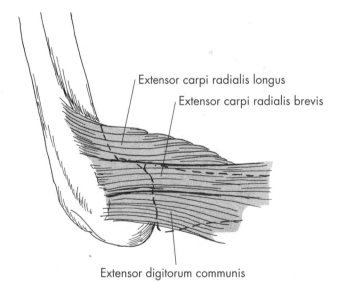

Figure 2-4 Lateral extensor wad. (Redrawn from Tullos H: *Instr Course Lect*, 1991.)

throwing the club head down at the ball with the right arm rather than pulling the club through with the left arm and trunk. This unorthodox swing causes stress at the flexor pronator group. "Swimmer's elbow" (also

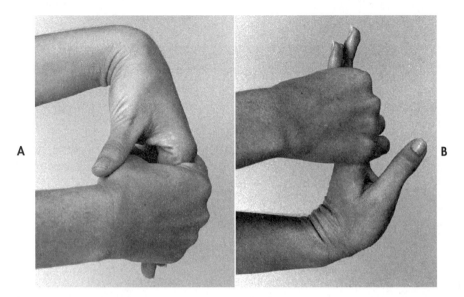

Figure 2-5 **A**, Wrist extensor stretching. Grasp the hand and slowly flex the wrist down until sustained stretch is felt. Hold for 10 seconds. Repeat 5 times per session, several times a day. **B**, Wrist flexor stretching. Grasp the hand and slowly extend the wrist until a sustained stretch is felt. Hold for 10 seconds. Repeat 5 times per session, several times a day.

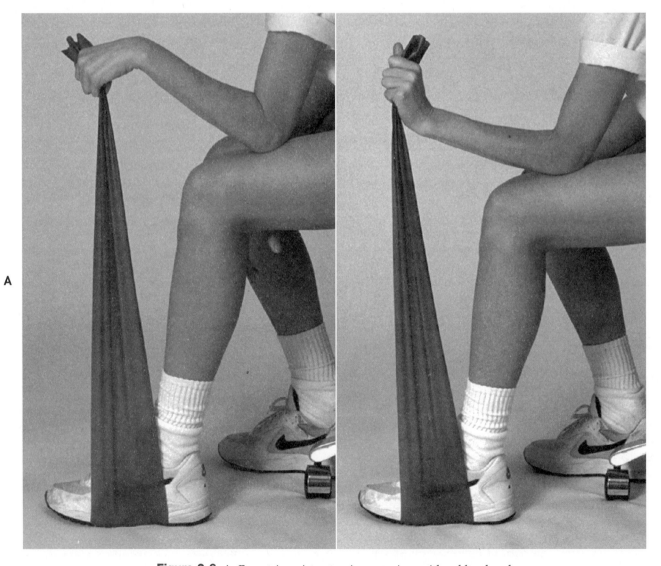

Figure 2-6 **A**, Eccentric wrist extension exercises with rubber band.

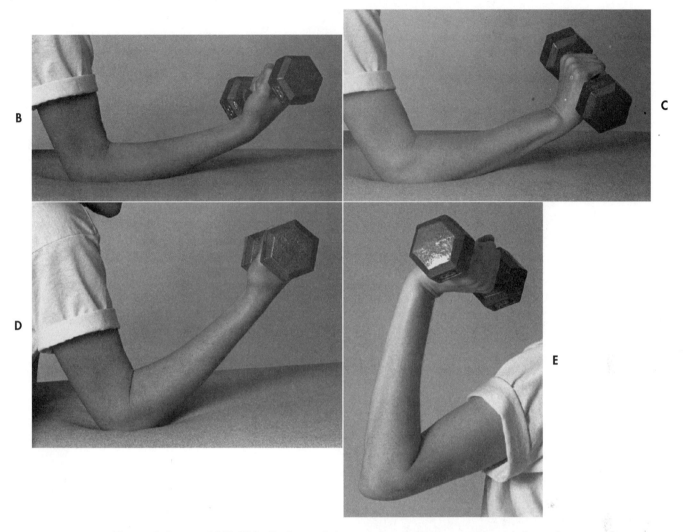

Figure 2-6—cont'd B, Wrist flexion-resistive training. **C**, Wrist extension-resistive training. **D**, Elbow flexion-resistive training. **E**, Elbow extension-resistive training.

medial epicondylitis) results from improper pull-through mechanics in the backstroke. Symptoms of medial epicondylitis include pain at the muscle group origin with resisted wrist flexion, pronation, or both. Weakness, commonly a result of pain, also may be detected in grasping activities.

General Rehabilitation Considerations
Progressive rehabilitation for epicondylitis proceeds through three sequential stages. In the *first (acute) phase*, the primary goal is to decrease inflammation and pain of the involved muscular origin. Submaximal conditioning may begin in this phase if the exercises do not cause pain. Recommended treatment methods for pain and inflammation include cryotherapy, whirlpool, HVGS, friction massage, and phonophoresis. Iontophoresis using an antiinflammatory such as dexamethasone also may be considered. It is important to avoid painful movements, like gripping activities, that aggravate the area.

The *second (subacute) phase* involves active strength-

ening and introduction to functional activities. Both concentric and eccentric strengthening are used in the involved muscle groups. As with other elbow disorders, it is important to include shoulder strengthening if deficiencies are noted. Gradual exposure to stressful activities is begun toward the end of this phase and is increased only if activities can be performed without pain.

The goal of the *third (final) phase* is to return the athlete to their sport and/or high level–work related activities. This is achieved through increased strengthening and endurance exercises, while maintaining joint flexibility.

A general outline of rehabilitation includes *gentle stretching exercises* initiated through wrist flexion, extension, and rotation (Fig. 2-5). These are held for 10 seconds and repeated for 5 to 10 repetitions. Vigorous stretching is avoided until the patient is pain free.

When the injury results from eccentric overload, *eccentric strengthening* is important to prevent recurrence (Fig. 2-6, *A*). Resistive training includes wrist flexion

Extensors   Flexors

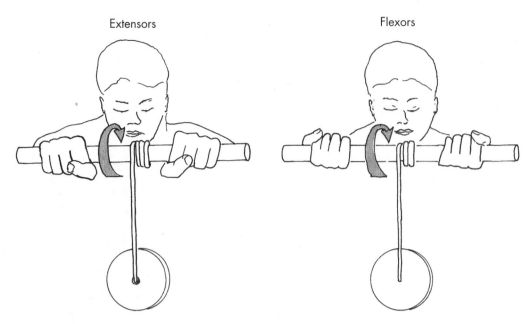

Figure 2-7 Wrist flexors and extensors. The patient rolls up a string with a weight tied on the end. The weight may be progressively increased. Flexors are worked with the palms up, extensors with the palms down. (From Galloway M, DeMaio M, Mangine R: Rehabilitative techniques in the treatment of medial and lateral epicondylitis, *Orthopedics* 15(9):1089, 1992.)

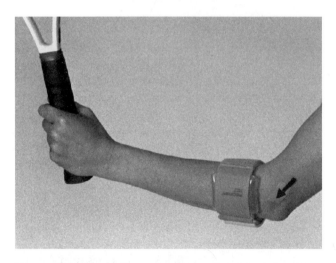

Figure 2-8 Aircast T-pneumatic arm band is secured just distal to the medial epicondyle. Arm band worn with normal daily activity, as well as with repetitive activities in work or sports. (From Aircast Corporation, Box T, Summit, New Jersey 07901.)

and extension in addition to forearm pronation and supination. This should be in a pain-free range (Figs. 2-6, *B-E*, and 2-7).

Equipment modifications that may be helpful include increasing the grip size of a racquet, decreasing string tension, and choosing a racquet with good vibration absorption characteristics (graphite, ceramic, composites). There is some disagreement on grip size in the literature, and recent studies have suggested that grip size may be less important than previously thought.

Lateral counterforce bracing is believed to diminish the magnitude of muscle contraction, decreasing muscle tension in the region of the damaged musculocutaneous unit (Fig. 2-8). Counterforce bracing should be used as a supplement to, not a replacement for, muscular strengthening exercises.

Epicondylitis is a common and often lingering pathologic condition. For this reason, it is critical that the rehabilitation process is progressed with minimal or no pain. The stressful components of high-level activity usually can be alleviated by altering the frequency, intensity, or duration of play.

REHABILITATION PROTOCOL

Epicondylitis WILK AND ANDREWS

Phase 1—Acute Phase
- Goals:
  Decrease inflammation/pain.
  Promote tissue healing.
  Retard muscular atrophy.
- Cryotherapy.
- Whirlpool.
- Stretching to increase flexibility.
  Wrist extension/flexion.
  Elbow extension/flexion.
  Forearm supination/pronation.
- Isometrics
  Wrist extension/flexion.
  Elbow extension/flexion.
  Forearm supination/pronation.
- HVGS.
- Phonophoresis.
- Friction massage.
- Iontophoresis (with an antiinflammatory such as dexamethasone).
- Avoid painful movements (such as gripping).

Phase 2—Subacute Phase
- Goals:
  Improve flexibility.
  Increase muscular strength and endurance.
  Increase functional activities and return to function.
- Emphasize concentric/eccentric strengthening.
  Concentrate on involved muscle group(s).
  Wrist extension/flexion (see Fig. 2-6, A).
  Forearm pronation/supination.
  Elbow flexion/extension.
- Initiate shoulder strengthening (if deficiencies are noted).
- Continue flexibility exercises.
- May use counterforce brace.
- Continue use of cryotherapy after exercise or function.
- Initiate gradual return to stressful activities.
- Gradually reinitiate previously painful movements.

Phase 3—Chronic Phase
- Goals:
  Improve muscular strength and endurance.
  Maintain/enhance flexibility.
  Gradually return to sport/high-level activities.
- Continue strengthening exercises (emphasize eccentric/concentric).
- Continue to emphasize deficiencies in shoulder and elbow strength.
- Continue flexibility exercises.
- Gradually diminish use of counterforce brace.
- Use cryotherapy as needed.
- Initiate gradual return to sport activity.
- Equipment modifications (grip size, string tension, playing surface).
- Emphasize maintenance program.

Galloway, DeMaio, and Mangine also divide their approach to patients with epicondylitis (medial or lateral) into three stages:
- The initial phase is directed toward reducing inflammation, preparing the patient for phase 2.
- The second phase emphasizes return of strength and endurance. Specific inciting factors are identified and modified.
- Phase 3 involves functional rehabilitation designed to return the patient to the desired activity level.

This protocol is also based on the severity of the initial symptoms and objective findings at initiation treatment.

Rehabilitation of the Elbow in Throwing Athletes

REHABILITATION RATIONALE

Slocum was one of the first to classify throwing injuries of the elbow into medial tension and valgus compression overload injuries.

■ *Valgus stress plus forced extension is the major pathologic mechanism of the thrower's elbow.*

Tension is produced on the medial aspect of the elbow. *Compression* is produced on the lateral aspect of the elbow. See the box for classification of these throwing injuries.

GENERAL REHABILITATION PRINCIPLES

Rehabilitation of the elbow joint complex in a throwing athlete requires a carefully directed program to ensure full restoration of motion and function. Fre-

REHABILITATION PROTOCOL

Evaluation-Based Rehabilitation Medial and Lateral Epicondylitis   GALLOWAY, DE MAIO, AND MANGINE

Rationale: Patients begin a rehabilitation protocol based on their symptoms and objective physical findings. The initial phase of each protocol is directed toward restoring ROM at the wrist and elbow. Phase 2 involves strength training and a structured return to activity.

	Protocol 1 (Severe Symptoms)	Protocol 2 (Mild/Moderate Symptoms)	Protocol 3 (Symptoms Resolved)
When	• Pain at rest • Point tenderness • Pain with minimally resisted wrist extension • Swelling • Grip strength difference (GSD) >50% • >5° motion loss at wrist/elbow	• Pain with activity only • Minimal point tenderness • Minimal pain with resisted wrist flexion/extension • GSD >50% • No motion loss	• No pain with daily activity • No referred pain • Full ROM • GSD <10%
Evaluation	• Duration of symptoms • Referred pain • Grip strength measurement • Elbow palpation • Motion measurement • History of injury or inciting activity • Differential diagnosis	• Duration of symptoms • Referred pain • Grip strength measurement • Elbow palpation • Motion measurement • History of injury or inciting activity • Differential diagnosis	• Review initial injury or inciting activity • Identify requirements for returning to desired activity • Identify remaining functional deficits

Treatment	**Phase 1 (Reduce Inflammation)**
	• Rest
	• Passive ROM
	• Cold therapy
	• Medications
	
	Phase 2 (Rehabilitation)
	• Limit activity
	• Cold therapy
	• Stretching (static)
	• Strengthening (isometric)
	• Ultrasound
	• HVGS
	• Proceed to Protocol 2 when tolerating above
	• Surgical indications
		Phase 1 (Reduce Inflammation)
		• Rest
		• Passive ROM
		• Cold therapy
		• Medications
		
		Phase 2 (Rehabilitation)
		• Limit activity
		• Flexibility
		• Strengthening
		• Transverse friction massage
		• Cold therapy
		• HVGS
		• Ultrasound
		• Proceed to Protocol 3
			• Preactivity flexibility
			• Strengthening
			  -isokinetic
			  -isotonic
			• Modalities
			  -whirlpool
			  -ice after activity
			• Technique modification
			• Equipment modification
			• Counterforce bracing
			• Friction massage
			• Gradual return to activity

Goals	• Resolution of pain at rest • Tolerate stretching/strengthening with minimal discomfort • Improve ROM • Maintain cardiovascular conditioning	• No pain with daily activity • No pain with stretching/progressive resistance exercises (PREs) • Full ROM • Prepare for functional rehabilitation • Maintain cardiovascular conditioning	• Pain-free return to activity • Prevent recurrence—maintenance program of stretching

Classification of Injuries of the Elbow in Throwing Athletes

Medial Stress
- Flexor muscle strain or tear.
- Avulsion of medial epicondyle.
- Attenuation or tear of the medial collateral ligament.
- Ulnar nerve traction.

Lateral Compression
- Hypertrophy of the radial head and capitellum.
- Avascular necrosis of the capitellum.
- Osteochondral fractures of the radial head or capitellum.

Forced Extension
- Olecranon osteophyte formation on the tip of the olecranon process.
- Loose body formation.
- Scarring and fibrous tissue deposition in the olecranon fossa.

TABLE 2-1 Joint Mobilization Grades of Oscillation

Grade 1	Small amplitude, beginning portion of motion; used to neuromodulate pain and improve joint lubrication; minimal stretch on capsule.
Grade 2	Large amplitude, performed midrange of motion; used to neuromodulate pain and improve joint lubrication; moderate stress to capsule.
Grade 3	Large amplitude, performed midrange to end-range; used to stretch the capsule; moderate stress.
Grade 4	Small amplitude, performed at end-range; used to produce pronounced stretch on capsule and ligaments.

From Maitland GD: *Vertebral manipulation,* London, 1977, Butterworths.

quently after surgery, motion is lost as a result of the elbow's high degree of joint congruency, capsular anatomy, and soft tissue changes. To obtain full function without complications, a sequential, progressive treatment program must be developed. This program requires that specific criteria be met at each stage before advancement to the next one. The final goal is to return the athlete to the sport as quickly and as safely as possible.

Several key principles should be considered during the rehabilitation of a throwing athlete with an elbow disorder. First, the effects of immobilization must be minimized. Second, healing tissue must never be overstressed. Third, the patient must fulfill specific criteria before progressing from one phase to the next during the rehabilitation process. Fourth, the rehabilitation program must be based on current clinical and scientific research. Fifth, the rehabilitation program should be adaptable to each patient and the patient's specific goals. Finally, these basic treatment principles should be followed throughout the rehabilitation process.

Elbow rehabilitation in throwing athletes generally follows a four-phase progression. It is important that certain criteria be met at each level before advancement is made to the next stage. This allows athletes to progress at their own pace based on tissue-healing constraints.

Phase 1 involves regaining motion lost during postsurgical immobilization. Pain, inflammation, and muscle atrophy also are treated.

Common regimens for inflammation and pain involve modalities such as cryotherapy, HVGS, ultrasound, and whirlpool. Joint mobilization techniques also can be used to help minimize pain and promote motion.

To minimize muscular atrophy, submaximal isometric exercises for elbow flexors and extensors, as well as for the forearm pronators and supinators, are started early. Strengthening of the shoulder also should begin relatively early to prevent functional weakness. Care should be taken early in the rehabilitation program to restrict ER movements that may place valgus stress on the medial structures of the elbow.

Elbow flexion contracture is common after an elbow injury or surgery when ROM is not treated appropriately. Prevention of these contractures is the key. Early ROM is vital to nourish the articular cartilage and promote proper collagen fiber alignment. A gradual increase in and early restoration of full passive elbow extension are essential to prevent flexion contraction. Several popular techniques to improve limited ROM are joint mobilization, contract-relax stretching, and low-load, long-duration stretching for the restoration of full elbow extension.

Joint mobilizations can be performed to the humeroulnar, humeroradial, and radioulnar joints. Limited elbow extension tends to respond to posterior glides of the ulna on the humerus. The grade of the mobilization depends on the phase of rehabilitation in effect (Table 2-1).

Another technique to restore full elbow extension is *low-load, long-duration stretching*. A good passive overpressure stretch can be achieved by having the patient hold a 2- to 4-lb weight or use an elastic band with the upper extremity resting on a fulcrum just proximal to the elbow joint to allow for greater extension. This stretch should be performed for 10 to 12 minutes to incorporate a long-duration, low-intensity stretch. Stretching of this magnitude has been found to elicit a plastic collagen tissue response, resulting in permanent soft tissue elongation. It is important to note that if the intensity of this stretch is too great, pain and/or a protective muscle response may result, which could inhibit collagen fiber elongation.

Phase 2, or the "intermediate phase," consists of improving the patient's overall strength, endurance, and elbow mobility. To progress to this phase, the patient must demonstrate full elbow ROM (0 to 135 degrees), minimal or no pain or tenderness, and a "good" (4/5) muscle grade for the elbow flexor and extensor groups. During this phase, isotonic strengthening exercises are emphasized for the entire arm and shoulder complex.

Phase 3 is the advanced strengthening phase. The primary goal in this phase is to prepare the athlete for the return to functional participation and initiation of throwing activities. A total arm-strengthening program is used to improve the power, endurance, and neuromuscular control of the entire limb. Advancement to phase 3 requires demonstration of full, pain-free ROM, no pain or tenderness, and 70% strength compared to the contralateral side.

Plyometric exercises are most beneficial in this phase; these drills closely simulate functional activities, such as throwing and swinging, and are performed at higher speeds. They also teach the athlete to transfer energy and stabilize the involved area. Plyometrics use a stretch-shortening cycle of muscle, thus using eccentric/concentric muscle extension. For instance, greater emphasis is placed on the biceps musculature in this phase of rehabilitation because it plays a vital role eccentrically during the deceleration and follow-through phases of the throwing motion by preventing hyperextension. One specific plyometric activity involves exercise tubing. Starting with the elbow flexed and the shoulder in 60 degrees of flexion, the patient releases the isometric hold, initiating an eccentric phase. As full extension is approached, the athlete quickly flexes the elbow again, going into a concentric phase. The eccentric activity produces a muscular stretch, thus activating the muscle spindles and producing a greater concentric contraction.

The primary targets for strengthening in this phase are the biceps, triceps, and wrist flexor/pronator muscles. The biceps, the wrist flexors, and pronators greatly reduce valgus stresses on the elbow during the throwing motion. Other key muscle groups stressed in this phase include the triceps and rotator cuff. The triceps are used in the acceleration phase of the throwing motion, while attention to the rotator cuff helps to establish the goal of total arm strengthening.

To improve shoulder strength, the throwing athlete is introduced to a set of submaximal isotonic exercises known as the "Thrower's Ten" program (Table 2-2.)

■ *Rehabilitation of an injured elbow is different from any other rehabilitation program for throwing athletes. Initially, elbow extension ROM must be obtained to prevent elbow flexion contracture. Next, valgus stress needs to be minimized through the conditioning of elbow and wrist flexors, as well as the pronator muscle group. Finally, the shoulder, especially the rotator cuff musculature, must be included in the rehabilitation process. The rotator cuff is vital to the throwing pattern and, if not strengthened, can lead to future shoulder problems.*

Phase 4, the final stage of the rehabilitation program for the throwing athlete, is "return to activity." This stage uses a progressive interval throwing program (see the box) to gradually increase the demands on the upper extremity by controlling throwing distance, frequency, and duration.

TABLE 2-2 **"Thrower's Ten" Program**

1. Dumbbell exercises for the deltoid and supraspinatus musculature.
2. Prone horizontal shoulder abduction.
3. Prone shoulder extension.
4. IR at 90 degrees of abduction of the shoulder with tubing.
5. ER at 90 degrees of abduction of the shoulder with tubing.
6. Elbow flexion/extension exercises (exercise tubing).
7. Serratus anterior strengthening—progressive push-ups.
8. Diagonal D2 pattern for shoulder flexion and extension with exercise tubing.
9. Press-ups.
10. Dumbbell wrist extension/flexion and pronation/supination.

Interval Throwing Program
PHASE 1

45-Foot Phase
Step 1: A. Warm-up throwing
B. 45 feet (25 throws)
C. Rest 15 minutes
D. Warm-up throwing
E. 45 feet (25 throws)
Step 2: A. Warm-up throwing
B. 45 feet (25 throws)
C. Rest 10 minutes
D. Warm-up throwing
E. 45 feet (25 throws)
F. Rest 10 minutes
G. Warm-up throwing
H. 45 feet (25 throws)

60-Foot Phase
Step 3: A. Warm-up throwing
B. 60 feet (25 throws)
C. Rest 15 minutes
D. Warm-up throwing
E. 60 feet (25 throws)
Step 4: A. Warm-up throwing
B. 60 feet (25 throws)
C. Rest 10 minutes
D. Warm-up throwing
E. 60 feet (25 throws)
F. Rest 10 minutes
G. Warm-up throwing
H. 60 feet (25 throws)

90-Foot Phase
Step 5: A. Warm-up throwing
B. 90 feet (25 throws)
C. Rest 15 minutes
D. Warm-up throwing
E. 90 feet (25 throws)
Step 6: A. Warm-up throwing
B. 90 feet (25 throws)
C. Rest 10 minutes
D. Warm-up throwing
E. 90 feet (25 throws)
F. Rest 10 minutes
G. Warm-up throwing
H. 90 feet (25 throws)

120-Foot Phase
Step 7: A. Warm-up throwing
B. 120 feet (25 throws)
C. Rest 15 minutes
D. Warm-up throwing
E. 120 feet (25 throws)

Step 8: A. Warm-up throwing
B. 120 feet (25 throws)
C. Rest 10 minutes
D. Warm-up throwing
E. 120 feet (25 throws)
F. Rest 10 minutes
G. Warm-up throwing
H. 120 feet (25 throws)

150-Foot Phase
Step 9: A. Warm-up throwing
B. 150 feet (25 throws)
C. Rest 15 minutes
D. Warm-up throwing
E. 150 feet (25 throws)
Step 10: A. Warm-up throwing
B. 150 feet (25 throws)
C. Rest 10 minutes
D. Warm-up throwing
E. 150 feet (25 throws)
F. Rest 10 minutes
G. Warm-up throwing
H. 150 feet (25 throws)

180-Foot Phase
Step 11: A. Warm-up throwing
B. 180 feet (25 throws)
C. Rest 15 minutes
D. Warm-up throwing
E. 180 feet (25 throws)
Step 12: A. Warm-up throwing
B. 180 feet (25 throws)
C. Rest 10 minutes
D. Warm-up throwing
E. 180 feet (25 throws)
F. Rest 10 minutes
G. Warm-up throwing
H. 180 feet (25 throws)
Step 13: A. Warm-up throwing
B. 180 feet (25 throws)
C. Rest 10 minutes
D. Warm-up throwing
E. 180 feet (25 throws)
F. Rest 10 minutes
G. Warm-up throwing
H. 180 feet (25 throws)
Step 14: Begin throwing off the
mound or return to re-
spective position

Interval Throwing Program
PHASE 2

Stage 1: Fastball Only
Step 1: Interval throwing
    15 throws off mound 50%
Step 2: Interval throwing
    30 throws off mound 50%
Step 3: Interval throwing
    45 throws off mound 50%
Step 4: Interval throwing
    60 throws off mound 50%
Step 5: Interval throwing
    30 throws off mound 75%
Step 6: 30 throws off mound 75%
    45 throws off mound 50%
Step 7: 45 throws off mound 75%
    15 throws off mound 50%
Step 8: 60 throws off mound 75%

Stage 2: Fastball Only
Step 9: 45 throws off mound 75%
    15 throws in batting practice

Step 10: 45 throws off mound 75%
    30 throws in batting practice
Step 11: 45 throws off mound 75%
    45 throws in batting practice

Stage 3
Step 12: 30 throws off mound 75%
    warm-up
    15 throws off mound 50%
    breaking balls
Step 13: 30 throws off mound 75%
    30 breaking balls 75%
    30 throws in batting practice
Step 14: 30 throws off mound 75%
    60 to 90 throws in batting practice
    25% breaking balls
Step 15: Simulated game: progressing by 15 throws per workout

Use interval throwing to 120-foot phase as a warm-up. All throwing off the mound should be done in the presence of the pitching coach to stress proper throwing mechanics. Use a speed gun to aid in effort control.

REHABILITATION PROTOCOL

Isolated Subcutaneous Ulnar Nerve Transposition
WILK AND ANDREWS

Phase 1—Immediate Postoperative Phase
- Goals:
  Allow soft tissue healing of relocated nerve.
  Decrease pain and inflammation.
  Retard muscular atrophy.

1 week
- Posterior splint at 90 degrees of elbow flexion with wrist free for motion (sling for comfort).
- Compression dressing.
- Exercises: gripping exercises, wrist ROM, shoulder isometrics.

2 weeks
- Remove posterior splint for exercise and bathing.
- Progress elbow ROM (passive ROM 15 to 120 degrees).
- Initiate elbow and wrist isometrics.
- Continue shoulder isometrics.

Phase 2—Intermediate Phase
- Goals:
  Restore full pain-free ROM.
  Improve strength, power, endurance of upper extremity musculature.
  Gradually increase functional demands.

3 weeks
- Discontinue posterior splint.
- Progress elbow ROM, emphasize full extension.

- Initiate flexibility exercises for wrist extension/flexion, forearm supination/pronation, elbow extension/flexion.
- Initiate strengthening exercises for wrist extension/flexion, forearm supination/pronation, elbow extensors/flexors, shoulder program.

6 weeks
- Continue all exercises listed above.
- Initiate light sport activities.

Phase 3—Advanced Strengthening Phase
- Goals:
  Increase strength, power, and endurance.
  Gradually initiate sports activities.

8 weeks
- Initiate eccentric exercise program.
- Initiate plyometric exercise drills.
- Continue shoulder and elbow strengthening and flexibility exercises.
- Initiate interval throwing program.

Phase 4—Return to Activity Phase
- Goals:
  Gradually return to sports activities.

12 weeks
- Return to competitive throwing.
- Continue Thrower's Ten exercise program (see p. 82).

Arthroplasty (Posterior Decompression) of the Elbow

REHABILITATION RATIONALE

The most common indication for arthroscopic elbow posterior decompression arthroplasty is the presence of a posterior compartment osteophyte, which often is caused by valgus extension overload activities, such as throwing a baseball. The primary goal after arthroplasty, as after any arthroscopic elbow procedure, is to reestablish full elbow and wrist ROM as soon as possible. Frequent osseous structure pain and inflammation, however, often slow the return of elbow extension. Progression of motion should be based on the amount of pain, inflammation, and soft tissue healing. Motion should be at least 15 to 90 degrees 10 days after surgery, reaching 10 to 100 degrees at 2 weeks. By 20 to 25 days after surgery, the patient should have full ROM of the elbow.

REHABILITATION PROTOCOL

Elbow Arthroplasty (Posterior Compartment/Valgus Extension Overload)

Phase 1—Immediate Motion Phase
- Goals:
  Improve motion, regain full ROM.
  Decrease pain and inflammation.
  Retard muscular atrophy.

1 to 4 days
- Perform ROM to tolerance (extension/flexion and supination/pronation).
  Often full elbow extension is not possible because of pain.
- Use gentle overpressure into extension.
- Begin wrist flexion/extension stretches.
- Begin gripping exercises (putty).
- Begin isometrics:
  Wrist extensors/flexors.
  Elbow extensors/flexors.
- Use compression dressing, ice 4 to 5 times daily.

5 to 10 days
- Perform ROM exercises to tolerance (at least 20 to 90 degrees).
- Use overpressure into extension.
- Use joint mobilization to reestablish ROM.
- Continue wrist flexion/extension stretches.

- Continue isometrics.
- Continue use of ice and compression to control swelling.

11 to 14 days
- Perform ROM exercises to tolerance (at least 10 to 100 degrees).
- Use overpressure into extension (3 to 4 times daily).
- Continue joint mobilization techniques.
- Initiate light dumbbell program (PREs) biceps, triceps.
  Wrist flexors/extensors, supinators/pronators.
- Continue use of ice after exercise.

Phase 2—Intermediate Phase
- Goal:
  Improve strength, power, and endurance.

2 to 4 weeks
- Perform full ROM exercises (4 to 5 times daily).
- Use overpressure into elbow extension.
- Continue PRE program for elbow and wrist musculature.
- Initiate shoulder program (especially external rotators, rotator cuff).

- Continue joint mobilization.
- Continue use of ice after exercise.

4 to 7 weeks
- Continue all exercises listed above.
- Initiate light upper body program.
- Continue use of ice after activity.

Phase 3—Advanced Strengthening Program.
- Goals:
  Improve strength, power, and endurance.
  Gradually return to functional activities.
- Criteria to begin phase 3:
  Full nonpainful ROM.
  Strength at least 75% of contralateral side.
  No pain or tenderness.

8 to 12 weeks
- Continue PRE program for elbow and wrist.
- Continue shoulder program.
- Continue stretching for elbow and shoulder.
- Initiate interval program and gradual return to sports activities.

REHABILITATION PROTOCOL

Elbow Arthroscopy

Phase 1—Immediate Motion Phase
- Goals:
  Regain full, pain-free wrist and elbow ROM.
  Decrease pain and inflammation.
  Retard muscular atrophy.

1 to 2 days
- Remove bulky dressing; replace with elastic dressing.
- Initiate wrist and elbow ROM exercises.
- Initiate putty/gripping exercises.
- Begin flexibility exercises: wrist extension/flexion, supination/pronation.
- Begin elbow active ROM and active-assisted ROM (motion to tolerance).
- Begin isometric strengthening exercises (shoulder, elbow, and wrist).

3 to 7 days
- Continue active ROM, and active-assisted ROM elbow (full ROM at day 7).
- Begin isotonic strengthening for wrist and elbow musculature (1 lb).

8 to 14 days
- Continue all exercises listed above.
- Continue ROM (0 to 125 degrees); emphasize full elbow extension.

Phase 2—Intermediate Phase
- Goals:
  Improve muscular strength, power, and endurance.
  Normalize joint arthrokinematics.

3 weeks
- Initiate elbow eccentric strengthening program.
- Initiate shoulder strengthening exercises.
- Continue ROM exercises for elbow.

Phase 3—Advanced Strengthening Phase
- Goals:
  Continue to increase strength and endurance.
  Prepare athlete for gradual return to functional activities.
- Criteria to progress to advanced phase:
  Full, nonpainful ROM.
  No pain or tenderness.
  Isokinetic test that fulfills criteria to throw.
  Satisfactory clinical exam.

5 weeks
- Continue all strengthening and flexibility exercises (Thrower's Ten Program, p. 82).
- Initiate interval throwing (phase 1, p. 83).

Phase 4—Return to Activity Phase
- Goals:
  Gradually return to functional activities.
  Continue strengthening exercises for upper extremity.

7 weeks
- Initiate competitive sports activities.
- Continue Thrower's Ten Program.
- Continue flexibility exercises (especially elbow extension stretches).
- Continue forearm supination/pronation.
- Continue all wrist/elbow exercises.

Isolated Fracture of the Radial Head

REHABILITATION RATIONALE

Mason's classification of radial head fractures is the most widely accepted and useful for treatment (Fig. 2-9). Rehabilitation is based on this classification (Table 2-3).

TREATMENT

Nondisplaced type I fractures require little or no immobilization. Active and passive ROM may be begun immediately after injury to promote full ROM. Conditioning in the form of elbow flexion and extension, supination and pronation isometrics, and wrist and shoulder isotonics can be implemented immediately (usually within the first week) after injury. Stress to

TABLE 2-3 Mason's Classification of Radial Head Fractures

Type	Description
Type I	Nondisplaced fracture Often missed on radiograph Positive posterior fat pad sign
Type II	Marginal radial head fractures with displacement, depression, or angulation
Type III	Comminuted fracture of the entire head
Type IV	Concomitant dislocation of elbow or other associated injuries

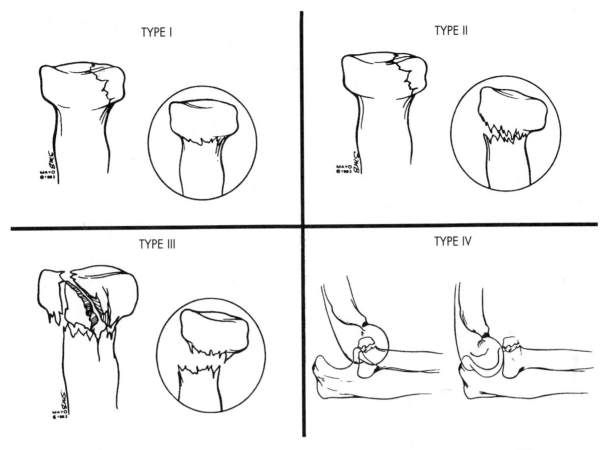

TYPE I   TYPE II

TYPE III   TYPE IV

Figure 2-9 Mason classification of radial head fractures. (From Broberg MA, Morrey BF: Results of treatment of fracture dislocations of the elbow, *Clin Orthop* 216:109, 1987.)

TABLE 2-4 **Treatment of Radial Head Fractures in Athletes**	
Type	**Treatment**
• Type I (nondisplaced)	Minimal immobilization and early motion
• Type II	ORIF* and early motion
• Type III	ORIF and early motion if possible
• Type IV (comminuted)	Radial head resection; check distal joint (Essex-Lopresti injury); guarded prognosis for return to sports

*Open reduction and internal fixation

the radial head is minimized. Three to 6 weeks of active elbow flexion and extension may be used, along with wrist isotonics.

Types II and III fractures usually require open reduction internal fixation. Frequently, immobilization is required for a brief time, followed by active and passive ROM exercises.

Type IV comminuted fractures frequently require stabilization of the elbow joint and excision of fragments and usually cause some functional limitation. Full ROM rarely returns and chronic elbow pain often persists.

Treatment for types I, II, III, and IV fractures is described in Table 2-4.

REHABILITATION PROTOCOL

Radial Head Fracture

Type I fracture or type II or III fracture treated with ORIF.

Phase 1—Immediate Motion Phase
- Goals:
  Decrease pain and inflammation.
  Regain full wrist and elbow ROM.
  Retard muscular atrophy.

1 week
- Begin elbow active ROM and active-assisted ROM; minimal accepted ROM (15 to 105 degrees) by 2 weeks.
- Begin putty/gripping exercises.
- Begin isometric strengthening exercises (elbow and wrist).
- Begin isotonic strengthening exercises for wrist.

Phase 2—Intermediate Phase
- Goals:
  Maintain full elbow ROM.
  Progress elbow strengthening exercises.
  Gradually increase functional demands.

3 weeks
- Initiate shoulder strengthening exercises; concentrate on rotator cuff.
- Continue ROM exercises for elbow (full flexion/extension).

3 weeks —cont'd
- Initiate light resistance elbow flexion/extension (1 lb).
- Initiate active-assisted ROM and passive ROM supination/pronation to tolerance.

6 weeks
- Continue active-assisted ROM and passive ROM supination/pronation to full range.
- Progress shoulder program.
- Progress elbow strengthening exercises.

Phase 3—Advanced Strengthening Phase
- Goals:
  Maintain full elbow ROM.
  Increase strength, power, endurance.
  Gradually initiate sporting activities.

7 weeks
- Continue active-assisted ROM and passive ROM to full supination/pronation.
- Initiate eccentric elbow flexion/extension.
- Initiate plyometric exercise program.
- Continue isotonic program forearm, wrist, and shoulder.
- Continue until 12 weeks.

Elbow Arthroplasty

REHABILITATION RATIONALE

Elbow arthroplasty may be indicated for the following conditions:
- Pain, instability, and bilateral ankylosis, such as in patients with advanced stage 3 or 4 rheumatoid arthrosis that is unresponsive to medical management.
- Failed interpositional or anatomic arthroplasty.
- Failed prosthetic arthroplasty.
- Arthrodesis in poor functional position.
- After en bloc resection for tumor.
- Degenerative arthrosis after failed debridement and loose body excision.
- Rheumatoid arthrosis in which synovectomy and radial head excision have failed.

Contraindications to elbow arthroplasty include the following:
- Active infection.
- Absent flexors or flail elbow from motor paralysis.
- Noncompliant patient with respect to activity limitations.
- Inadequate posterior skin quality.
- Inadequate bone stock or ligamentous instability with resurfacing implants.
- Neurotrophic joint.

Elbow prostheses are classified as semiconstrained (loose-hinge or sloppy-hinge), nonconstrained (minimally constrained), or fully constrained. Fully constrained prostheses are no longer used because of their unacceptable failure rate.

REHABILITATION PROTOCOL
Total Elbow Replacement*

3 days	• Remove bulky dressing and replace with light compressive dressing. • Begin active ROM exercises for the elbow and forearm 6 times a day for 10 to 15 minutes.	6 weeks	• Discontinue elbow extension splint during the day if elbow stability is adequate. • ROM exercises may now be performed with elbow away from body.

■ *Active ROM exercises should be performed with the elbow close to the body to avoid excessive stretch of the reconstructed elbow collateral ligaments.*

	• Fit an elbow extension splint to be worn between exercise sessions and at night.	8 weeks	• Discontinue elbow extension splint at night. • Initiate gradual, gentle strengthening exercises for hand and forearm. Light resistance may be begun to the elbow. • Perform therapy within the patient's comfort level.
2 weeks	• Passive ROM exercises may be initiated to the elbow. • Functional electrical stimulation (FES) may be initiated to stimulate biceps, triceps, or both.		

*From Cannon NM: *Diagnosis and treatment manual for physicians and therapists,* ed 3, 1991, The Hand Rehabilitation Center of Indiana, PC.

Bibliography

Andrews JR, Schemmel SP, Whiteside JA: Evaluation, treatment, and prevention of elbow injuries in throwing athletes. In *The upper extremity in sports medicine,* St. Louis, 1990, Mosby.

Andrews JR, Whiteside JA: Common elbow problems in the athlete, *J Orthop Sports Phys Ther* 17(6):289, 1993.

Bennet JB, Tullos HS: Acute injuries to the elbow. In *The upper extremity in sports medicine,* St. Louis, 1990, Mosby.

Broberg MA, Morrey BF: Results of treatment fracture dislocations of the elbow, *Clin Orthop* 216:109, 1987.

Cannon, N: *Diagnosis and treatment manual for physicians and therapists,* Indianapolis, 1991, Hand Center.

Galloway M, DeMaio M, Mangine R: Rehabilitative techniques in the treatment of medial and lateral epicondylitis, *Orthopedics* 15(9):1089, 1992.

Maitland GD: *Vertebral manipulation,* London, 1977, Butterworths.

Morrey BF: Biomechanics of the elbow and forearm, *Orthop Sports Med* 17:840, 1994.

Seto JL et al: Rehabilitation following ulnar collateral ligament reconstruction of athletes. *J Orthop Sports Phys Ther* 14:100, 1991.

Tullos HS, Bennett J, Shephard D: Adult elbow dislocations mechanism of instability, *Instr Course Lect* 35:69, 1986.

Wilk KE: Rehabilitation of the elbow complex. In Andrews JR, Soffer S, editors: *Elbow arthroscopy,* Philadelphia, 1994, Mosby.

Wilk KE, Arrigo CA, Andrews JR: Rehabilitation of the elbow in the throwing athlete, *J Orthop Sports Phys Ther* 17:305, 1993.

Wilk KE et al: Stretch-shortening drills for the upper extremities: theory and clinical application, *J Orthop Sports Phys Ther* 17(5):225, 1993.

CHAPTER THREE

Rehabilitation of the Shoulder

FRANK W. JOBE, MD

DIANE MOYNE SCHWAB, PT

KEVIN E. WILK, PT

JAMES R. ANDREWS, MD

General Principles

The glenohumeral joint is inherently unstable, exhibiting the greatest amount of motion of any joint in the body (Fig. 3-1). The humeral head is stabilized through a complex array of both static (passive) and dynamic (active) stabilizers. These mechanisms provide the necessary balance between functional mobility and stability (see the box).

During the rehabilitation of athletes involved in throwing or overhead activities, dynamic functional stability is improved in various ways.

- Pylometrics
- Eccentrics
- Proprioception
- Neuromuscular control
- Force couple efficiency
- Scapular stability
- Stretching

The low success rate in returning these athletes to competition after surgical decompression reinforces the importance and desirability of both prevention of injury and nonoperative management.

Impingement Syndrome

PROGRESSIVE STAGES OF IMPINGEMENT (NEER AND HAWKINS)

(See the box on p. 93.)

Neer demonstrated that the functional arc of the shoulder is forward, not lateral, and impingement occurs predominantly against the anterior edge of the acromion and the coracoacromial ligament.

■ *Both structural and functional factors may contribute to subacromial impingement.*

A common problem in overhead athletes (such as throwers, tennis players, and swimmers) is shoulder pain caused by impingement of the rotator cuff tendons underneath the coracoacromial arch (Tables 3-1 and 3-2).

Mechanisms of Glenohumeral Joint Stability

Passive	Active
Joint geometry	Compression of joint surfaces
Limited joint volume	Dynamic ligament tension
Adhesion/cohesion of joint surfaces	Neuromuscular control
Ligamentous restraints	
Soft tissue barrier	
Glenoid labrum	

■ *Shoulder impingement may be primary or secondary. Differentiating primary impingement from secondary impingement is crucial to proper management and rehabilitation. If secondary impingement is managed as "classic" impingement (repeated subacromial injections, acromioplasty), the underlying instability problem will not be adequately corrected.*

SECONDARY IMPINGEMENT

Secondary impingement is a relative decrease in the subacromial space caused by *instability* of the glenohumeral joint or by functional scapulothoracic instability. Secondary impingement caused by glenohumeral instability often is triggered by weakness of the rotator cuff mechanism and the biceps tendon, leading to overload of the passive restraints during throwing and resulting in glenohumeral laxity. The active restraints of the glenohumeral joint (the rotator cuff and biceps tendon) attempt to stabilize the humeral head; however, they eventually fatigue and weaken, with resultant abnormal translation of the humeral head and mechanical impingement of the rotator cuff by the coracoacromial arch (Fig. 3-2).

In throwing athletes, secondary impingement may be caused by subacromial impingement due to functional scapular instability (Fig. 3-2). Weakness of the scapulothoracic muscles leads to abnormal positioning of the scapula. Disruption of the scapulohumeral

rhythm occurs, leading to impingement of the rotator cuff under the coracoacromial arch, because humeral elevation is not synchronized with scapular elevation and upward rotation. With this disruption, the acromion is not elevated sufficiently to allow unrestricted passage of the rotator cuff under the coracoacromial arch.

Because of these factors, rehabilitation should be directed at strengthening both the rotator cuff and the scapular rotators to establish proper scapulohumeral rhythm. Rotator cuff strengthening decreases im-

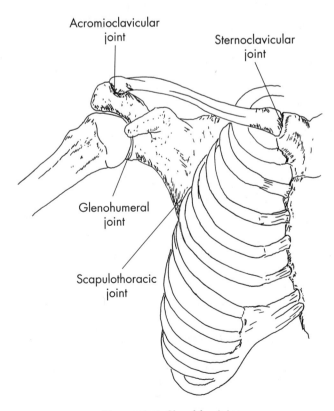

Figure 3-1 Shoulder joint.

Progressive Stages of Impingement

Stage 1: Edema and Inflammation

Typical age	Less than 25 years, but may occur at any age
Clinical course	Reversible lesion
Physical signs	• Tenderness to palpation over the greater tuberosity of the humerus
	• Tenderness along anterior ridge of acromion
	• Painful arc of abduction between 60 to 120 degrees, increased with resistance at 90 degrees
	• Positive impingement sign
	• Shoulder range of motion (ROM) may be restricted with significant subacromial inflammation

Stage 2: Fibrosis and Tendonitis

Typical age	25 to 40 years
Clinical course	Not reversible by modification of activity
Physical signs	Stage 1 signs plus the following:
	• Greater degree of soft tissue crepitus may be felt because of scarring in the subacromial space
	• Catching sensation with lowering of arm at approximately 100 degrees
	• Limitation of active and passive ROM

Stage 3: Bone Spurs and Tendon Ruptures

Typical age	Greater than 40 years
Clinical course	Not reversible
Physical signs	Stages 1 and 2 signs plus the following:
	• Limitation of ROM, more pronounced with active motion
	• Atrophy of infraspinatus
	• Weakness of shoulder abduction and external rotation
	• Biceps tendon involvement
	• Acromioclavicular joint tenderness

TABLE 3-1 Structural Factors That May Increase Subacromial Impingement

Structure	Abnormal Characteristics
Acromioclavicular joint	Congenital anomaly
	Degenerative spur formation
Acromion	Unfused acromion
	Degenerative spurs on undersurface
	Malunion/nonunion of fracture
Coracoid	Congenital anomaly
	Abnormal shape after surgery or trauma
Rotator cuff	Thickening of tendon from calcific deposits
	Tendon thickening after surgery or trauma
	Upper-surface irregularities from partial or complete tears
Humerus	Increased prominence of greater tuberosity from congenital anomalies or malunions

Modified from Matsen FA III, Arntz CT: Subacromial impingement. In Rockwood CA Jr, Matsen FA III, editors: *The shoulder*, Philadelphia, 1990, WB Saunders.

TABLE 3-2 Functional Factors That May Increase Subacromial Impingement

Structure	Abnormal Characteristics
Scapula	Abnormal position from thoracic kyphosis or acromioclavicular joint separation
	Abnormal motion from trapezius/serratus anterior paralysis or limited motion at scapulothoracic joint
	Functional scapulothoracic instability from scapulothoracic muscle weakness or fatigue
	Disruption of scapulohumeral rhythm because of serratus anterior fatigue or weakness
Rotator cuff	Loss of humeral head depressor mechanism from:
	C5-C6 radiculopathy
	Suprascapular nerve palsy
	Partial-/full-thickness rotator cuff tears
	Rupture of long head of biceps brachii
Glenohumeral joint increased capsule	Posterior capsular tightness that may lead to superior migration of humeral head in shoulder flexion
	Capsular laxity

Modified from Matsen FA III, Arntz CT: Subacromial impingement. In Rockwood CA Jr, Matsen FA III, editors: *The shoulder*, Philadelphia, 1990, WB Saunders.

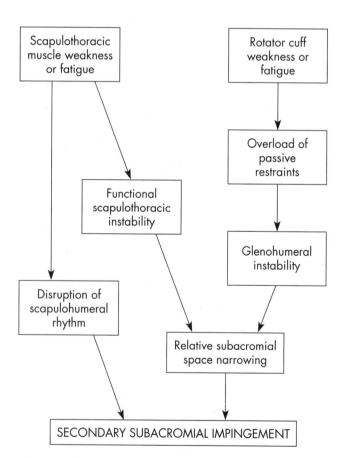

Figure 3-2 Development of secondary shoulder impingement.

pingement by improving humeral head depression and preventing excessive superior migration of the humeral head during arm elevation. Scapular rotator strengthening ensures that the scapula follows the humerus, providing dynamic stability and synchronization of the scapulohumeral rhythm.

PRIMARY IMPINGEMENT

Primary impingement, as described by Neer, is impingement of the rotator cuff beneath the coracoacromial arch. This is a *mechanical* impingement that may result from subacromial crowding (see Table 3-1).

■ *Instability of the glenohumeral joint is **absent** in primary impingement.*

IMPINGEMENT IN THE OVERHEAD ATHLETE

Overhead athletes repetitively subject their shoulder joints to high microtrauma stresses, the accumulative effects of which may lead to a spectrum of shoulder injuries. These athletes usually exhibit adaptive

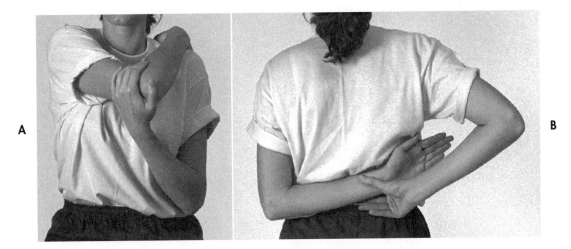

Figure 3-3 A, Crossed-arm adduction for posterior capsular stretching. **B,** The posterior capsule should be stretched to achieve full internal rotation.

changes in motion because of the repetitive stresses, and these adaptations often result in acquired laxity anteriorly and a loss of flexibility in the posterior muscles and posterior capsule. Because posterior capsular tightness often causes anterosuperior migration of the humeral head, contributing to impingement, posterior capsular stretching is useful (Fig. 3-3).

■ *Anterior capsular stretching should be avoided or carefully evaluated to prevent exacerbation of preexisting anterior capsular instability.*

Jobe divides overhand or throwing athletes with anterior shoulder pain into four groups (see the box on p. 97) based on clinical signs of instability and/or impingement (Figs. 3-4 and 3-5).

Biomechanics of Throwing

The overhead throwing motion has been divided into the following six stages (Fig. 3-6):
- Stage 1 Begins with wind up and ends as the ball leaves the nondominant hand
- Stage 2 Early cocking as the ball is released from the glove hand, the shoulder abducts, externally rotates, and terminates as the forward foot contacts the ground
- Stage 3 Late cocking proceeds as the dominant shoulder achieves maximum external rotation
- Stage 4 Acceleration begins with internal humeral rotation and ends with ball release
- Stage 5 Deceleration begins after ball release and constitutes 30% of the time required to dissipate the excess kinetic energy of the throwing motion
- Stage 6 Follow-through completes the remaining 70% of this time frame and ends when all motion is complete

Pain in the late cocking phase can be felt *anteriorly* and *superiorly* secondary to anterior subluxation of the humerus, with aggravated impingement of the rota-

tor cuff as the humeral head moves superiorly. In the late cocking and early acceleration phases, initial symptoms may be posterior, probably secondary to posterior capsular and rotator cuff strain as the glenohumeral joint attempts to balance the occult anterior laxity.

The role of the biceps in throwing is controversial, but recent evidence suggests that the biceps plays an integral role in overhead function. It appears that the biceps brachii plays a significant role in deceleration of the pitching arm and in anterior stability of the glenohumeral joint. Keating et al. showed that the subscapularis contributes 53% of the rotator cuff movement, making it perhaps the most important muscle in humeral head stabilization.

General Rehabilitation Principles in Throwing Athletes (Hawkins and Litchfield)

Functional Plane of Motion

Rehabilitation of the shoulder should be performed in functional planes of motion. Most exercises are done anterior to the scapular plane or in the scapular plane. This generally is a pain-free range. Exercises in the coronal plane should be avoided because this is a nonfunctional motion and often exacerbates impingement.

Short Lever Arm

Early in the rehabilitation program, especially in athletes with pain, passive and active movements should be initiated with the elbow flexed to decrease torque around the shoulder. During the resisted and strengthening phases of rehabilitation, loads should be applied with the arms close to the body and the elbows flexed to shorten the lever arm. Electromyogram (EMG) analysis has documented high levels of supraspinatus activity with straight-arm resisted exercises in scapular-plane rehabilitation. This long lever arm

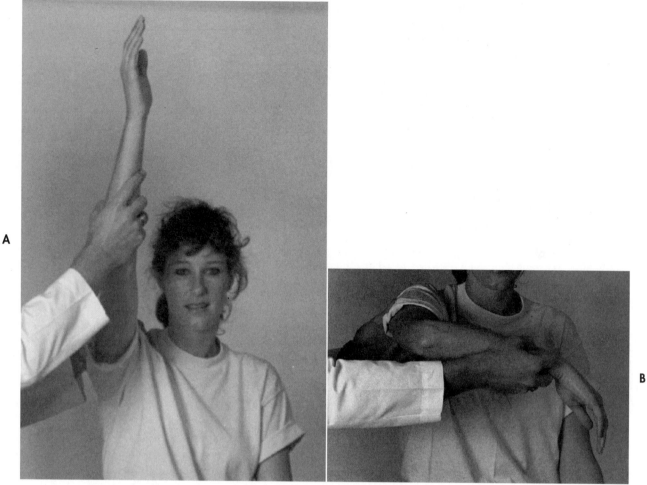

Figure 3-4 A, Impingement test. Evidence of rotator cuff disease or impingement syndrome can be demonstrated with the Neer impingement sign. In a positive Neer test, the patient's pain is reproduced when the arm is forced into elevation, which jams the greater tuberosity against the anterior/inferior surface of the acromion. **B,** Impingement sign.

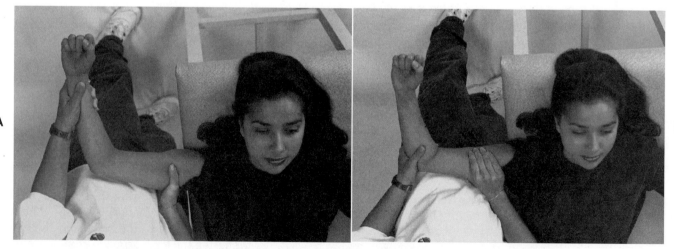

Figure 3-5 A, Anterior apprehension test by abduction and external rotation of the arm while pushing anteriorly on the humeral head. **B,** Relocation test. The patient with instability may have reduced apprehension by pushing the humeral head posteriorly.

Anterior Shoulder Pain in the Throwing Athlete: Four Groups Based on Clinical Signs

Group 1
Patient
- Pure impingement
- No instability
- Usually more than 35 years of age

Exam
- Positive impingement signs
- Negative apprehension signs
- With anesthesia, stable joint

Group 2
Patient
- Primary instability because of chronic labral microtrauma
- Secondary impingement

Exam
- Positive impingement signs
- Pain, but no apprehension with apprehension maneuver
- Pain relieved with relocation test
- With anesthesia, unstable shoulder (often subtle)

Group 3
Patient
- Instability due to hyperelasticity
- Subsequent impingement
- Age variable

Exam
- Positive impingement signs
- Pain, but no apprehension with apprehension maneuver
- Relief of pain with relocation test
- Hyperelasticity indicated by increased elbow hyperextension, positive thumb-forearm apposition test (ability to place thumb on forearm)

Group 4
Patient
- Pure instability (subluxation)
- No impingement
- Typical history of single traumatic event (e.g., anterior subluxation during football practice)

Exam
- Negative impingement signs
- Pain with apprehension testing
- Relief of pain with relocation test

Modified from Jobe FW et al: *The shoulder in sports*. In Rockwood CS Jr, Matsen FA III, editors: *The shoulder*, Philadelphia, 1990, WB Saunders.

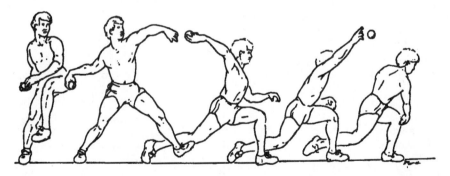

Figure 3-6 Five stages of the overhand throwing motion: stage 1, wind-up; stage 2, early cocking; stage 3, late cocking; stage 4, acceleration; and stage 5, follow-through. (From Glousman RE et al: Dynamic EMG analysis of the throwing shoulder with glenohumeral instability, *J Bone Joint Surg* 70A:220, 1988.)

often induces pain and should be avoided by bending the elbow of the athlete with painful shoulders.

Deceleration Musculature

Conditioning and eccentric strengthening should be included for the muscles prominent in the deceleration phase of throwing (i.e., latissimus dorsi, biceps brachii). The shoulder encounters enormous stresses in this phase.

Scapular Platform

A stable scapular platform and synchronization of the scapulohumeral rhythm are important in any rehabilitation or conditioning program.

Stretching

Most overhead athletes have limited internal rotation, a tight posterior capsule, and excessive external rotation. Historically, shoulder stretching has been done in many directions; however, stretching of the anterior capsule and exacerbation of underlying anterior subluxation or instability is unwise. Increasing internal rotation and eliminating posterior capsular tightness have been shown to increase the athlete's performance. A rigorous posterior capsular stretching program is indicated. (See Fig. 3-3.)

Progression of Exercise Program

The rehabilitation program should gradually increase forces and loading rates in a manner that reproduces the athlete's specific functional demands.

Prophylactic Shoulder Conditioning

To maximize performance and avoid injury, the maintenance program should decrease posterior capsular tightness and improve eccentric strength of the shoulder and scapular muscles.

Rotator Cuff Tendonitis and Tears in Throwing Athletes

In throwing athletes, rotator cuff tendonitis may be caused by mechanical abrasion, overuse, excessive anterior translation of the humeral head within the glenohumeral joint space, or a combination of these factors. Considerations in the choice of a rehabilitation protocol include (1) the degree of shoulder stability, (2) the duration of the condition (acute or chronic), (3) the strength and endurance of the shoulder girdle musculature, (4) the performance requirements of the athlete's sport, and (5) the flexibility of the soft tissues around the shoulder.

REHABILITATION PROTOCOL

Repair (Deltoid Splitting) of Type I Rotator Cuff Injury (Small Tear [Less Than 1 cm]) WILK AND ANDREWS

Phase 1—Protective Phase (week 0 to 6)
GOALS
- Gradual return to full ROM
- Increase shoulder strength
- Decrease pain

0 to 3 weeks
- Fit sling for comfort (1 to 2 weeks).
- Perform pendulum exercises.
- Initiate active-assisted ROM exercises (L-bar exercise).
  Employ ROM exercises in a nonpainful range, with a gentle and gradual increase of motion to tolerance.
- Use rope and pulley for flexion (only).
- Perform elbow ROM, hand gripping.
- Begin isometrics (submaximal, subpainful isometrics):
  Abductors
  External rotators
  Internal rotators
  Elbow flexors
  Shoulder flexors
- Use pain-control modalities (ice, high-voltage galvanic stimulation [HVGS]).

3 to 6 weeks
- Progress all exercises (continue all above exercises).
- Perform active-assisted ROM L-bar exercises ER/IR (shoulder at 45 degrees abduction).
- Begin surgical tubing ER/IR (arm at side).
- Initiate humeral head stabilization exercises.

Phase 2—Intermediate Phase (7 to 12 weeks)
GOALS
- Full, nonpainful ROM
- Improve strength and power
- Increase functional activities; decrease residual pain

7 to 10 weeks
- Perform active-assisted ROM exercises (L-bar):
  Flexion to 170 to 180 degrees
  Perform ER/IR at 90 degrees abduction of shoulder:
    ER to 75 to 90 degrees
    IR to 75 to 85 degrees
  Perform ER exercises with 0 degrees abduction:
    ER to 30 to 40 degrees
- Perform strengthening exercises for shoulder.
  Perform exercise tubing ER/IR with arm at side.
  Use isotonics dumbbell exercises for the following:
    Deltoid
    Supraspinatus
    Elbow flexors
    Scapular muscles
- Use upper body ergometer.
- Full ROM is the goal of weeks 8 to 10.

10 to 12 weeks
- Continue all above exercises.
- Initiate isokinetic strengthening (scapular plane).

REHABILITATION PROTOCOL—cont'd

Phase 2—Intermediate Phase (7 to 12 weeks)—cont'd

10 to 12 weeks —cont'd
- Initiate side-lying ER/IR exercises (dumbbell).
- Initiate neuromuscular scapulae control exercises.

Phase 3—Advanced Strengthening Phase (weeks 13 to 21)

GOALS
- Maintain full, nonpainful ROM
- Improve shoulder complex strength
- Improve neuromuscular control
- Gradual return to functional activities.

13 to 18 weeks
- Begin active stretching program for the shoulder.
  Use active-assisted ROM L-bar flexion, ER/IR.
- Perform capsular stretches.
- Initiate aggressive strengthening program (isotonic program):
  Shoulder flexion
  Shoulder abduction
  Supraspinatus
  ER/IR
  Elbow flexors/extensors
  Scapular muscles
- Perform an isokinetic test (modified neutral position) at week 14:
  ER/IR at 180 and 300 degrees per second
- Begin general conditioning program.

18 to 21 weeks
- Continue all exercises listed above.
- Initiate interval sport program.

Phase 4—Return to Activity Phase (21 to 26 weeks)

GOALS
- Gradual return to recreational sport activities

21 to 26 weeks
- Perform isokinetic test (modified neutral position).
- Continue to comply to interval sport program.
- Continue basic ten program (p. 114) for strengthening and flexibility.

REHABILITATION PROTOCOL

Repair (Deltoid Splitting) of Type II Rotator Cuff Injury (Medium to Large Tear [Greater Than 1 cm and Less Than 5 cm]) WILK AND ANDREWS

Phase 1—Protective Phase (0 to 6 weeks)

GOALS
- Gradual increase in ROM
- Increase shoulder strength
- Decrease pain and inflammation

0 to 3 weeks
- Fit brace or sling (physician determines).
- Begin pendulum exercises.
- Perform active-assisted ROM exercises (L-bar exercise):
  Flexion to 125 degrees
  ER/IR (shoulder at 40 degrees abduction) to 30 degrees
- Perform passive ROM to tolerance.
- Use rope and pulley—flexion.
- Perform elbow ROM and hand-gripping exercises.
- Begin submaximal isometrics:
  Flexors
  Abductors
  ER/IR
  Elbow flexors
- Use ice and pain modalities.

3 to 6 weeks
- Discontinue brace or sling.
- Continue all exercises listed above.
- Perform active-assisted ROM exercises:
  Flexion to 145 degrees
  ER/IR (performed at 65 degrees abduction) range to tolerance

Phase 2—Intermediate Phase (7 to 14 weeks)

GOALS
- Full, nonpainful ROM (10 weeks)
- Gradual increase in strength
- Decrease pain

7 to 10 weeks
- Perform active-assisted ROM L-bar exercises:
  Flexion to 160 degrees
  ER/IR (performed at 90 degrees shoulder abduction) to tolerance (greater than 45 degrees)

Continued

Repair (Deltoid Splitting) of Type II Rotator Cuff Injury (Medium to Large Tear [Greater Than 1 cm and Less Than 5 cm]) WILK AND ANDREWS

Phase 2—Intermediate Phase (7 to 14 weeks)—cont'd

7 to 10 weeks —cont'd
- Perform strengthening exercises:
  Use exercise tubing ER/IR, arm at side.
  Initiate humeral head stabilizing exercise.
  Initiate dumbbell strengthening exercises for the following:
    Deltoid
    Supraspinatus
    Elbow flexion/extension
    Scapular muscles

10 to 14 weeks
- Continue all exercises listed above (full ROM by 10 to 12 weeks).
- Begin isokinetic strengthening (scapular plane).
- Begin side-lying ER/IR exercises (dumbbell).
- Begin neuromuscular control exercises for scapular.
  NOTE: Patient must be able to elevate arm without shoulder and scapular hiking before initiating isotonics; if unable, maintain on humeral head stabilizing exercises.

Phase 3—Advanced Strengthening Phase (15 to 26 weeks)
GOALS
- Maintain full, nonpainful ROM
- Improve strength of shoulder
- Improve neuromuscular control
- Gradual return to functional activities

15 to 20 weeks
- Continue active-assisted ROM exercise with L-bar:
  Flexion, ER, IR
- Perform self-capsular stretches.
- Begin aggressive strengthening program:
  Shoulder flexion
  Shoulder abduction (to 90 degrees)
  Supraspinatus
  ER/IR
  Elbow flexors/extensors
  Scapular muscles
- Begin conditioning program.

21 to 26 weeks
- Continue all exercises listed above.
- Use isokinetic test (modified neutral position) for ER/IR at 180 and 300 degrees per second.
- Begin interval sport program.

Phase 4—Return to Activity Phase (24 to 28 weeks)
GOALS
- Gradual return to recreational sport activities

24 to 28 weeks
- Continue all strengthening exercises.
- Continue all flexibility exercises.
- Continue progression on interval programs.

Repair (Deltoid Splitting) of Type III Rotator Cuff Injury (Large to Massive Tear [Greater Than 5 cm])
WILK AND ANDREWS

Phase 1—Protective Phase (0 to 8 weeks)

0 to 4 weeks
- Fit brace or sling (determined by physician).
- Begin pendulum exercises.
- Perform passive ROM to tolerance:
  Flexion
  ER/IR (shoulder at 45 degrees abduction)
- Perform elbow ROM.
- Perform hand gripping exercises.
- Initiate continuous passive motion (CPM).
- Use submaximal isometrics:
  Abductors
  ER/IR
  Elbow flexors
- Use ice and pain modalities.

- Perform gentle active-assisted ROM with L-bar at 2 weeks.

4 to 8 weeks
- Discontinue brace or sling.
- Perform active-assisted ROM with L-bar:
  Flexion to 100 degrees
  ER/IR (shoulder 45 degrees abduction) 40 degrees
- Continue pain modalities.

Phase 2—Intermediate Phase (8 to 14 weeks)
GOALS
- Establish full ROM (12 weeks)
- Gradually increase strength
- Decrease pain

REHABILITATION PROTOCOL—cont'd

Phase 2—Intermediate Phase (8 to 14 weeks)—cont'd

8 to 10 weeks
- Perform active-assisted ROM L-bar exercises:
  Flexion to tolerance
  ER/IR (shoulder 90 degrees abduction) to tolerance
- Begin isotonic strengthening:
  Deltoid to 90 degrees
  ER/IR side-lying
  Supraspinatus
  Biceps/triceps
  Scapular muscles

10 to 14 weeks
- Continue all exercises listed above (full ROM by 12 to 14 weeks).
- Begin neuromuscular control exercises.
  If patient is unable to elevate arm without shoulder hiking (scapulothoracic substitution), maintain on humeral head stabilizing exercises.

Phase 3—Advanced Strengthening Phase (15 to 26 weeks)

GOALS
- Maintain full, nonpainful ROM
- Improve strength of shoulder
- Improve neuromuscular control
- Gradual return to functional activities

15 to 20 weeks
- Continue active-assisted ROM exercise with L-bar:
  Flexion, ER, IR
- Perform self-capsular stretches.
- Begin aggressive strengthening program:
  Shoulder flexion
  Shoulder abduction (to 90 degrees)
  Supraspinatus
  ER/IR
  Elbow flexors/extensors
  Scapular strengthening
- Begin conditioning program.

21 to 26 weeks
- Continue all exercises listed above.
- Use isokinetic test (modified neutral position) for ER/IR at 180 and 300 degrees per second.
- Begin interval sport program.

Phase 4—Return to Activity Phase (24 to 28 weeks)

GOAL
- Gradual return to recreational sport activities

24 to 28 weeks
- Continue all strengthening exercises.
- Continue all flexibility exercises.
- Continue progression on interval program.

REHABILITATION PROTOCOL

Rotator Cuff Tendonitis and Tears in Throwing Athletes
JOBE AND SCHWAB

Phase 1

REDUCE INFLAMMATION
- Modify or refrain from activity that aggravates the problem.
- Provide modalities for pain relief.

ROM
- Pay careful attention to the posterior capsule so that the humeral head sits back in the fossa and does not slide anteriorly or superiorly.

ACTIVE STRENGTHENING
- Perform internal rotation (IR) and external rotation (ER) with the arm at the side.
- Use elastic tube for resistance.
- Limit range of ER if necessary to reduce discomfort.
- If pain continues, change exercise to isometric mode.

- If still painful, adjust shoulder position to permit a small amount of abduction (towel roll or small pillow under the arm).
- Progress to free weights as pain decreases and strength increases.
- Perform IR on involved side with a bolster under the lateral chest wall to decrease joint compression; limit excursion.
- Begin supraspinatus exercise when 90 degrees of elevation in the scapular plane is possible.
- Alternate supraspinatus exercise with shoulder flexion and abduction.

Continued

REHABILITATION PROTOCOL—cont'd

Rotator Cuff Tendonitis and Tears in Throwing Athletes
JOBE AND SCHWAB

Phase 1—cont'd **ACTIVE STRENGTHENING —cont'd**	• Perform shoulder extension prone or bending forward from the waist; do not move behind the plane of the body. • Use strong shoulder extensors, as depressors of the humeral head; resist upward migration of the head and reduce the change of further impingement. • Use shoulder shrugs *only* for patients with *secondary* impingement *without* generalized tissue laxity.
ENDURANCE TRAINING	• Begin after ROM is reestablished. • Use of an arm ergometer is best. • Ensure short-duration, low-intensity, frequent rest.
Phase 2 **ROM**	• Use posterior cuff and capsule stretch as necessary. • Active ROM is preferable, but aggressive stretching may be warranted if healing is progressing but motion is not.
ISOKINETIC TRAINING	• Only if no pain is present. • High-speed (over 200 degrees per second). • Perform IR and ER standing with dynamometer, head tilted.

ECCENTRIC STRENGTHENING	• Use rotator cuff. • Use posterior shoulder girdle, including horizontal adduction. • Use military press. • Perform push-ups, beginning with wall push-ups. Emphasize protraction and serratus activity. During the eccentric phase do not lower the trunk below the level of the elbows.
SKILL RETRIEVAL	• Most important part to the patient. • Begin with low intensity. • If pain occurs, retreat to previous level until it resolves.
CONDITIONING	• Forearm, wrist, and hand on ipsilateral side tend to weaken from disuse during the period of active shoulder pathology. • For lower extremities and trunk, use exercises such as lunges, squats, trunk flexibility exercises. • Regain cardiovascular fitness.
Phase 3 **ISOKINETIC TRAINING**	• Add flexion and extension, abduction and adduction. • Test as necessary.
ENDURANCE	• Initiate longer and more intense workouts on arm ergometer.
SKILL RETRIEVAL	• Make refinements in intensity and coordination.

REHABILITATION PROTOCOL

Throwing Athletes After Operative Repair of Rotator Cuff: Anterior Capsular Repair   JOBE AND SCHWAB

Timing depends on the specifics of surgery and the pathologic condition: full-thickness tears, excessive joint laxity, and inadequate joint space.

Phase 1 **ROM (ROTATOR CUFF REPAIR)**	• Perform gentle passive ROM only for first months after open repair. • Fit a sling for comfort. • Maintain arm at side for IR and ER.
ROM (ANTERIOR CAPSULAR LABRAL RECONSTRUCTION)	• Fit a pillow abduction splint for up to 2 weeks. • Perform active exercises in splint: Shoulder elevation Elbow flexion and extension Wrist motion Ball squeezes
STRENGTHENING	• Initiate at appropriate time for each procedure (surgeon's orders).

REHABILITATION PROTOCOL—cont'd

Phase 1—cont'd
STRENGTHENING —cont'd

- Begin isometrically: IR and ER, flexion, abduction, extension.
- Use only pain-free motion for strengthening.
- Add active-resistive exercises later with arm at side and use elastic tube for IR and ER, bend forward and work on extension, horizontal abduction in supine position from scapular plane.

Phase 2
ROM

- Continue and become more aggressive if full motion unavailable; hang from overhead bar.

STRENGTHENING

- IR and ER: increase resistance of elastic bands; progress to free weights in side-lying position; use bolster for IR.
- Flexion: include work for anterior deltoid, some exercises in 110-125-degree range.
- Abduction: limit to 90 degrees.
- Supraspinatus: in pain-free range only.
- Horizontal abduction: prone, limit motion to plane of trunk, watch for substitution of scapular adductors and trunk rotators.

Phase 3
ROM
STRENGTHENING

- Perform full active and passive.
- Perform eccentric rotator cuff exercises.
- Include elbow, wrist, and hand.
- Use military press with arm in front of chest.
- Perform push-ups with scapular protraction, beginning with wall push-ups.

ISOKINETIC EXERCISE

- Begin when patient can lift 5 to 10 lbs. in ER and 15 to 20 lbs. in IR.
- Ensure pain free exercise only.
- High-speed (200 degrees).

ENDURANCE

- Use arm ergometer to level of performance required.

CONDITIONING

- Encompass whole body.

Phase 4
ISOKINETIC TESTING

- Involved arm must be 90% of uninvolved.
- Then progress to sport-specific program (see following pages for pitchers and other throwers).

REHABILITATION PROTOCOL

Pitchers' Throwing Program JOBE AND SCHWAB

Step 1
- Toss the ball (no wind-up) against a wall on alternate days.
- Start with 25 to 30 throws, build up to 70 throws and gradually increase throwing distance.

Number of Throws	Distance (feet)
20	20 (warm-up)
25 to 40	30 to 40
10	20 (cool-down)

Step 2
- Toss the ball (playing catch with easy wind up) on alternate days.

Number of Throws	Distance (feet)
10	20 (warm-up)
10	30 to 40
30 to 40	50
10	20 to 30 (cool-down)

Continued

REHABILITATION PROTOCOL—cont'd

Pitchers' Throwing Program　JOBE AND SCHWAB

Step 3
- Continue to increase throwing distance while still tossing the ball with an easy wind-up.

Number of Throws	Distance (feet)
10	20 (warm-up)
10	30 to 40
30 to 40	50 to 60
10	30 (cool-down)

Step 4
- Increase throwing distance to maximum of 60 feet.
- Continue tossing the ball with an occasional throw at no more than half speed.

Number of Throws	Distance (feet)
10	30 (warm-up)
10	40 to 45
30 to 40	60 to 70
10	30 (cool-down)

Step 5
- Gradually increase distance to a maximum of 150 feet.

Phase 5-1

Number of Throws	Distance (feet)
10	40 (warm-up)
10	50 to 60
15 to 20	70 to 80
10	50 to 60
10	40 (cool-down)

Phase 5-2

Number of Throws	Distance (feet)
10	40 (warm-up)
10	50 to 60
20 to 30	80 to 90
20	50 to 60
10	40 (cool-down)

Phase 5-3

Number of Throws	Distance (feet)
10	40 (warm-up)
10	60
15 to 20	100 to 110
20	60
10	40 (cool-down)

Phase 5-4

Number of Throws	Distance (feet)
10	40 (warm-up)
10	60
15 to 20	120 to 150
20	60
10	40 (cool-down)

Step 6
- Progress to throwing off the mound.
- Try to use proper body mechanics, especially when throwing off the mound:
  Stay on top of the ball.
  Keep the elbow up.
  Throw over the top.
  Follow through with the arm and trunk.
  Use the legs to push.

Phase 6-1

Number of Throws	Distance (feet)
10	60 (warm-up)
10	120 to 150 (lobbing)
30	45 (off the mound)
10	60 (off the mound)
10	40 (cool-down)

Phase 6-2

Number of Throws	Distance (feet)
10	50 (warm-up)
10	120 to 150 (lobbing)
20	45 (off the mound)
20	60 (off the mound)
10	40 (cool-down)

Phase 6-3

Number of Throws	Distance (feet)
10	50 (warm-up)
10	60
10	120 to 150 (lobbing)
10	45 (off the mound)
30	60 (off the mound)
10	40 (cool-down)

Phase 6-4

Number of Throws	Distance (feet)
10	50 (warm-up)
10	120 to 150 (lobbing)
10	45 (off the mound)
40 to 50	60 (off the mound)
10	40 (cool-down)

If phase 6-4 is completed without pain or discomfort and the pitcher is throwing at approximately ¾ speed, pitcher can proceed to Step 7—"Up/Down Bullpens"—which simulates a game situation. The pitcher rests between series of pitches to reproduce the rest period between innings.

REHABILITATION PROTOCOL—cont'd

Step 7 Up/Down Bullpens (½ to ¾ speed)

Day 1

Number of Throws	Distance (feet)
10 warm-up throws	120 to 150 (lobbing)
10 warm-up throws	60 (off the mound)
40 pitches	60 (off the mound)
Rest 10 minutes	
20 pitches	60 (off the mound)

Day 2—Off

Day 3

Number of Throws	Distance (feet)
10 warm-up throws	120 to 150 (lobbing)
10 warm-up throws	60 (off the mound)
30 pitches	60 (off the mound)
Rest 10 minutes	
10 warm-up throws	60 (off the mound)
20 pitches	60 (off the mound)
Rest 10 minutes	
10 warm-up throws	60 (off the mound)
20 pitches	60 (off the mound)

Day 4—Off

Day 5

Number of Throws	Distance (feet)
10 warm-up throws	120 to 150 (lobbing)
10 warm-up throws	60 (off the mound)
30 pitches	60 (off the mound)
Rest 8 minutes	
20 pitches	60 (off the mound)
Rest 8 minutes	
20 pitches	60 (off the mound)
Rest 8 minutes	
20 pitches	60 (off the mound)

The pitcher is now ready to begin a normal routine, from throwing batting practice to pitching in the bullpen. The trainer or physical therapist can and should adjust this program as needed. Each step may take more or less time than listed, and the the trainer, physical therapist, and physician should monitor the program. The pitcher should work hard, but should not overdo it.

REHABILITATION PROTOCOL

Throwing Program for Catchers, Infielders, and Outfielders
JOBE AND SCHWAB

General
- Repeat each step 3 times.
- All throws should have an arc or "hump."
- The maximum distance thrown by infielders and and catchers is 120 feet.
- The maximum distance thrown by outfielders is 200 feet.

Step 1
- Toss the ball with no wind-up.
- Stand with feet shoulder-width apart and face the player throwing toward.
- Concentrate on rotating and staying on top of the ball.

Number of Throws	Distance (feet)
5	20 (warm-up)
10	30
5	20 (cool-down)

Step 2
- Stand sideways to the person throwing toward.
- Keep feet shoulder-width apart.

- Close up and pivot onto back foot when throwing.

Number of Throws	Distance (feet)
5	30 (warm-up)
5	40
10	50
5	30 (cool-down)

Step 3
- Repeat the position in step 2.
- Step toward the target with front leg and follow through with back leg.

Number of Throws	Distance (feet)
5	50 (warm-up)
5	60
10	70
5	50 (cool-down)

Continued

REHABILITATION PROTOCOL—cont'd

Throwing Program for Catchers, Infielders, and Outfielders
JOBE AND SCHWAB

Step 4
- Assume the pitcher's stance.
- Lift and stride with lead leg.
- Follow through with back leg.

Number of Throws	Distance (feet)
5	60 (warm-up)
5	70
10	80
5	60 (cool-down)

Step 5
- Outfielders: Lead with glove-side foot forward.
  Take one step, crow hop, and throw the ball.
- Infielders: Lead with glove-side foot forward.
  Take a shuffle step and throw the ball.
  Throw the last 5 throws in a straight line.

Number of Throws	Distance (feet)
5	70 (warm-up)
5	90
10	100
5	80 (cool-down)

Step 6
- Repeat the throwing technique in Step 5.
- Assume playing position.
- Infielders and catchers do not throw more than 120 feet.

- Outfielders do not throw more than 150 feet (mid-outfield).

Number of Throws	Infielders/Catchers	Outfielders
5	80 (warm-up)	80 (warm-up)
5	80 to 90	90 to 100
5	90 to 100	110 to 125
5	110 to 120	130 to 150
5	80 (cool-down)	80 (cool-down)

Step 7
- Assume playing position.

Number of Throws	Infielders/Catchers	Outfielders
5	80 (warm-up)	80 to 90 (warm-up)
5	80 to 90	110 to 130
5	90 to 100	150 to 175
5	110 to 120	180 to 200
5	80 (cool-down)	90 (cool-down)

Step 8
- Repeat Step 7.
- Use a Fungo bat to hit to infielders and outfielders while in their normal playing positions.

REHABILITATION PROTOCOL

Arthroscopic Subacromial Decompression—Intact Rotator Cuff   WILK AND ANDREWS

This evaluation-based rehabilitation protocol is used for patients who have a stable shoulder (intact rotator cuff) after arthroscopic shoulder decompression (Fig. 3-7, p. 108).

Phase 1—Immediate Motion Phase (Days 1 to 14)
GOALS
- Prevent negative effects of immobilization.
- Regain full, pain-free ROM.
- Retard muscular atrophy.
- Reduce pain and inflammation.

- Begin pendulum exercises to promote early motion and minimize pain (Fig. 3-8).
- Begin active-assisted exercises with T-bar:
  Shoulder flexion (Fig. 3-9)
  Shoulder extension (Fig. 3-10)
  IR and ER (Fig. 3-11)
  Begin rotation exercises at 0 degrees of abduction; progress to 45 degrees of abduction, eventually gaining 90 degrees of abduction.
  Carefully monitor progression.

REHABILITATION PROTOCOL—cont'd

Phase 1—Immediate Motion Phase (Days 1 to 14)—cont'd

GOALS—cont'd
- Begin capsular stretching for anterior, posterior, and inferior capsule, using opposite arm and hand to create overpressure.
- Use modalities to control pain and inflammation:
  - Ice
  - HVGS
  - Ultrasound
  - Nonsteroidal antiinflammatory drugs (NSAIDs)

Phase 2—Intermediate Phase (2 to 6 weeks)

CRITERIA FOR PROGRESSION TO PHASE 2
- Minimal pain and tenderness
- Nearly complete motion
- Good (⅘) strength

GOALS
- Normalize full, pain-free motion and shoulder arthrokinematics.
- Improve muscular strength.
- Improve neuromuscular control.
- Eliminate residual inflammation and pain.
- Continue active-assisted exercises with more aggressive stretching at all end ranges.
- Use joint mobilization techniques for capsular restriction, especially the posterior capsule.
- ■ *Posterior capsular tightness causes superior and anterior humeral head elevation during shoulder elevation, contributing to impingement. Emphasize stretching of this portion of the capsule.*
- Begin strengthening: progress from isometric (Figs. 3-12, 3-13, 3-14, and 3-15) to isotonic dumbbell exercises:
  - Shoulder abduction to 90 degrees
  - Supraspinatus (scaption: empty can) (Fig. 3-16)
  - Shoulder flexion to 90 degrees
  - Side-lying IR and ER (Fig. 3-17)
  - Elbow flexion and extension

- Perform scapular stabilizing exercises: emphasize scapular movements through manual resistance during neuromuscular control exercises:
  - Scapular retraction (rhomboideus, middle trapezius)
  - Scapular protraction (serratus anterior)
  - Scapular depression (latissimus dorsi, trapezius, serratus anterior)
- Begin submaximal isokinetics in the plane of the scapular or in the modified neutral position late in this phase.
- ■ *Rathburn and Macnab have shown that with the arm adducted (at the side), a zone of avascularity exists in the supraspinatus. With abduction, vascularity improves. Thus, Wilk and Andrews recommend that rotator cuff exercises be performed with the arm slightly abducted.*
- Begin proprioceptive neuromuscular facilitation exercises in the D₂ flexion/extension pattern with isometric holds (rhythmic stabilization).

Phase 3—Dynamic Strengthening (6 to 12 weeks)

CRITERIA FOR PROGRESSION TO PHASE 3
- Full, painless ROM
- No pain or tenderness
- 70% strength of contralateral shoulder
- Stable shoulder on clinical exam (negative impingement)

Continued

Arthroscopic Subacromial Decompression—Intact Rotator Cuff   WILK AND ANDREWS

When	Immediate Motion Phase 7-14 days	Intermediate Phase 2-6 weeks	Dynamic Strengthening Phase 6-12 weeks	Return To Activity 12-16 weeks
Criteria for progression	• Stable Shoulder	• Minimal pain • Nearly complete ROM • Strength at least 4/5 (good)	• Painless full ROM • No pain • Strength 70% of contralateral side • No impingement by exam	• Full painless ROM • No pain • Muscle strength that fulfills criteria for sport (isometric/isokinetic) • Satisfactory PE
Signs	• Inflammation • Pain • Loss of ROM • Weakness	• Pain • ROM • Weakness • Poor neuromuscular control		• Isokinetic dynamometer 85% contralateral side

Rx	• Passive & active assisted motion exercises
	   -pendulum
	   -T-bar
	• Capsular stretches
	• Strengthening
	   -submaximal
	   -isometrics
	• Modalities
	   -ice
	   -high voltage galvanic stim
	• NSAIDS
		• Active assisted ROM
		• Active ROM
		• Aggressive stretching
		• Strengthening
		   -isotonic dumbbell
		   -submaximal
		   -isokinetics
		• Neuromuscular control exercises
		   -PNF
		• Cardiovascular fitness
			• Aggressive stretching
			• Strengthening
			   -constant loading (eccentric & concentric)
			   -isokinetics
			   -manual resistance
			   -plyometrics
			• Neuromuscular control exercises
				• Interval program

Goals	• Prevent effects of immobilization • Full, painless ROM • Prevent atrophy • Reduce pain & inflammation	• Normalize full ROM • Regain & improve strength • Improve neuromuscular control • Eliminate pain & inflammation	• Improve strength, power, endurance • Improve neuromuscular control • Prepare for gradual return to functional activities	• Unrestricted activity • Maintain normal motion & function

Figure 3-7 Evaluation-based rehabilitation protocol: rehabilitation after arthroscopic shoulder decompression. The protocol is based on four phases: 1, immediate motion phase of 7 to 14 days; 2, intermediate phase of 2 to 6 weeks; 3, dynamic strengthening phase of 6 to 12 weeks; and 4, return to activity phase of 12 to 16 weeks. (From Wilk KE, Andrews JR: *Orthopedics* 16(3):349, 1993.)

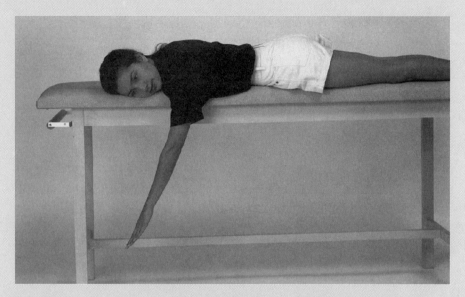

Figure 3-8 Pendulum exercise performed in the prone position to provide ROM to the glenohumeral joint and also to neuromodulate pain.

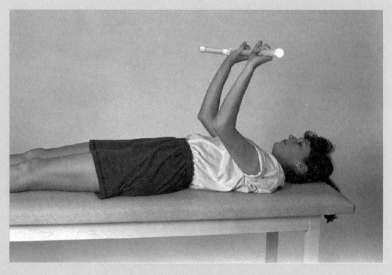

Figure 3-9 Active assisted flexion performed with an L-bar. Note hand placement of external rotation.

Continued

Arthroscopic Subacromial Decompression—Intact Rotator Cuff WILK AND ANDREWS

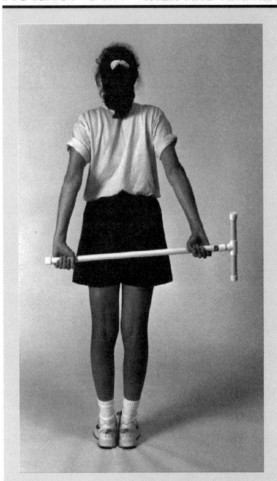

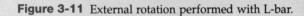

Figure 3-10 Active assisted extension with L-bar.

Figure 3-11 External rotation performed with L-bar.

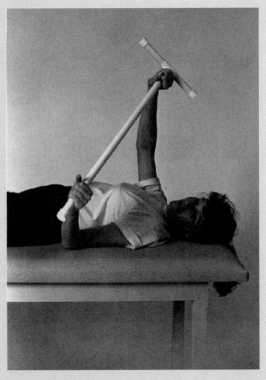

REHABILITATION PROTOCOL—cont'd

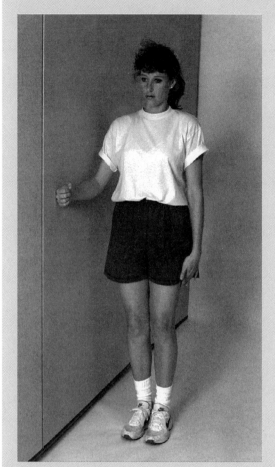

Figure 3-12 Submaximal isometrics for the external rotation musculature.

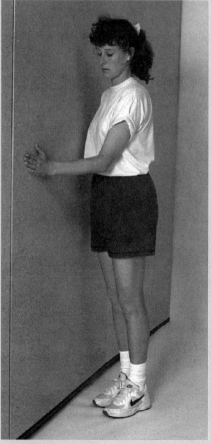

Figure 3-13 Submaximal isometrics for the internal rotator musculature.

Continued

Arthroscopic Subacromial Decompression—Intact Rotator Cuff   WILK AND ANDREWS

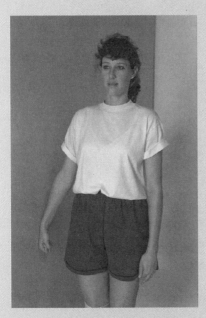

Figure 3-14 Submaximal isometrics for the shoulder abductors.

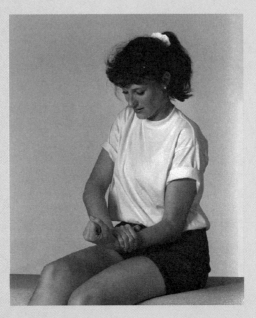

Figure 3-15 Submaximal isometric contraction for the elbow flexors.

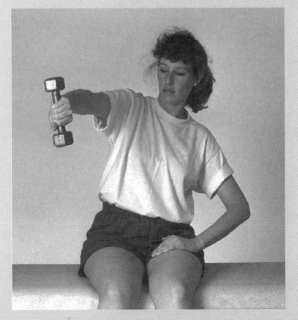

Figure 3-16 Isotonic resistance exercise for the supraspinatus muscle (scaption).

REHABILITATION PROTOCOL—cont'd

Phase 3—Dynamic Strengthening (6 to 12 weeks)—cont'd

GOALS
- Improve shoulder complex strength, power, endurance
- Improve neuromuscular control and shoulder proprioception
- Prepare for gradual return to functional activities

WARNING SIGNALS
- Loss of motion (especially IR)
- Lack of strength progression (especially abductors)
- Continued pain (especially night pain)

- Begin fundamental shoulder exercises (see the boxes) to ensure progressive improvement in shoulder strength. These exercises are chosen because of the observed high EMG activity of the shoulder and scapulothoracic musculature.

STRENGTHENING:
- Progress isokinetics, manual resistive, and eccentric exercises.
- For competitive athletes who require enhanced strength and who are exposed to large deceleration stresses, begin a plyometric program:
  Plyometric drills with eccentric loading phase before concentric response phase
  Plyoball, exercise tubing, and/or wall (Fig. 3-18)

Phase 4—Return to Activity (12 to 16 weeks)

CRITERIA FOR PROGRESSION TO PHASE 4
- Full, painless ROM
- No pain or tenderness
- Muscular strength (isokinetic/ isometric) that fulfills established criteria
- Satisfactory clinical exam

GOALS
- Progressive return to unrestricted activity
- Maintenance of normal shoulder strength and motion

- Continue fundamental shoulder exercises (p. 114).
- Begin interval program (see box and Tables 3-3, 3-4, and 3-5):
  Throwing athletes, tennis and golf athletes
  Progressive, systematic interval program before returning to demands of sport
  For throwing athletes, monitor the number of throws, distance, intensity, and types of throws, and progress to enhance a return to competition.

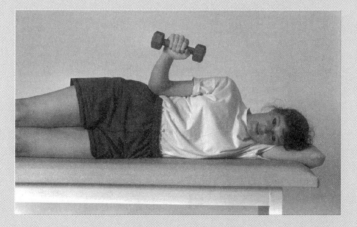

Figure 3-17 External rotation strengthening with weights.

Continued

REHABILITATION PROTOCOL—cont'd

Arthroscopic Subacromial Decompression—Intact Rotator Cuff WILK AND ANDREWS

Fundamental Shoulder Exercises ("Basic Ten")

1. Rope and pulley flexion
2. L-bar flexion stretches
3. L-bar external rotation stretches
4. L-bar internal rotation stretches
5. External/internal rotation strengthening
6. Lateral raises to 90 degrees
7. Empty can
8. Passive ROM—horizontal abduction
9. Biceps curls
10. Self capsular stretches

Throwers' Ten Program

1. Diagonal pattern D_2 extension and flexion
2. External/internal rotation at 0 degrees abduction
3. Shoulder abduction (palm down) to 90 degrees
4. Scaption with internal rotation
5. Prone horizontal abduction (neutral rotation); prone horizontal abduction (full external rotation, 100 degrees abduction)
6. Press-ups
7. Prone rowing
8. Push-ups
9. Elbow flexion/extension
10. Wrist flexion/extension; supination/pronation

Modified from Wilk KE et al: *Preventive and rehabilitative exercises for the shoulder and elbow*, ed 3, Birmingham, 1993, American Sports Medicine Institute.

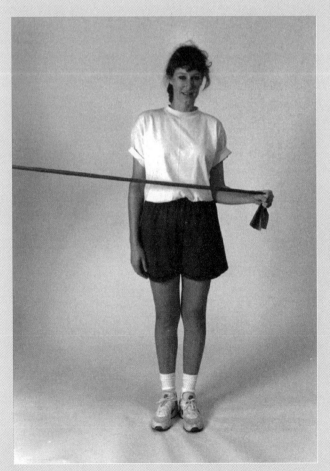

Figure 3-18 With the elbow close to the body and flexed 90 degrees, the shoulder is externally rotated against the resistance of the band.

REHABILITATION PROTOCOL—cont'd

Interval Throwing Program Following Arthroscopic Subacromial Decompression

45-Foot Phase

Step 1: A) Warm-up throwing
B) 45 feet (25 throws)
C) Rest 15 minutes
D) Warm-up throwing
E) 45 feet (25 throws)

Step 2: A) Warm-up throwing
B) 45 feet (25 throws)
C) Rest 10 minutes
D) Warm-up throwing
E) 45 feet (25 throws)
F) Rest 10 minutes
G) Warm-up throwing
H) 45 feet (25 throws)

60-Foot Phase

Step 3: A) Warm-up throwing
B) 60 feet (25 throws)
C) Rest 15 minutes
D) Warm-up throwing
E) 60 feet (25 throws)

Step 4: A) Warm-up throwing
B) 60 feet (25 throws)
C) Rest 10 minutes
D) Warm-up throwing
E) 60 feet (25 throws)
F) Rest 10 minutes
G) Warm-up throwing
H) 60 feet (25 throws)

90-Foot Phase

Step 5: A) Warm-up throwing
B) 90 feet (25 throws)
C) Rest 15 minutes
D) Warm-up throwing
E) 90 feet (25 throws)

Step 6: A) Warm-up throwing
B) 90 feet (25 throws)
C) Rest 10 minutes
D) Warm-up throwing
E) 90 feet (25 throws)
F) Rest 10 minutes
G) Warm-up throwing
H) 90 feet (25 throws)

120-Foot Phase

Step 7: A) Warm-up throwing
B) 120 feet (25 throws)
C) Rest 15 minutes
D) Warm-up throwing
E) 120 feet (25 throws)

Step 8: A) Warm-up throwing
B) 120 feet (25 throws)
C) Rest 10 minutes
D) Warm-up throwing
E) 120 feet (25 throws)
F) Rest 10 minutes
G) Warm-up throwing
H) 120 feet (25 throws)

150-Foot Phase

Step 9: A) Warm-up throwing
B) 150 feet (25 throws)
C) Rest 15 minutes
D) Warm-up throwing
E) 150 feet (25 throws)

Step 10: A) Warm-up throwing
B) 150 feet (25 throws)
C) Rest 10 minutes
D) Warm-up throwing
E) 150 feet (25 throws)
F) Rest 10 minutes
G) Warm-up throwing
H) 150 feet (25 throws)

180-Foot Phase

Step 11: A) Warm-up throwing
B) 180 feet (25 throws)
C) Rest 15 minutes
D) Warm-up throwing
E) 180 feet (25 throws)

Step 12: A) Warm-up throwing
B) 180 feet (25 throws)
C) Rest 10 minutes
D) Warm-up throwing
E) 180 feet (25 throws)
F) Rest 10 minutes
G) Warm-up throwing
H) 180 feet (25 throws)

Step 13: A) Warm-up throwing
B) 180 feet (25 throws)
C) Rest 10 minutes
D) Warm-up throwing
E) 180 feet (25 throws)
F) Rest 10 minutes
G) Warm-up throwing
H) 180 feet (50 throws)

Step 14:
Begin throwing off the mound or return to respective position.

From Wilk RE, Andrews JR: Rehabilitation following arthroscopic subacromial decompression, *Orthopedics* 16(3):349, 1993.

Continued

REHABILITATION PROTOCOL—cont'd

Arthroscopic Subacromial Decompression—Intact Rotator Cuff WILK AND ANDREWS

TABLE 3-3 Interval Golf Program

	Monday	Wednesday	Friday
First week	10 putts 10 chips 5' rest 15 chips	15 putts 15 chips 5' rest 25 chipping	20 putts 20 chips 5' rest 20 putts 20 chips 5' rest 10 chips 10 short irons
Second week	20 chips 10 short irons 5' rest 10 short irons	20 chips 15 short irons 10' rest 15 short irons 15 chips putting	15 short irons 10 medium irons 10' rest 20 short irons 15 chips
Third week	15 short irons 15 medium irons 10' rest 5 long irons 15 short irons 15 medium irons 10' rest 20 chips	15 short irons 10 medium irons 10 long irons 10' rest 10 short irons 10 medium irons 5 long irons 5 wood	15 short irons 10 medium irons 10 long irons 10' rest 10 short irons 10 medium irons 10 long irons 10 wood
Fourth week	15 short irons 10 medium irons 10 long irons 10 drives 15' rest Repeat	Play 9 holes	Play 9 holes
Fifth week	9 holes	9 holes	18 holes

Flexing exercises before hitting
Use ice after play
(') abbreviation for minutes
chips = pitching wedge
short irons = W, 9, 8
medium irons = 7, 6, 5
long irons = 4, 3, 2
woods = 3, 5
drives = driver
From Wilk RE, Andrews JR: Rehabilitation following arthroscopic subacromial decompression, *Orthopedics* 16(3):349, 1993.

REHABILITATION PROTOCOL—cont'd

TABLE 3-4 Interval Tennis Program*

First Week	Second Week	Third Week	Fourth Week
Monday			
12 FH	25 FH	30 FH	30 FH
8 BH	15 BH	25 BH	30 BH
10-minute rest	10-minute rest	10 OH	10 OH
13 FH	25 FH	10-minute rest	10-minute rest
7 BH	15 BH	30 FH	Play 3 games
		25 BH	10 FH
		10 OH	10 BH
			5 OH
Wednesday			
15 FH	30 FH	30 FH	30 FH
8 BH	20 BH	25 BH	30 BH
10-minute rest	10-minute rest	15 OH	10 OH
15 FH	30 FH	10-minute rest	10-minute rest
7 BH	20 BH	30 FH	Play set
		25 BH	10 FH
		15 OH	10 BH
			5 OH
Friday			
15 FH	30 FH	30 FH	30 FH
10 BH	25 BH	30 BH	30 BH
10-minute rest	10-minute rest	15 OH	10 OH
15 FH	30 FH	10-minute rest	10-minute rest
10 BH	15 BH	30 FH	Play 1½ sets
	10 OH	15 OH	10 FH
		10-minute rest	10 BH
		30 FH	3 OH
		30 BH	
		15 OH	

*FH = forehand ground stroke; BH = backhand ground stroke; OH = overhead shot.
Ice after each day of play.
From Wilk RE, Andrews JR: Rehabilitation following arthroscopic subacromial decompression, *Orthopedics* 16(3):349, 1993.

Continued

TABLE 3-5 **Isokinetic Criteria for Return to Throwing***		
1. Bilateral compression	ER	98% to 105%
2. Bilateral compression	IR	105% to 115%
3. Bilateral compression	ABD	98% to 103%
4. Bilateral compression	ADD	110% to 125%
5. Unilateral ratio	ER/IR	66% to 70%
6. Unilateral ratio	ABD/ADD	78% to 85%
7. Peak torque/body weight ratio	ER	18% to 22%
8. Peak torque/body weight ratio	IR	28% to 32%
9. Peak torque/body weight ratio	ABD	24% to 30%
10. Peak torque/body weight ratio	ADD	32% to 38%

*All data represent 180% test speed
Modified from Wilk KE, Andrews JR, Arrigo CA: The abductor and adductor strength characteristics of professional baseball pitchers, *Am J Sports Med* 23(3):307, 1995.

Shoulder Instability

REHABILITATION RATIONALE

Shoulder instability may be based on several factors, including the direction and degree of the instability, as well as the time of onset and the frequency of dislocation (see the box).

Traumatic Anterior Shoulder Instability

The most common cause of instability in the shoulder is traumatic anterior dislocation of the shoulder. The shoulder dislocates because it is forced into abduction and external rotation, overcoming the capsular labral restraints. After traumatic anterior shoulder dislocation, patients frequently experience intermittent subluxations. *Subluxation* is defined as increased excursion of the humeral head on the glenoid fossa without complete dislocation. Individuals who sustain an initial dislocation before the age of 20 years as a result of minimal trauma have the highest risk of recurrent dislocation. Rowe and Sakellarides reported a 92% recurrence rate in individuals age 20 years or younger at the time of initial dislocation.

■ *Age at dislocation appears to be a more important factor than length of immobilization, specific rehabilitation program, or degree of initial trauma.*

Although no data have documented the concept that a long immobilization period decreases the risk of recurrence, it seems reasonable to immobilize the shoulder briefly, to allow healing of traumatized tissues, in conjunction with a strengthening program to strengthen the dynamic shoulder stabilizers. Patients older than 40 years of age at initial dislocation probably should be immobilized for a briefer period than are younger patients, because the recurrence rate in this age group is low, and longer immobilization is more likely to lead to shoulder stiffness. Immobilization is continued only until pain subsides, typically in 7 to 10 days.

Although the essential pathologic lesion in younger patients (less than 25 years of age) may be disruption or stretching of the anterior capsule and ligamentous structures, weakening of the rotator cuff tendons is more common in patients more than 40 years of age. Rotator cuff tear should be suspected in patients older than 40 years, especially if persistent pain or weakness does not improve within 2 weeks of reduction.

Shoulder Instability			
Direction	**Degree**	**Onset**	**Frequency**
Anterior	Dislocation	Traumatic	Acute
Posterior	Subluxation	Atraumatic	Recurrent
Inferior	Micro	Voluntary	Fixed
Multi-directional		Involuntary	

Patients *without* a Bankart lesion respond more favorably to rehabilitation. Rockwood et al. reported that only 12% of patients with traumatic instability responded favorably to a rehabilitation program, compared with 80% of patients with atraumatic instability.

Rehabilitation after acute shoulder dislocation has the following objectives:
- Avoidance of redislocation during rehabilitation by avoiding positions of hyperflexion, external rotation, and shoulder abduction combined with external rotation
- Reestablishment of good motion
- Progressive strengthening of the dynamic stabilizers of the shoulder
- Plyometric and sports-specific exercises to prepare the athlete for safe return to normal sports activities
- A decrease in the risk of future recurrent dislocation

REHABILITATION PROTOCOL

Acute Traumatic Anterior Shoulder Dislocation

- Immobilize young patients in a sling for 4 to 6 weeks. Patients older than 40 years are immobilized only until pain subsides.
- Begin active ROM exercises of elbow, wrist, and hand.
- Avoid positions of extreme adduction and ER during immobilization, as well as for 3 months after removal of sling.
- After immobilization is discontinued, gradually progress through rehabilitation program that emphasizes strengthening of the rotator cuff and scapular musculature (see p. 122).

- Prerequisites for return to sports and overhead activities include full ROM, return of strength, and absence of pain.
- When the patient returns to athletic activities, a harness that limits abduction may be used to help avoid recurrent injury.
- If progress in therapy is slow, an arthrogram or magnetic resonance imaging (MRI) should be obtained to rule out a rotator cuff pathologic condition, especially in older patients.

REHABILITATION PROTOCOL

Anterior Capsular Shift Procedure: Regular WILK AND ANDREWS

The goal of this rehabilitation protocol is to return the patient/athlete to activity or sport as quickly and safely as possible, while maintaining a stable shoulder. The program is based on muscle physiology, biomechanics, anatomy, and the healing process following anterior capsular shift surgery, in which an incision is made into the ligamentous capsule of the shoulder, the capsule is pulled tighter, and is sutured together. The ultimate goal is a functional, stable shoulder and a pain-free return to the presurgery functional level.

Phase 1—Protection Phase (0 to 6 weeks)
GOALS   Allow healing of sutured capsule
         Begin early protected ROM
         Retard muscle atrophy
         Decrease pain and inflammation

0 to 2 weeks
- Precautions:
  Sleep in immobilizer for 4 weeks
  No overhead activities for 6 weeks
  Wean from immobilizer and fit sling as soon as possible (determined by orthopaedist or therapists), approximately 3 to 4 weeks
- Begin gripping exercises with putty.
- Perform elbow flexion/extension and pronation/supination.
- Begin pendulum exercises (nonweighted).
- Perform rope and pulley active-assisted exercises:
  Shoulder flexion to 90 degrees
  Shoulder abduction to 60 degrees

Continued

Anterior Capsular Shift Procedure: Regular   WILK AND ANDREWS

Phase 1—Protection Phase (0 to 6 weeks)—cont'd

0 to 2
weeks—
cont'd

- Perform T-bar exercises:
  ER to 15 to 20 degrees with arm ab-ducted at 40 degrees
  Shoulder flexion/extension
- Perform active ROM, cervical spine.
- Begin isometrics:
  Flexors, extensors, ER, IR, abduction
- Criteria for hospital discharge:
  Shoulder active-assisted ROM: flexion 90 degrees, abduction 45 degrees, ER 45 degrees
  Minimal pain and swelling
  "Good" proximal and distal muscle power

2 to 4
weeks

- Goals:
  Gradually increase ROM
  Normalize arthrokinematics
  Improve strength
  Decrease pain and inflammation

- Perform ROM exercises:
  T-bar active-assisted exercises
  ER to 25 degrees at 45 degrees shoulder abduction
  IR to 65 degrees at 45 degrees shoulder abduction
  Shoulder flexion/extension to tolerance
  Shoulder abduction to tolerance
  Shoulder horizontal abduction/adduction
  Rope and pulley flexion/extension (Fig. 3-19)
  All exercises are performed to tolerance; take to point of pain and/or resistance and hold.
- Begin gentle self-capsular stretches
- Initiate gentle joint mobilization to rees-tablish normal arthrokinematics:
  Scapulothoracic joint
  Glenohumeral joint
  Sternoclavicular joint

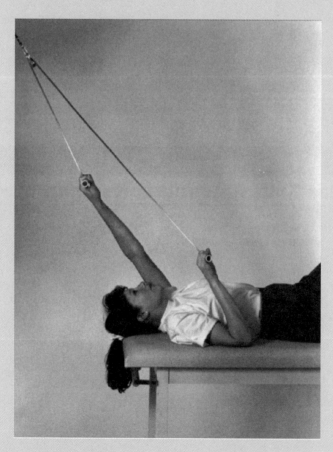

Figure 3-19 Supine elevation using overhead pulley.

REHABILITATION PROTOCOL—cont'd

Phase 1—Protection Phase (0 to 6 weeks)—cont'd

2 to 4 weeks—cont'd	• Perform strengthening exercises: Isometrics May begin tubing for ER/IR at 0 degrees • Begin conditioning program for trunk, lower extremities, cardiovascular system. • Use modalities, ice, and NSAIDs to decrease pain and inflammation.
4 to 6 weeks	• Continue all exercises to tolerance. • Perform ROM exercises: T-bar active-assisted exercises ER to 25 to 35 degrees at 45 degrees of shoulder abduction ER to 5 to 10 degrees at 90 degrees of shoulder abduction IR to 75 degrees at 90 degrees of shoulder abduction Continue all others to tolerance.

Phase 2—Intermediate Phase (6 to 12 weeks)

GOALS	• Full, nonpainful ROM by 10 to 12 weeks • Normalize arthrokinematics • Increase strength • Improve neuromuscular control
6 to 8 weeks	• Begin ROM exercises: T-bar active-assisted exercises at 90 degrees abduction Continue all exercises listed above. Gradually increase ROM to full ROM at week 12. Continue self-capsular stretches. Continue joint mobilization. • Perform strengthening exercises: Begin isotonic dumbbell program: Side-lying ER (see Fig. 3-17) Side-lying IR Shoulder abduction Supraspinatus Latissimus dorsi Rhomboids Biceps curl Triceps curl Shoulder shrugs Push-ups into chair (serratus anterior) Continue tubing at 0 degrees for ER/IR (see Fig. 3-18). • Begin neuromuscular control exercises for scapulothoracic joint.
8 to 10 weeks	• Continue all exercises. • Begin tubing exercises for rhomboids, latissimus dorsi, biceps, and triceps. • Begin aggressive stretching and joint mobilization if needed.

Phase 3—Dynamic Strengthening Phase (12 to 20 weeks)

12 to 17 weeks

GOALS:	• Improve strength, power, and endurance • Improve neuromuscular control • Prepare athlete to begin throwing
CRITERIA TO ENTER PHASE 3	• Full, nonpainful ROM (patient *must* fulfill this criteria) • No pain or tenderness • Strength 70% or more of contralateral side
EMPHASIS	• High-speed, high-energy strengthening exercises • Eccentric exercises • Diagonal patterns
12 weeks	• Perform thrower's ten exercises (p. 114). • Perform tubing exercises: IR/ER at 0 degrees abduction (arm at side) Rhomboids Latissimus dorsi Biceps Diagonal patterns D₂ extension Diagonal patterns • Perform dumbbell exercises for supraspinatus and deltoid. • Initiate serratus anterior strengthening (push-ups/floor). • Perform trunk, lower strengthening exercises. • Perform neuromuscular exercises. • Begin self-capsular stretches.
17 to 20 weeks	• Continue all exercises. • Emphasize gradual return to recreational activities.

Phase 4—Return to Activity (20 to 28 weeks)

GOALS	• Progressive increase in activities to prepare for full functional return
CRITERIA TO PROGRESS TO PHASE 4	• Full ROM • No pain or tenderness • Isokinetic test that fulfills criteria to throw • Satisfactory clinical exam
20 to 24 weeks	• Begin interval throwing programs (p. 115) if patient is a recreational athlete. • Continue tubing exercises (phase 3). • Continue ROM exercises.

REHABILITATION PROTOCOL

Anterior Capsular Shift (Accelerated) WILKS AND ANDREWS

Phase 1—Protection Phase (0 to 4 weeks)

GOALS
- Allow healing of sutured capsule
- Begin early protected ROM
- Retard muscular atrophy
- Decrease pain and inflammation

0 to 2 weeks
- Precautions:
  Sleep in immobilizer for 4 weeks.
  Do not permit any overhead activities for 6 weeks.
  Wean from immobilizer and fit sling as soon as possible (determined by orthopaedist or therapist).
  Exercises
- Begin gripping exercises with putty.
- Perform elbow flexion/extension and pronation/supination.
- Perform pendulum exercises (non-weighted).
- Perform rope and pulley active-assisted exercises:
  Shoulder flexion to 90 degrees
  Shoulder abduction to 60 degrees
- Perform T-bar exercises:
  ER to 15 degrees with arm abducted at 30 degrees
  Shoulder flexion/extension to tolerance
- Perform active ROM, cervical spine.
- Begin isometrics:
  Flexors, extensors, ER, IR, abduction
- Criteria for hospital discharge:
  Shoulder active assisted ROM: flexion 90 degrees, abduction 45 degrees, ER 25 degrees
  Minimal pain and swelling
  "Good" proximal and distal muscle power

2 to 4 weeks
- Goals:
  Gradually increase ROM.
  Normalize arthrokinematics.
  Improve strength.
  Decrease pain and inflammation.
- Perform ROM exercises:
  T-bar active-assisted exercises
  ER at 30 degrees, abduction to 45 degrees
  IR at 30 degrees, abduction to 45 degrees

Shoulder flexion/extension to tolerance
Shoulder abduction to tolerance
Shoulder horizontal abduction/adduction
Rope and pulley flexion/extension
Perform *all* exercises to tolerance; take to point of pain and/or resistance and hold.
- Begin gentle self-capsular stretches.
- Initiate gentle joint mobilization to reestablish normal arthrokinematics:
  Scapulothoracic joint
  Glenohumeral joint
  Sternoclavicular joint
- Perform strengthening exercises:
  Isometrics
  May begin tubing for ER/IR at 0 degrees.
- Begin conditioning program for trunk, lower extremities, cardiovascular system.
- Use modalities, ice, and NSAIDs to decrease pain and inflammation.

5 to 6 weeks
- Perform active-assisted ROM flexion to tolerance.
- Perform IR/ER at 45 degrees abduction to tolerance.
- Begin IR/ER at 90 degrees abduction to tolerance.
- Begin isotonic (light weight) strengthening.
- Continue gentle joint mobilization (grade 3).

Phase 2—Intermediate Phase (7 to 12 weeks)

GOALS
- Full, nonpainful ROM by 8 to 10 weeks
- Normalize arthrokinematics
- Increase strength
- Improve neuromuscular control

7 to 10 weeks
- Perform ROM exercises:
  T-bar active-assisted exercises
  Continue all exercises
  Gradually increase ROM to full ROM at 8 to 10 weeks
  Continue self-capsular stretches.
  Continue joint mobilization.

REHABILITATION PROTOCOL—cont'd

Phase 2—Intermediate Phase (7 to 12 weeks)—cont'd

7 to 10 weeks—cont'd	• Perform strengthening exercises: Begin isotonic dumbbell program: Side-lying ER Side-lying IR Shoulder abduction Supraspinatus Latissimus dorsi Rhomboids Biceps curl Triceps curl Shoulder shrugs Push-ups into chair (serratus anterior) Continue tubing at 0 degrees for ER/IR. • Begin neuromuscular control exercises for scapulothoracic joint.
10 to 12 weeks	• Continue all exercises. • Begin tubing exercises for rhomboids, latissimus dorsi, biceps, and triceps. • Begin aggressive stretching and joint mobilization if needed.

Phase 3—Dynamic Strengthening Phase (12 to 20 weeks)

GOALS	• Improve strength, power, and endurance • Improve neuromuscular control • Prepare athlete to begin throwing
CRITERIA TO ENTER PHASE 3	• Full, nonpainful ROM (patient *must* fulfill this criteria) • No pain or tenderness • Strength 70% or more of contralateral side
EMPHASIS	• High-speed, high-energy strengthening exercises • Eccentric exercises • Diagonal patterns
12 weeks	• Perform thrower's ten exercises (p. 114).

	• Perform tubing exercises: IR/ER in 90 degrees of shoulder abduction/90 degrees of flexion of elbow (slow sets, fast sets) Rhomboids Latissimus dorsi Biceps Diagonal patterns D$_2$ extension Diagonal patterns D$_2$ flexion • Perform dumbbell exercises for supraspinatus and deltoid. • Practice serratus anterior strengthening (push-ups/floor). • Perform trunk, lower strengthening exercises. • Perform neuromuscular exercises. • Perform self-capsular stretches.
17 to 20 weeks	• Continue all exercises. • *Begin plyometrics for shoulder:* *ER at 90 degrees abduction* *IR at 90 degrees abduction* *D$_2$ extension plyometrics* *Biceps plyometrics* *Serratus anterior plyometrics*

Phase 4—Throwing Phase (20 to 26 weeks)

GOALS	• Progressive increase in activities to prepare for full functional return
CRITERIA TO PROGRESS TO PHASE 4	• Full ROM • No pain or tenderness • Isokinetic test that fulfills criteria to throw • Satisfactory clinical exam
20 weeks	• Begin interval throwing programs (p. 115). • Continue throwers ten exercises (p. 114). • Continue plyometric exercises.
24 weeks	• Progress interval throwing program, phase 2 (p. 115).
26 to 30 weeks	• Return to sports.

Anterior Capsular Labral Reconstruction in Throwing Athletes with Anterior Instability JOBE AND SCHWAB

Throwing athletes without complete dislocation are classified into one of the following four categories:
- Pure impingement with no underlying or antecedent instability
- Instability with secondary impingement
- General ligamentous laxity with instability secondary to this laxity
- Traumatic incident leading to instability

Athletes in the last three categories who do not respond to a specific program of conservative care are candidates for anterior capsular labral reconstruction. Rehabilitation emphasizes strengthening of the dynamic stabilizers and restoration of structural flexibility. Timing of the rehabilitation sequence depends on the degree of laxity, the presence or absence of impingement, and the specifics of labral repair or reconstruction.

Full ROM is not a prerequisite for beginning the strengthening program; full strength is not necessary to begin the endurance training. Because the plan is an interactive one, it is divided into "sections" rather than "phases," which have sequential timing connotations.

Section 1—Regaining Motion
- Perform active shoulder ROM on the first postoperative day:
  Take arm out of sling, lifting up and out.
  Use active assisted if active alone is not possible.
- Begin active elbow and wrist flexion and extension.
- Squeeze a ball on the first postoperative day.
- Add exercises for shoulder motion after sling is removed:
  Goal is full ROM by 2 months.
  Understand what "full" is for different patients (dominant and nondominant may not be the same).
  After 2 months it is very difficult to gain additional motion.

Section 2—Strengthening
- Isometric exercises; begin as soon as splint is removed; use multiple angles:
  IR
  ER
  Flexion
  Abduction
  Extension
- Isotonic exercises: begin at week 1:
  IR and ER: arm at side and use elastic resistance or tubing
  Extension: prone or standing while bending forward; keep elbow straight; do not move behind the plane of the trunk
  Horizontal adduction: begin 2 weeks later; use scapular plane for starting position; do not finish behind this plane

- Progressive strengthening:
  Rotators:
  Increase resistance of elastic bands
  Move onto side-lying position and use free weights, begin with 1 lb
  Supraspinatus in pain-free range only:
  Begin with just the weight of the arm and increase by .5- to 1-lb increments only
  Anterior deltoid:
  Active abduction to 90 degrees only
  Add segments of work above 110 degrees
  Horizontal abduction:
  Prone or standing leaning forward from waist
  Do not move behind the plane of the trunk
  Do not be fooled by scapular adduction and trunk rotation mimicking horizontal abduction
  Eccentric work:
  Begin 3 months postoperatively
  Accentuate rotator cuff
  Serratus anterior:
  Begin with wall push-ups, move on to hands and knee push-ups, and then to full push-ups
  Emphasize scapular protraction at the end of each push
- Isokinetic training:
  Begins when patient can lift 5 to 10 lbs in ER and 15 to 20 lbs in IR without pain

Section 3—Improving Endurance
- Begin early with low resistance for ROM.
- Start with easy 5-minute program:
  1 minute forward
  1-minute rest
  1 minute backward
  1-minute rest
  1 minute forward
- Increase gradually in 1-minute increments.
- Add sprint and interval training workouts.

Section 4—Sport-Specific Rehabilitation
- Begin at about 4 months postoperatively.
- Involved shoulder should have 70% of uninvolved shoulder strength (test isokinetic fashion).
- See appropriate tables for timing for pitchers and other throwers (rotator cuff section).
- If patient has pain, decrease:
  Number of throws
  Speed of throws
  Distance of throws
  Number of days spent practicing
- Keep speed below ¾ of maximum until about 7 months postoperatively; full speed is not reasonable until about 1 year postoperatively.

Anterior Capsulolabral Reconstruction (Open Procedure) in Throwing Athletes WILK AND ANDREWS

Phase 1—Immediate Motion Phase (0 to 7 weeks)

0 to 2 weeks
- Fit sling for comfort for 1 week.
- Use immobilization brace for 4 weeks during sleep only.
- Gentle active-assisted ROM exercises with T-bar:
  Flexion to tolerance (0 to 120 degrees)
  ER at 20 degrees abduction to tolerance (maximum 15 to 20 degrees)
  IR at 20 degrees abduction to tolerance (maximum 45 degrees)
- Perform rope and pulley exercises.
- Perform ROM exercises for hand and elbow.
- Initiate isometrics (ER, IR, abduction, biceps).
- Squeeze ball.
- Perform elbow flexion/extension.
- Use ice.

3 to 4 weeks
- Perform active-assisted ROM exercises with T-bar:
  Flexion to tolerance (maximum 120 to 140 degrees)
  ER at 45 degrees abduction (acceptable 20 to 30 degrees)
  IR at 45 degrees abduction (acceptable 45 to 60 degrees)
- Begin light isotonics for shoulder musculature:
  Adduction
  Supraspinatus
  ER/IR
  Biceps
- Begin scapular strengthening exercises:
  Rhomboids
  Trapezius
  Serratus anterior

5 to 6 weeks
- Progress all active-assisted ROM with T-bar:
  Flexion (maximum 160 degrees)
  ER/IR at 90 degrees abduction
  ER to 45 to 60 degrees
  IR to 65 to 95 degrees
- Upper body ergometer (UBE) arm at 90 degrees abduction
- Use diagonal patterns, manual resistance.
- Progress all strengthening exercises.

Phase 2—Intermediate Phase (8 to 14 weeks)

8 to 10 weeks
- Progress to full ROM:
  Flexion to 180 degrees
  ER to 90 degrees
  IR to 85 degrees
- Perform isokinetic strengthening exercises (neutral position).
- Progress all strengthening exercises.
- Perform scapular strengthening exercises.

10 to 14 weeks
- Continue all flexibility exercises, self-capsular stretches.
- Begin throwers ten program (p. 114)
- UBE 90 degrees abduction.
- Use diagonal pattern (manual resistance).

Phase 3—Advanced stage (4 to 6 months)
- Continue all flexibility exercises:
  ER/IR stretches
  Flexion stretch
  Self-capsular stretches
- Continue throwers' ten program.
- Perform isokinetics ER/IR (90/90 position)
- Use isokinetics test (throwers' series).
- Perform plyometric exercises.
- Begin interval throwing program (see rotator cuff section) if surgeon approves.

Phase 4—Return to Activity (6 to 9 months)
- Continue all strengthening exercises, including throwers' ten program.
- Continue all stretching exercises.

Arthroscopic Anterior Capsulolabral Reconstruction in Overhead Athletes WILK AND ANDREWS

Phase 1—Restricted Motion–Maximal Protection Phase (0 to 6 weeks)

0 to 2 weeks
- Fit sling for comfort for 2 weeks.
- Ensure immobilization in brace for 4 weeks during sleep only.
- Perform gentle active-assisted ROM with T-bar:
  Forward flexion 0 to 60 degrees
  ER at 20 degrees abduction (maximal motion 0 degrees)
  IR at 20 degrees abduction (maximal motion 45 degrees)
  Do *not* abduct and externally rotate shoulder during first 4 weeks.
- Perform ROM exercises for elbow and hand.
- Begin isometrics; submaximal, subpainful contraction:
  ER, IR, abduction, biceps with arm at side (0 degrees abduction)
- Squeeze ball.
- Use ice, modalities for pain control.

3 to 4 weeks
- Discontinue use of sling.
- Continue use of immobilization during sleep.
- Continue gentle active-assisted ROM with T-bar:
  Flexion 0 to 90 degrees
  ER at 20 degrees abduction (maximal motion 15 degrees)
  IR at 20 degrees abduction (maximal motion 65 degrees)
- Continue isometrics.
- Continue elbow and hand motion exercises.

5 to 6 weeks
- Discontinue use of immobilization during sleep.
- Gradually progress all ROM exercises with T-bar:
  Flexion (0 to 135 degrees)
  ER at 45 degrees abduction (maximal motion 30 degrees)
  IR at 45 degrees abduction (maximal motion 60 degrees)
- Begin light-weight isotonic shoulder exercises (IR/ER, abduction, supraspinatus, biceps, triceps).
- Begin light-weight isotonic scapular strengthening (retroactive, protraction, elevation, depression).
- Begin UBE at 70 degrees abduction.

Phase 2—Moderate Protection Phase (7 to 14 weeks)

7 to 9 weeks
- Progress all motion exercises:
  Flexion (0 to 180 degrees)
  ER at 90 degrees abduction (maximal motion 75 degrees)
  IR at 90 degrees abduction (maximal motion 85 degrees)
- Continue isotonic strengthening program.
- Begin diagonal strengthening program.
- Continue all scapular strengthening.
- Begin isokinetic exercises (neutral position).
- Begin exercise tubing (ER/IR at 0 degrees abduction).

10 to 14 weeks
- Continue and progress all exercises: goal is full ROM by 12 to 14 weeks.
- Begin manual resistance exercise program.

Phase 3—Minimal Protection Phase (15 to 21 weeks)

15 to 18 weeks
- Continue all flexibility exercises, capsular stretches to maintain full ROM.
- Begin throwers' ten program (p. 114).
- Begin light swimming.
- Begin exercises in the 90 degrees position.

18 to 24 weeks
- Continue flexibility exercises.
- Begin internal throwing program (see rotator cuff section) when:
  Full nonpainful ROM
  Strength 90% of contralateral side
  No pain or tenderness
  Satisfactory clinical exam
- Continue throwers' ten program.
- Begin plyometric exercise program.

Phase 4—Advanced Strengthening Phase (22 to 26 weeks)
- Begin aggressive strengthening program for shoulder and scapular musculature.
- Continue throwers' ten program.
- Continue plyometric program.
- Progress interval throwing program.

Phase 5—Return to Activity (7 to 9 months)
- Continue all strengthening exercises.
- Continue all stretching exercises.
- Begin unrestricted throwing.

Prosthetic Shoulder Arthroplasty

REHABILITATION RATIONALE

Rehabilitation after shoulder arthroplasty depends on multiple factors, including the status of the soft tissues around the shoulder (intact or torn rotator cuff, size of tear, security of repair), the quality of the bone, the stability of the implant and the fixation technique used, any concomitant injuries or systemic illness, and the expectations of the patient.

Neer suggests dividing patients into two groups: (1) those who can participate in a reasonably *normal rehabilitation program* (such as patients with osteoarthritis), and (2) those with deficiencies of bone or muscle who must be placed in a *limited-goals rehabilitation program*. In the normal rehabilitation program, motion is begun early to prevent the formation of function-threatening adhesions or to retard their maturation. In the limited-goals group, rehabilitation is aimed at maintaining joint stability and obtaining a lesser ROM with reasonable muscle control. In this limited-goals setting, the initiation of exercises is delayed somewhat and the extent of passive or assisted early motion is reduced. Elevation usually is limited to 90 degrees and ER to 20 degrees. These limited arcs of movement allow more scar formation and greater joint mobility than in a more aggressive rehabilitation program.

A typical rehabilitation program is performed five times daily for 15 to 20 minutes each session. The exercises are patient assisted and should be safe and easily understood so they can be performed reliably at home.

REHABILITATION PROTOCOL

Shoulder Arthroplasty in Patients with Intact Rotator Cuff (No Tissue Deficiency)   (NEER, MODIFIED)

■ *Patients with a tenuous repair of the rotator cuff are not permitted active forward elevation, active ER, or assisted IR until 6 weeks after surgery.*

Phase 1

1 day
- Begin active wrist, finger, and elbow exercises.
- Use immobilization in sling-and-swathe (for tenuous rotator cuff cuff repairs, an abduction brace may be used).

2 to 6 days
- Begin passive or assisted gentle motion of shoulder. Many of the exercises are done supine to provide a feeling of safety and to allow gravity assistance beyond 90 degrees.

- Caution patient to avoid active flexion or abduction of and leaning on operated extremity during daily activities.
- Begin pendulum in circles (clockwise, counterclockwise). Initially, pendulums may be done with elbow flexed. On day 4 or 5, remove the sling during exercises.
- Begin assisted ER, first with the uninvolved hand and eventually with a dowel stick (see Fig 3-11).
- Begin assisted flexion exercise while supine (Fig. 3-20). Lifting power is provided by the uninvolved arm. Flexion is performed with the elbow flexed. The patient grasps the wrist of the operated arm with the uninvolved hand and reaches first for the forehead and then progressively overhead.

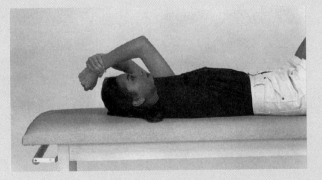

Figure 3-20 Supine assisted flexion, lifting with the uninvolved arm.

Continued

REHABILITATION PROTOCOL

Shoulder Arthroplasty in Patients with Intact Rotator Cuff (No Tissue Deficiency) (NEER, MODIFIED)

Phase 2
7 to 9 days

- Perform straight elbow pendulum exercises.
- Begin hyperextension exercises. Both hands grasp the dowel stick and the operated extremity is guided into hyperextension. Hyperextension with a dowel stick makes IR easier.
- Begin IR exercises. The patient grasps the wrist of the operated extremity behind the low back and tries to slide the hand upward (see Fig. 3-3, B). To get the involved hand behind the back initially, the fingers are used to "walk" around the hip.

- Begin pulley exercises for forward flexion only. Patient faces the pulley and increases motion in flexion. Give a pulley to the patient for use at home.

Phase 3
14 to 16 days

- Begin horizontal ER (supine). This is possible only if 120 to 140 degrees of flexion has been obtained. The patient lies supine and, with clasped hands, raises the arms in flexion (Fig. 3-21), slides the clasped hands down behind the neck, and separates the elbows (Fig 3-22).
- Begin active-assisted ROM in abduction with dowel stick (supine) and/or pulley.
- Continue pendulum exercises in all planes.

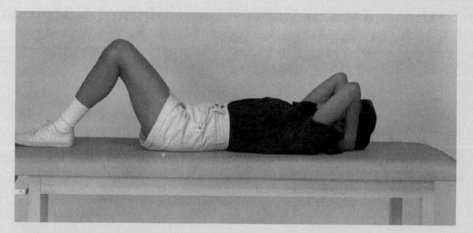

Figure 3-21 Horizontal external rotation. Note clasped hands behind back of head.

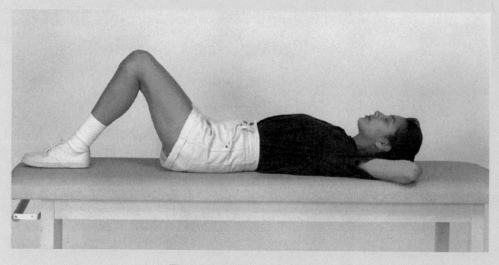

Figure 3-22 Separate elbows.

REHABILITATION PROTOCOL—cont'd

Phase 3—cont'd

17 to 21 days
- Add isometric exercises for IR, ER, abduction, and extension. These isometric exercises are performed with the elbow flexed at 90 degrees and held close to the body, with a door jamb, wall, or opposite hand providing assistance. Each position is held for 5 seconds.
- Continue active-assisted ROM exercises.

Phase 4

6 weeks
- Perform active strengthening and stretching of any remaining limitations of ROM.

- Emphasize anterior deltoid and subscapularis strengthening.
- When active shoulder flexion can be performed easily in the supine position, encourage active flexion in the sitting position. Resistance can be added.
- Progress resistance for forward flexion, IR, ER.
- Work on any focal deficiencies.
- Continue therapy as outpatient and at home until ROM, strength, and function are completely restored.

REHABILITATION PROTOCOL

Shoulder Arthroplasty: Intact Rotator Cuff Rehabilitation
WILK AND ANDREWS

Phase 1—Immediate Motion Phase (0 to 4 weeks)

GOALS
- Increase passive ROM
- Decrease shoulder pain
- Retard muscular atrophy and prevent rotator cuff shutdown

EXERCISES
- Use CPM machine.
- Perform passive ROM exercises:
  Flexion (0 to 90 degrees)
  ER (at 30 degrees abduction) 0 to 30 degrees
  IR (at 30 degrees abduction) 0 to 35 degrees
- Perform pendulum exercises.
- Perform elbow and wrist ROM exercises.
- Perform grasping exercises for hand.
- Use ice and modalities for pain control.
- Begin isometrics (ER, IR, abduction) on day 10.
- Use electrical muscle stimulation (if needed).
- Begin use of rope and pulley at week 2.
- Begin active-assisted ROM (ER, IR, flexion) with T-bar at week 2.

Phase 2—Active Motion Phase (4 to 10 weeks)

GOALS
- Improve shoulder strength
- Improve ROM
- Increase functional activities
- Decrease pain

EXERCISES
- Use rope and pulley (flexion).
- Perform pendulum exercises.
- Perform active ROM (supine flexion).
- Perform seated flexion (short arc 45 to 90 degrees)
- Perform seated abduction.
- Begin exercise tubing ER/IR at 4 weeks.
- Use dumbbell for biceps/triceps.
- Practice scapulothoracic strengthening.
- Perform joint mobilization.

Phase 3—Strengthening Phase

CRITERIA FOR PROGRESSION TO PHASE 3
- Passive ROM: flexion 0 to 160 degrees
  ER 0 to 75 degrees
  IR 0 to 80 degrees
- Strength (ER, IR, abduction) ⅗ of uninvolved extremity

GOALS
- Improve strength of shoulder musculature
- Neuromuscular control of shoulder complex
- Improve functional activities

EXERCISES
- Use exercise tubing: IR/ER.
- Practice dumbbell strengthening:
  Abduction
  Supraspinatus
  Scapulothoracic
- Perform stretching exercises.
- Perform T-bar exercises.
- Perform rope and pulley exercises.

REHABILITATION PROTOCOL

Total Shoulder Arthroplasty: Tissue-Deficient Group
WILK AND ANDREWS

The goal of the rehabilitation process is to provide greater joint stability to patients, while decreasing their pain and improving their functional status. The goal of the tissue-deficient group (bone loss, muscle loss) is joint stability and less joint mobility.

Phase 1—Immediate Motion Phase (0 to 4 weeks)

GOALS
- Increase passive ROM
- Decrease shoulder pain
- Retard muscular atrophy

EXERCISES
- Use CPM
- Perform passive ROM:
  Flexion 0 to 90 degrees
  ER (at 30 degrees abduction) 0 to 20 degrees
  IR (at 30 degrees abduction) 0 to 30 degrees
- Perform pendulum exercises.
- Perform ROM of elbow and wrist.
- Perform gripping exercises.
- Use isometrics:
  Abductors
  ER/IR
- Begin use of rope and pulley at 2 weeks.
- Perform active-assisted ROM exercises (when able).

Phase 2—Active Motion Phase (4 to 12 weeks)

GOALS
- Improve shoulder strength
- Improve ROM
- Decrease pain/inflammation
- Increase functional activities

EXERCISES
- Begin active-assisted ROM exercises with L-bar at 4 to 5 weeks or when tolerable:
  Flexion
  ER
  IR
- Continue use of rope and pulley (flexion).

- Continue pendulum exercises.
- Perform active ROM exercises:
  Seated flexion (short arc 45 to 90 degrees)
  Supine flexion (full available range)
  Seated abduction (0 to 90 degrees)
  Exercise tubing IR/ER (4 to 6 weeks)
  Dumbbell biceps/triceps
  Gentle joint mobilization (6 to 8 weeks)

Phase 3—Strengthening Phase

CRITERIA FOR PROGRESSION TO PHASE 3
- Passive ROM: Flexion 0 to 120 degrees
  ER of 30 to 40 degrees at 90 degrees abduction
  IR of 45 to 55 degrees at 90 degrees abduction
- Strength level (ER, IR, abduction) $\frac{4}{5}$ of involved extremity
  Note: *Some patients will never enter this phase.*

GOALS
- Improve strength of shoulder musculature
- Improve and gradually increase functional activities

EXERCISES
- Continue exercise tubing (ER/IR).
- Practice dumbbell strengthening:
  Abduction
  Supraspinatus
  Flexion
- Perform stretching exercise.
- Perform L-bar stretches:
  Flexion
  ER
  IR

Adhesive Capsulitis

REHABILITATION RATIONALE

Adhesive capsulitis is characterized by a marked loss of active and passive shoulder motion caused by inflammation and adherence of the capsule to the anatomic neck of the humerus and to itself at the inferior axillary fold. Joint volume is decreased to less than 10 to 12 ml (normal is 20 ml).

The criteria for diagnosis of a "frozen shoulder" are not universally accepted, but the following general criteria are applicable: (1) decreased glenohumeral motion and loss of synchronous shoulder girdle motion, (2) restricted elevation (less than 135 or 90 degrees depending on the author), (3) external rotation 50% to 60% of normal, and (4) arthrogram findings of 5 to 10 cc volume with obliteration of normal axillary fold.

Routine radiographic examination typically reveals no significant pathologic condition. Lundberg, however, noted that 50% of patients with adhesive capsulitis had osteopenia on radiographic evaluation. Shoulder arthrography is considered the gold standard of radiographic evaluation. Because it is invasive, it is not advocated for routine use if patients have a classic history and physical examination.

Rockwood and Matsen listed eight categories of conditions that should be considered in the differential diagnosis of frozen shoulder (see box).

Neviasier described the following four stages of adhesive capsulitis determined at arthroscopic examination: (1) mild synovitis at inferior recess, (2) acute synovitis with adhesions of the dependent folds of the synovial lining, (3) maturation of adhesions, and (4) chronic adhesions.

Risk Factors

Patients with diabetes mellitus are especially susceptible to adhesive capsulitis: 10% to 19% in diabetic patients compared with 2% to 5% in the general population. As many as 77% of diabetic patients with frozen shoulder have bilateral involvement. Patients who have taken insulin for more than 10 years are much more likely to have permanent disability than are other patients, despite proper treatment.

Primary Versus Secondary Frozen Shoulder

■ *Frozen shoulder may be considered primary, or idiopathic, when it develops spontaneously, and is considered secondary when an underlying, precipitating pathologic condition is present (e.g., fracture).*

Primary frozen shoulder is a unique condition that typically is unilateral and rarely recurs in the same shoulder. Subsequent involvement of the contralateral shoulder occurs in up to 20% of patients.

Three classic stages in clinical course of primary (idiopathic) frozen shoulder have been described:
1. Painful (or freezing) phase:
   lasts 2 to 9 months
   gradual onset of diffuse shoulder pain, gradual loss of glenohumeral motion
   patient uses arm less and less to avoid pain
   patient begins to substitute scapulothoracic motion when using the arm
2. Stiffening (or frozen) phase
   lasts 4 to 12 months
   shoulder movement often restricted in characteristic pattern, with loss of ER, IR and abduction
3. Thawing phase
   highly variable time course
   gradual regaining of shoulder motion
Secondary Frozen Shoulder
Secondary frozen shoulder results from a known precipitating event (e.g., upper extremity fracture).

Differential Diagnosis of Frozen Shoulder

Trauma
Fractures of shoulder region
Other fractures anywhere in upper extremity
Shoulder dislocation, especially a missed posterior dislocation
Hemarthrosis of shoulder secondary to contusion

Other Soft Tissue Disorders about the Shoulder
Tendonitis of rotator cuff
Tendonitis of long head of biceps
Subacromial bursitis
Impingement
Shoulder-hand syndrome
Fibrositis
Soft tissue neoplasm
Suprascapular nerve entrapment
Thoracic outlet syndrome
Neuralgic amyotrophy—Parsonage-Turner syndrome
Polymyalgia rheumatica

Joint Disorders
Degenerative arthritis of acromioclavicular joint
Degenerative arthritis of glenohumeral joint
Inflammatory arthritis—monarticular/polyarticular
Septic arthritis
Neuropathic arthritis, e.g., syringomyelia, diabetes
Crystalline arthritis—gout, pseudogout
Hemophilic arthritis
Osteochondromatosis

Bone Disorders
Avascular necrosis—osteonecrosis
Metastatic tumor
Primary bone tumor, including multiple myeloma
Paget's disease
Osteomalacia
Hyperparathyroidism

Cervical Spine Disorders
Cervical spondylosis
Cervical disc herniation
Neoplasm
Infection

Intrathoracic Disorders
Diaphragmatic irritation
Pancoast tumor
Myocardial infarction
Esophagitis

Abdominal Disorders
Gastric ulcer
Cholecystitis or cholelithiasis
Subphrenic abscess

Psychogenic

From Rockwood CA, Matsen FA: *The Shoulder*, Philadelphia, 1990, WB Saunders.

The dominant arm usually is involved, and earlier presentation for medical treatment is associated with a better prognosis than for primary frozen shoulder.

■ *The underlying, precipitating pathologic condition must be treated.*

Treatment

The goals of treatment are to obtain pain relief and to restore ROM of the shoulder. Treatment is based on the clinical findings and the *stage of disease* at the time of presentation and is continually modified according to the patient's response to various modalities.

■ *Best treatment is prevention through patient education to avoid prolonged shoulder immobilization.*

Binder et al. found that 50% of patients with frozen shoulders received no advice from their primary care physicians about the need for early shoulder motion.

REHABILITATION PROTOCOL

Adhesive Capsulitis: Patients Presenting Early in Clinical Course   ROCKWOOD AND MATSEN

1 day
- Prescribe NSAIDs.
- Begin pendulum exercises for 1 to 2 minutes every 1 to 2 hours while awake.
- If pain awakens patient, perform exercises for 1 to 2 minutes.

2 weeks
- If pain persists, inject 10 mg intraarticularly of triamcinolone through a posterior approach (Fig. 3-23).

- If relief is obtained with injection but pain recurs, it is permissible to give one more injection.
- Once pain has been relieved, begin stretching exercises are (see next protocol).

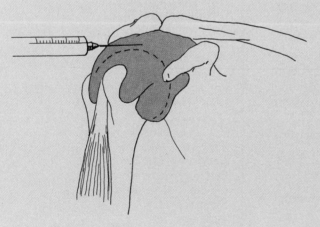

Figure 3-23 Subacromial injection.

REHABILITATION PROTOCOL

Adhesive Capsulitis: Patients Presenting Later in Clinical Course ROCKWOOD AND MATSEN

For patients with moderate to marked stiffness and pain that are primarily at the *end* of the ROM, begin a stretching program at the *initial visit*.

Phase 1
STRETCHING
- Use pendulum exercises and hot packs or bath to warm up for stretching exercises.
- Concentrate on passive forward elevation and ER.
- Perform forward elevation stretch by assisted elevation of the affected arm to reach up to a solid object that is just beyond reach. Patients stand on tiptoes, then lower themselves to maintain a moderate stretch, adjusted to tolerance, for 20 to 30 seconds. Lower the affected arm using the opposite arm to avoid a painful free fall. Repeat 5 times every several hours.
- Perform ER stretch with the arm at the side and the elbow flexed at 90 degrees. Carefully monitor this exercise. Patient rotates the trunk with the hand fixed on the side of a door frame to stretch the anterior structures, allowing progressive ER. A sustained stretch of 30 to 60 seconds 8 to 10 times a day is recommended.

STRENGTHENING
- Once stretching exercises are underway, begin strengthening within the limits of the newly achieved ROM.
- First practice forward elevation strengthening with progression of resistance or load only when 10 repetitions are done without difficulty. Use the supine position first, lifting up to 3 kg. Then use the sitting position with weight dropped to 250 gm and slowly progress to 10 kg as tolerated.
- Do ER strengthening using a Theraband (elastic resistance) looped around the wrist with the elbow flexed at a right angle. Do 5 repetitions, held for 5 seconds each session, progressing resistance as tolerated.

Phase 2
- Plot the examination and progress at the next visit with the physician (usually 2 to 3 weeks later).
- Review and refine exercises.
- Add stretching into IR. Perform this initially with stretching into extension using a dowel stick behind the back.
- When 15 to 20 cm of clearance behind the back is possible, discontinue the stick. The good arm is used to pull the hand of the affected arm up the back, progressively obtaining more IR.
- A towel in the hand, passed over the opposite shoulder and pulling the affected hand, accomplishes the same goal. (See Fig 3-22.)
- Now begin strengthening using elastic resistance looped over a door handle. The patient rotates the arm across the opposite chest wall and holds for 5 seconds for 5 repetitions.
- As ROM improves, add further resistance to the strengthening program in all directions.

Many patients discontinue their exercises when they achieve 150 degrees of forward elevation, 45 degrees of ER, and IR to the level of the twelfth thoracic spinous process. Patients should be encouraged to continue exercises 3 to 5 minutes twice daily for 3 more months.
- May begin stretching in abduction. This has been avoided up to this point to prevent impingement type of pain. Earlier in the protocol the humeral head cannot glide inferiorly to clear the coracoacromial arch.

Failure to Progress

Continued Pain

Reexamine and search for other causes of pain; evaluation should include (1) arthrogram to rule out rotator cuff tear if pain is exacerbated by resisted ER or abduction, (2) evaluation of compliance and increased direct supervision if compliance is poor, and (3) modification of the rehabilitation program or a different therapist.

Manipulation

Occasionally a patient who does not progress with a supervised stretching program requires manipulation under anesthesia. Timing of manipulation is controversial. Advocates suggest manipulation for those patients who do not obtain 90 degrees of passive forward elevation and show little progress after several months of physical therapy.

Manipulation is begun in abduction with stabilization of the scapula to achieve as much motion as possible. Gradual and judicious use of pressure should be observed to avoid possible complications (fracture, rotator cuff damage, brachial plexus stretch). The amount of pushing depends on the quality of bone and soft tissue of the specific patient. After manipulation, 20 mg of triamcinolone acetonide is injected intraarticularly.

A gentle ROM program begins on the day of manipulation for forward elevation and ER, including the use of a pulley for stretching.

Continue exercises in the hospital for 3 to 5 days, until a home exercise program is possible. Neviaser recommends that the arm be supported at 90 degrees of abduction at night for 3 weeks after manipulation and during the day while in the hospital. This is combined with early ROM exercises.

Contraindications to manipulation include (1) frozen shoulder resulting from shoulder dislocation or fracture of the proximal humerus, (2) moderate osteopenia on radiographs, (3) patient's inability to cooperate with required exercise program after manipulation, and (4) acute or irritable phase of frozen shoulder (relative contraindication).

Risks of manipulation under anesthesia include fracture or dislocation of the humerus, tearing of the rotator cuff, hemarthrosis, and traction injuries to the brachial plexus.

Other Techniques

Brisement (distension arthrography) has been reported to have a beneficial effect for patients with moderate shoulder restriction. We have not had favorable results with this technique.

Arthroscopy is contraindicated for lysis of old adhesions because such adhesions are extracapsular.

Physiotherapy modalities, such as application of heat or ice, short-wave diathermy, and ultrasound, have not been shown to have benefit on their own, but may be useful adjuncts for selected patients.

Open release has been advocated for shoulders that have contraindications to manipulation under anesthesia or that have not improved after manipulation.

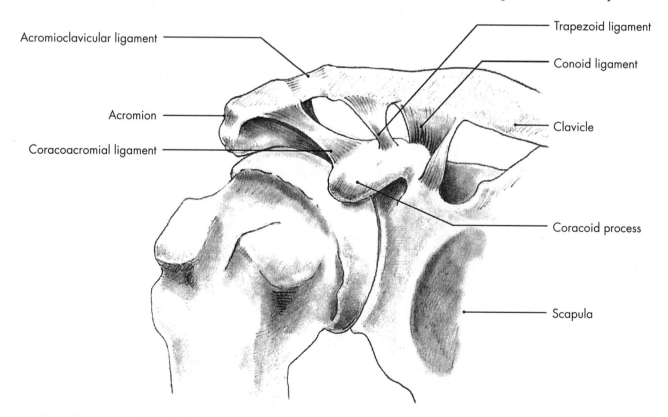

Figure 3-24 Acromioclavicular joint and surrounding structures (anterior view).

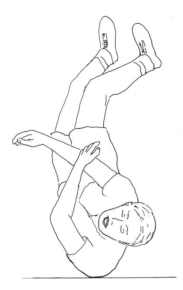

Figure 3-25 The most common mechanism of acromioclavicular joint injury is a direct force that occurs from a fall on the point of the shoulder. (Redrawn from Rockwood CA, Green DP, editors: *Fractures in adults,* ed 2, Philadelphia, 1984, JB Lippincott.)

At open release, the coracohumeral ligament, inferior capsule, and inferior portion of the subscapularis are surgically released. We have no experience with this technique.

Acromioclavicular Joint Injury

REHABILITATION RATIONALE

Anatomy

The acromioclavicular joint is a diarthrodial joint with a fibrocartilaginous intraarticular disc. Two significant ligamentous structures are associated with the joint: the acromioclavicular ligaments, which provide horizontal stability (Fig. 3-24), and the coracoclavicular ligaments, which are the main supensory ligament of the upper extremity, providing vertical stability to the joint.

Recent studies show that only 5 to 8 degrees of motion of the acromioclavicular joint is possible in any plane.

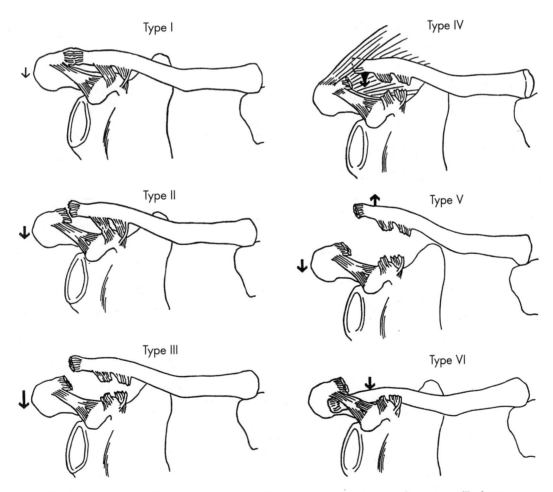

Type I

Type II

Type III

Type IV

Type V

Type VI

Figure 3-26 Classification of injuries to the acromioclavicular joint ligaments. (Redrawn and modified from Rockwood CA, Green DP, editors: *Fractures in adults,* ed 2, Philadelphia, 1984, JB Lippincott.)

The most common mechanism of injury of the acromioclavicular joint is a direct force from a fall on the point of the shoulder (Fig. 3-25, p. 135).

Rockwood classifies acromioclavicular joint injuries into six types (Fig. 3-26, p. 135).

Type I
- Mild sprain of the acromioclavicular ligament
- No disruption of acromioclavicular or coracoclavicular ligaments

Type II
- Disruption of acromioclavicular joint
- Acromioclavicular joint wider because of disruption (less than 4 mm or 40% difference)
- Sprained but *intact* coracoclavicular ligaments with coracoclavicular space essentially the same as the normal shoulder on radiographs
- Downward force (weight) may disrupt acromioclavicular ligament, but *not* the coracoacromial ligament

Type III
- Coracoclavicular and acromioclavicular ligaments disrupted
- Shoulder complex displaced inferiorly

- Coracoclavicular interspace 25% to 100% greater than in normal shoulder, or 4 mm distance (especially with weights applied)

Type IV
- Clavicle is displaced posteriorly through fibers of trapezius
- Acromioclavicular ligament and coracoclavicular ligaments disrupted
- Deltoid and trapezius muscles detached from distal clavicle

Type V
- Vertical separation of clavicle is greatly separated from scapula over a type III injury (100% to 300% more than normal shoulder)

Type VI
- Clavicle is dislocated inferiorly under the coracoid process

Types I and II injuries are treated conservatively, as are type III injuries in nonactive, nonlaboring patients. Most types of IV, V, and VI injuries require open reduction and internal fixation, as do type III injuries in more active individuals.

REHABILITATION PROTOCOL

Acromioclavicular Joint Injuries ROCKWOOD AND MATSEN

Type I

1 day
- Apply ice to shoulder for 24 to 48 hours.
- Fit sling for comfort up to 7 days.
- Perform active ROM for fingers, wrist, elbow every 3 to 4 hours.
- Gently maintain normal ROM with rest in sling as needed.
- Begin pendulum exercises on day 2 or 3.

7 to 10 days
- Symptoms typically subside.
- Discontinue sling.
- Do not permit any heavy lifting, stresses, or contact sports until full painless ROM and no point tenderness over acromioclavicular joint (usually at 2 weeks).

Type II

1 day
- Apply ice for 24 to 48 hours.
- Fit sling for comfort for 1 to 2 weeks.

7 day
- Begin gentle ROM exercises of shoulder and allow use of arm for dressing, eating, and activities of daily living (ADL).
- Discard sling at 7 to 14 days.
- Do not permit any heavy lifting, pushing, pulling, or contact sports for at least 6 weeks.

Type III

Nonoperative treatment indicated for inactive and nonlaboring patients:

1 day
- Discuss "bump" remaining on shoulder, natural history, surgical risks, and recurrence.
- Apply ice for 24 hours.
- Prescribe mild analgesics for several days.
- Place in a sling.
- Begin performing ADL at 3 to 4 days.
- Slowly progress to functional ROM with gentle passive ROM exercises at about 7 days.
- Patient typically has full ROM at 2 to 3 weeks with gentle ROM exercises.

Proximal Humeral Fractures

Codman described four segments of proximal humeral fractures: (1) the articular segment of the humeral head, (2) the greater tuberosity, (3) the lesser tuberosity, and (4) the humeral shaft. Neer classified fractures of the proximal humerus based on the identification of the four major fragments and their relationships to one other. When any of the four major segments is displaced more than 1 cm or angulated more than 45 degrees, the fracture is displaced. If no fragment is displaced, the fracture is a one-part fracture; 80% of proximal humeral fractures fall into this category. The primary concerns of this classification are the status of the blood supply of the humeral head and the relationship of the humeral head to the displaced parts and to the glenoid.

Bertoft et al. reported the greatest improvement in ROM after proximal humeral fractures occurred between 3 and 8 weeks after fracture. Return to normal function and motion may require 3 to 4 months. Bony healing is typically complete by 6 to 8 weeks in adults.

REHABILITATION PROTOCOL

Undisplaced Proximal Humeral Fractures ROCKWOOD AND MATSEN

Rockwood and Matsen advocate a three-phase protocol devised by Neer.

Phase 1

1 day
- Begin hand, wrist, and elbow active ROM.
- Support arm in a sling at the side or in a Velpeau position.
- A swath may be needed in the immediate postfracture period for immobilization and comfort.
- An axillary pad may be useful.
- Periodic views in two perpendicular planes are essential to establish that the fracture is clinically stable and is not displacing.

7 to 10 days
- Begin gentle ROM exercises if clinical situation is stable.
- Perform exercises 3 to 4 times a day for 20 to 30 minutes.
- Applying hot packs 20 minutes before exercise may be beneficial.
- Early in the program, an analgesic may be needed for pain control.
- First begin pendulum exercises (Codman) with arm rotation in inward and outward circles (Fig. 3-27).
- Begin supine ER with a stick (see Fig. 3-11). Support the elbow and distal humerus with a folded towel or sheet to create a sense of security for the patient; 15 to 20 degrees of abduction may aid in performing these exercises.

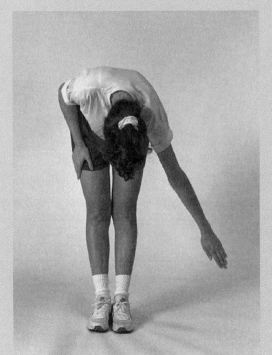

Figure 3-27 Pendulum exercise.

Continued

REHABILITATION PROTOCOL—cont'd

Undisplaced Proximal Humeral Fractures   ROCKWOOD AND MATSEN

Phase 1—cont'd

3 to 5 weeks
- Begin assisted forward elevation (Fig. 3-28).
- Perform pulley exercises (see Fig. 3-19).
- Perform ER with a stick (Fig. 3-29).
- Perform extension with a stick.
- Perform isometric exercises (Fig. 3-30).

Phase 2 (6 weeks to 2 months)

■ *Phase 2 exercises involve early active, resistive, and stretching exercises.*
- Begin supine active forward elevation as gravity is partially eliminated, thus making forward elevation easier (Fig. 3-31).

- Progress forward elevation to an erect position with a stick in the unaffected hand to assist the involved arm in forward elevation.
- As strength is gained, may perform unassisted active elevation while erect, with emphasis on keeping the elbow bent and the arm close to the midline.
- Use Therabands of progressive strengths for internal rotators; external rotators; and anterior, middle, and posterior deltoid (3 sets of 10 to 15 repetitions at each exercise session).
- Perform stretching for forward elevation on the top of a door or wall, and stretching in the door jamb for ER.

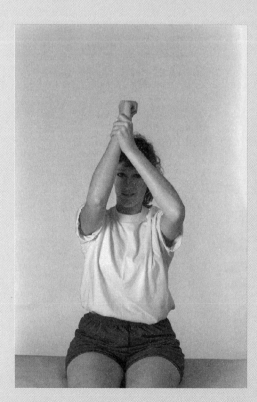

Figure 3-28 Active assisted forward elevation of the shoulder.

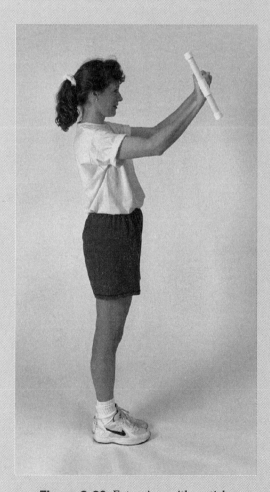

Figure 3-29 Extension with a stick.

REHABILITATION PROTOCOL—cont'd

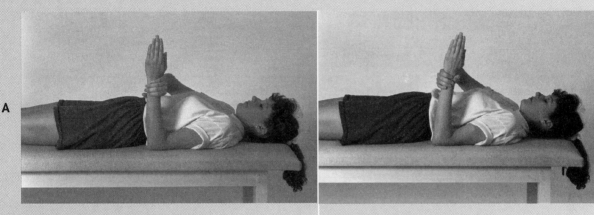

Figure 3-30 A, Placement of hand for isometric exercise of muscles of external rotation. **B,** Placement of the hand for isometric exercise of muscles of internal rotation. Exercises are performed with the patient supine.

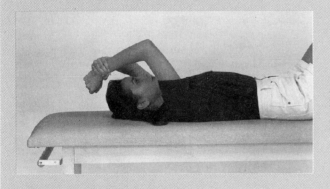

Figure 3-31 Assisted flexion exercise (supine). Lifting power is provided by the good arm. Early range of motion without stressing the deltoid and subscapularis repair is possible with this exercise.

Continued

REHABILITATION PROTOCOL—cont'd

Undisplaced Proximal Humeral Fractures ROCKWOOD AND MATSEN

Phase 2 (6 weeks to 2 months)—cont'd

- Raise arm over the head with the arms clasped.
- Perform ER and abduction of the arms with the hands placed behind the head.
- Help with IR by using the normal arm to pull the involved arm into IR (see Fig. 3-3, B).

Phase 3 (3 months)

- May use light weights after 3 months; start with 1 lb and increase in 1-lb increments with a 5-lb limit. If pain persists after using weights, eliminate or decrease weight.
- Replace Theraband with rubber tubing to increase resistance.
- Stretching on the end of the door and prone stretching for forward elevation are helpful.
- Perform functional activity for strength gain.

Bibliography

Andrews JR, Wilk KE, editors: *The athlete's shoulder*, New York, 1995, Churchill Livingstone.

Barrett WP et al: Total shoulder arthroplasty, *J Bone Joint Surg* 69A:865, 1987.

Bertoft ES, Lundh I, Ringquist I: Physiotherapy after fracture of the proximal end of the humerus, *Scand J Rehab Med* 16:11, 1984.

Binder AI et al: Frozen shoulder: a long-term prospective study, *Ann Rheum Dis* 43:361, 1984.

Braatz JH, Gogia PP: The mechanics of pitching, *J Orthop Sports Phys Ther* 9:56, 1987.

Brewster C, Schwab DR: Rehabilitation of the shoulder following rotator cuff injury or surgery, *J Orthop Sports Phys Ther* 18:2, 1993.

Codman EA: *The shoulder: rupture of the supraspinatus tendon and other lesions in or about the subacromial bursa*, Boston, 1934, Thomas Todd.

Cook DA, Heiner JP: Acromioclavicular joint injuries, *Orthop Rev* 19:6, 1990.

Craig EV: Total shoulder replacement, *Orthopedics* 11:1, 1988.

Craig EV, Hsu KC: Shoulder problems in weekend athletes, *Orthop Rev* 21:2, 1992.

Culham E, Peat M: Functional anatomy of the shoulder complex, *J Orthop Sports Phys Ther* 18:1, 1993.

Davies GJ, Dickoff-Hoffman S: Neuromuscular testing and rehabilitation of the shoulder complex, *J Orthop Sports Phys Ther* 18:2, 1993.

Dillman CJ, Fleisig GS, Andrews JR: Biomechanics of pitching, with emphasis upon shoulder kinematics, *J Orthop Sports Phys Ther* 18:2, 1993.

Gardner L, Miller J, Moore E: Postinjury shoulder rehabilitation program, *Surg Rounds Orthop* 4:28, 1990.

Glousman RE, Jobe FW: How to detect and manage the unstable shoulder, *J Musculoskel Med* 7:93, 1990.

Hawkins RJ, Kennedy JC: Impingement syndrome in athletes, *Am J Sports Med* 8:3, 1980.

Hawkins RJ, Mohtadi NG: Clinical evaluation of shoulder instability, *Clin Sports Med* 1:1, 1991.

Jobe FW, Bradley JP: Rotator cuff injuries in baseball: prevention and rehabilitation, *Sports Med* 6:378, 1988.

Jobe FW et al: Anterior capsulolabral reconstruction of the shoulder in athletes in overhand sports, *Am J Sports Med* 19:5, 1991.

Jobe FW, Jobe CM: Painful athletic injuries of the shoulder, *Clin Orthop* 173:117, 1983.

Jobe FW, Kvitne RS: Shoulder pain in the overhead or throwing athlete, *Orthop Rev* 18:9, 1989.

Jobe FW, Moynes DR, Brewster CE: Rehabilitation of shoulder joint instabilities, *Orthop Clin North Am* 18:3, 1987.

Jobe FW, Moynes DR: Delineation of diagnostic criteria and a rehabilitation program for rotator cuff injuries, *Am J Sports Med* 10:6, 1982.

Jobe FW, Pink M: Classification and treatment of shoulder dysfunction in the overhead athlete, *J Orthop Sports Phys Ther* 18:2, 1993.

Kamkar A, Irrgang JJ, Whitney SL: Nonoperative management of secondary shoulder impingement syndrome, *J Orthop Sports Phys Ther* 17:5, 1993.

Keating JF et al: The relative strengths of the rotator cuff muscles, *J Bone Joint Surg* 75B:137, 1993.

Leffert RD: The frozen shoulder, *Instr Course Lect* 34:19, 1985.

Lichfield R et al: Rehabilitation of the overhead athlete, *J Orthop Sports Phys Ther* 18:2, 1993.

Lloyd JA, Lloyd HM: Adhesive capsulitis of the shoulder, *South Med J* 76:7, 1983.

Lundberg BJ: The frozen shoulder, *Acta Orthop Scand* (suppl) 119:1, 1969.

Meister K, Andrews JR: Classification and treatment of rotator cuff injuries in the overhead athlete, *J Orthop Sports Phys Ther* 18:2, 1993.

Neer CS II: Impingement lesions, *Clin Orthop* 173:70, 1983.

Neviaser RJ, Neviaser TJ: Observations of impingement, *Clin Orthop* 254:60, 1990.

Pappas AM, Zawacki RM, McCarthy CF: Rehabilitation of the pitching shoulder, *Am J Sports Med* 13:4, 1990.

Rathbun JB, Macnab I: The microvascular pattern of the rotator cuff, *J Bone Joint Surg* 52B:540, 1970.

Rockwood CA, Matsen FA: *The shoulder*, Philadelphia, 1990, WB Saunders.

Rowe CR, Sakellarides HT: Factors related to recurrences of anterior dislocations of the shoulder, *Clin Orthop* 20:40, 1961.

Simon ER, Hill JA: Rotator cuff injuries: an update, *J Orthop Sports Phys Ther* 10:394, 1989.

Townsend H et al: EMG analysis of the glenohumeral muscles during a baseball rehabilitation program, *Am J Sports Med* 19:3, 1991.

Wilk KE et al: *Preventive and rehabilitative exercises for the shoulder and elbow*, ed 3, Birmingham, 1993, American Sports Medicine Institute.

Wilk KE et al: Plyometrics for the upper extremity: theory and clinical application, *J Orthop Sports Phys Ther* 17:225, 1993.

Wilk KE, Andrews JR: Rehabilitation following arthroscopic subacromial decompression, *Orthopedics* 16(3):349, 1993.

Wilk KE, Andrews JR, Arrigo CA: The abductor and adductor strength characteristics of professional baseball pitchers, *Am J Sports Med* 23(3):307, 1995.

Wilk KE, Andrews JR, Arrigo CA: The strength characteristics of the internal and external rotator muscles in professional baseball pitchers, *Am J Sports Med* 21:261, 1993.

Wilk KE, Arrigo C: Current concepts in the rehabilitation of the athletic shoulder, *J Orthop Sports Phys Ther* 18:1, 1993.

Wilk KE, Arrigo CA, Andrews JR, *Functional training for the overhead athlete* (Home Study Course: Sports physical therapy section), La Crosse, Wis, 1995, American Physical Therapy Association.

CHAPTER FOUR

Fractures of the Pelvis, Acetabulum, and Lower Extremity

THOMAS A. RUSSELL, MD

ANA K. PALMIERI, MD

Rehabilitation Rationale

The goals of successful treatment of lower extremity injuries are (1) restoration of functional range of motion (ROM) of all joints, (2) rehabilitation of all muscle-tendon units, and (3) unrestricted weight bearing. Rehabilitation of lower extremity injuries proceeds in stages based on the physiology of repair and the regeneration of the soft and hard tissues.

In the past 10 years, operative repair and stabilization of lower extremity fractures has been most frequently used to obtain these goals. This trend is due, in large part, to the belief that anatomic restoration of intraarticular fractures and functional stabilization of diaphyseal and metaphyseal fractures provide a stable platform for the healing of muscle-tendon units and allow an earlier ROM of the joints. Early rehabilitation decreases the time of immobilization and disability of the patient. Advances in interlocking intramedullary nailing and external fixation techniques have decreased complication rates and allowed a more aggressive approach to rehabilitation.

CLASSIFICATION

Classification systems have been devised for each specific fracture; the systems most often cited are discussed in the respective sections.

Two classification systems are used most often for soft tissue injuries: the *Tscherne* system for closed fractures and the *Gustilo and Anderson* system, with its later modification, for open fractures. Two other classification systems have been proposed more recently, the Mueller/AO classification and the Orthopaedic Trauma Association's modification of this classification, but these require time for validation and application to the literature.

The Tscherne classification serves primarily to alert the surgeon that significant crush and swelling of the soft tissue envelope may delay healing and lead to compartment syndromes or contractures (Table 4-1).

The Gustilo-Anderson classification of open fractures with subsequent modification helps to determine the relative risks of infection and nonunion (Table 4-2).

In 1984, Gustilo and Anderson reported infections in 4% of type IIIA fractures, in 52% of type IIIB, and 42% of type IIIC. Amputation rates were 0%, 16%, and 42%, respectively. In later reports (1985 and 1988), infection rates were decreased by the addition of gram-negative coverage to the antibiotic regimen. For closed fractures, most authors now recommend using 1 gm of either first-generation cephalosporin or vancomy-

TABLE 4-1 The Tscherne Classification of Soft Tissue Injuries in Closed Fractures

Grade 1 Soft tissue damage absent
Indirect forces
Torsion fractures

Grade 2 Superficial abrasion or contusion caused by fragment pressure from within
Mild-to-moderate fracture severity

Grade 3 Deep, contaminated abrasion associated with local skin or muscle contusion from direct trauma
Bumper injuries (pedestrian–motor vehicle)
Increased fracture severity with comminution or segmental injury

Grade 4 Skin extensively contused with crushed muscle
Muscle damage may be severe
Compartment syndromes common

TABLE 4-2 The Gustilo-Anderson Classification of Soft Tissue Injury in Open Fractures

Type I Wound less than 1 cm long
Minimal soft tissue damage, no signs of crush
Usually simple transverse or short oblique fracture with little comminution

Type II Wound more than 1 cm long
Slight-to-moderate crushing injury, no extensive soft tissue damage, flap, or avulsion
Moderate fracture comminution and contamination

Type III Extensive wound and soft tissue damage, including muscles, skin, and (often) neurovascular structures
Greater degree of fracture comminution and instability
High degree of contamination

IIIA Adequate soft tissue coverage of the fracture, despite extensive laceration, flaps, or high-energy trauma
This subtype includes highly comminuted or segmental fractures from high energy, regardless of the size of the wound. Type IIIA fractures do *not* require free flaps

IIIB Open fracture associated with extensive injury to or loss of soft tissue, with periosteal stripping and exposure of bone
Massive contamination and severe comminution
After debridement and irrigation, bone is exposed and requires a local flap or free flap

IIIC Any open fracture associated with an arterial injury that must be repaired, regardless of the extent of soft tissue injury
Open fractures with arterial injuries have projected amputation rates ranging from 25% to 90%

cin. For open fractures, the following protocol currently is recommended:

Type I fractures Give 2 gm cephalosporin (cefazolin or cephamandol) on admission; 1 gm every 8 hours for 48 to 72 hours.

Type II or III fractures Combine cephalosporin (as above) and aminoglycoside (tobramycin, gentamicin) for 3 days.
Tobramycin dosage is 1.5 mg/kg on admission and 3 to 5 mg/kg each day in divided doses for 3 days.
Monitor and adjust aminoglycoside levels.
Add penicillin if *Clostridia* contamination is possible (e.g., farmyard injury).

Reinstitute antibiotic coverage for 24 to 48 hours after wound closure.

■ *Prolonging antibiotic therapy for more than 3 days has been reported to be ineffective in preventing wound infection (Gustilo).*

FRACTURE STABILIZATION

Fracture stabilization generally should be obtained by the method that provides adequate stability with minimal damage to the vascularity of the soft tissues. Intraarticular fractures with any displacement require open reduction and internal fixation, and bone grafting is often necessary for subchondral support to mini-

mize the chance of joint incongruity. Metaphyseal and diaphyseal fractures usually are stabilized with intramedullary nailing, external fixation, plate-and-screw devices. Fracture stabilization in the lower extremity requires more fatigue-resistant implants and devices than does the upper extremity because of the increased demands of weight bearing and the larger size of the joints and muscle-tendon units involved.

Open fractures generally are treated with repeat debridements until a stable soft tissue envelope is achieved by delayed primary closure or skin graft or flap coverage of the wound, preferably by 5 to 7 days. Stabilization of fractures with Gustilo-Anderson type I soft tissue injuries generally is the same as for closed fractures. Types II and III soft tissue injuries usually require stabilization of the fracture with intramedullary nailing or external fixation. Plate-and-screw fixation generally is reserved for displaced intraarticular fractures. Often the best treatment of severe type IIIC injuries is amputation, although the surgeon must obviously make this decision based on the clinical findings.

Acute bone grafting, sometimes used for **closed** fractures with bone loss from impaction, such as tibial plateau or pilon fractures, is not recommended for open fractures. At 6 to 12 weeks, bone grafting may be indicated in open fractures if the soft tissue envelope is stable and free of drainage, especially in fractures with bone loss. This situation is more common with open tibial fractures than with femoral fractures.

Occasionally *dynamization* is recommended to transfer stress from the implant to the extremity when external fixation systems or static interlocking intramedullary nails are used for fracture stabilization. Dynamization of static interlocking nails usually is an outpatient surgical procedure consisting of removal of the interlocking screws from the *longest fragment* of the injured bone. Nail dynamization usually is performed at 6 to 12 weeks in the tibia and at 12 to 24 weeks in the femur. Dynamization should not be performed with unstable fractures that would permit loss of alignment and significant leg-length inequality. These problems occur primarily in proximal and distal third fractures where the nail diameter and intramedullary canal diameter are mismatched, permitting translational and rotational instability after removal of the interlocking screw. Bone grafting as a biologic stimulus is typically used in these unstable fractures where dynamization is contraindicated.

Active or passive dynamization of external fixation systems is more frequent. *Active dynamization,* as described by Kenwright and Goodship, involves controlled application of a cyclic load over a prescribed distance with a prescribed force. *Passive dynamization* is achieved by modifying the external fixator by allowing axial collapse with load bearing or sequential removal of components of the fixator to encourage more load bearing on the extremity. Passive dynamization has been shown to be primarily effective in closure of small gaps and is best applied early after injury.

Early stabilization of lower extremity fractures in patients with multiple injuries has been proven to reduce the incidence of pulmonary complications and to decrease the number of days in the intensive care unit and hospital.

DELAYED UNION AND NONUNION

Delayed union or nonunion of lower extremity fractures usually is indicated by symptoms of continued pain, continued inability to bear full weight on the extremity, and radiographic evidence of lack of callus and consolidation of the fracture lines. Most lower extremity fractures heal by 6 months. After 6 months, a fracture is described as a delayed union if it produces continued symptoms. Nonunion usually is indicated by 9 to 12 months of continued symptoms and radiographic signs. Once delayed union or nonunion is diagnosed, consideration should be given either to revising the mechanical construct or to using a biologic stimulus in the form of bone grafting or electrical stimulation. In fractures with bone loss or severe soft tissue injuries, early prophylactic bone grafting has been shown to reduce healing time by 20% to 30%.

Patients with certain metabolic abnormalities and diseases are more likely to have delayed healing, such as those with alcoholism, an incompetent or impaired immune system, a condition requiring immune suppression (transplant patients), concomitant systemic disease (diabetes mellitus, peripheral vascular disease), or malnutrition. Cure or treatment of the underlying disorder must be part of the treatment of the extremity injury.

INFECTION

Infection after lower extremity fractures may occur early or late. The infection must be aggressively treated with debridement, irrigation, and appropriate antibiotic therapy. Superficial infections may respond to local care and oral antibiotics. Deep infections require prompt diagnosis, surgical intervention, and intravenous antibiotics for prolonged periods.

GENERAL PRINCIPLES OF REHABILITATION

Rehabilitation after lower extremity fractures follows a general sequence of time-interval–dependent exercises and goals. Based on the relative average times of soft tissue and bony repair, the following four phases of rehabilitation are identified: **phase 1** (0 to 6 weeks), mobilization of adjacent joints and muscles and protected weight bearing for diaphyseal and metaphyseal fractures; **phase 2** (6 weeks to 3 months), strengthening and endurance exercises with progressive weight bearing; **phase 3** (3 to 6 months), progression to full unsupported weight bearing, agility and endurance training, reentry into work and recreational activities; and **phase 4** (more than 6 months), resumption of normal activities.

A general outline of exercises and activities is shown in the box.

Exercises and Activities After Lower Extremity Fractures

Open-Chain Exercises	Closed-Chain Exercises
Characteristics	**Characteristics**
Distal segment is free	Distal segment is not free
No weight bearing	Partial weight bearing
Motion is only distal to axis of motion	Motion is both distal and proximal to the axis of motion
Muscle contraction primarily concentric	Muscle contraction includes concentric, eccentric, isometric, and isotonic
Movements are usually isolated	Movements are functional. Can emphasize one muscle group, but entire kinetic chain works together
Load is artificial	Loads are physiological and through the entire kinetic chain
Velocity is predetermined	Variable velocity
Stabilization is often artificial (straps and belts)	Stabilization is a product of normal postural mechanisms
Usually in one cardinal plane of motion	Motion takes place in all planes of joints
Proprioceptive carry-over to functional activties questionable	Significant proprioceptive carry-over to functional activities
Exercises often limited by equipment	Exercises limited only by imagination
Exercises	**Exercises**
Isometrics	***Non–weight-bearing closed-chain exercises***
Straight leg raises	Hip machine for uninvolved leg
Knee ROM exercises	Sitting with knee flexed, performing towel slides
Terminal knee extension	
Stationary bicycle	***Partial weight-bearing (PWB) closed-chain exercises***
Proprioceptive neuromuscular facilitation (PNF)	PWB minisquats
Isokinetic exercise equipment	PWB wall sits
Weight equipment (in the seated position)	PWB lunges
	Proprioception emphasis using BAPS board
	Allow PWB ambulation when patient is 50% weight bearing
	Full weight-bearing closed-chain exercises
	Wall sits
	Minisquats with or without resistance
	Lunges
	Proprioception with BAPS board or Fitter treadmill (retro walking and forward walking)
	Pool
	Stair machines (forward and reverse stance)
	NordicTrack ski machines
	Agility drills
	Step-ups
	Sliding lunges

Acetabular Fractures

REHABILITATION RATIONALE

Letournel and Judet introduced the concept of column classification of acetabular fractures (Fig. 4-1). This concept considers the acetabulum to be made up of anterior and posterior columns and walls. These walls and columns architecturally resemble a circle surrounded by a triangle. Analysis of radiographs and computed tomograms allow fractures of the acetabulum to be grouped into five major patterns and five combined patterns. The first two basic patterns are *anterior* and *posterior wall* fractures, usually associated

with dislocation of the hip. *Anterior* and *posterior column* fractures are less common, may be associated with hip dislocations similar to wall fractures, and usually result in instability of the hip and major joint incongruity. A fracture line that traverses through the anterior and posterior columns is a *transverse* fracture. This pattern is relatively common, may be associated with central dislocation of the hip, and often requires open reduction and internal fixation if it involves the weight-bearing surface of the acetabulum.

The five combined patterns include *anterior wall and anterior column* fractures, *posterior wall and posterior column* fractures, *transverse with posterior wall* fractures,

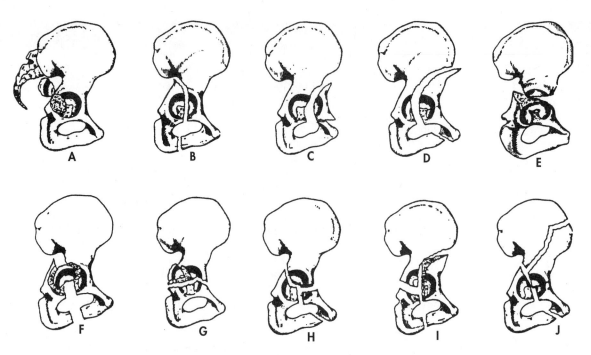

Figure 4-1 Letournel and Judet classification of acetabular fractures. **A,** Posterior wall. **B,** Posterior column. **C,** Anterior wall. **D,** Anterior column. **E,** Transverse. **F,** Posterior column and posterior wall. **G,** Transverse and posterior wall. **H,** T-shaped. **I,** Anterior and posterior hemitransverse. **J,** Complete both-column. (From Letournel E, Judet R: *Fractures of the acetabulum,* New York, 1981, Springer-Verlag.)

hemitransverse fractures, and *both-column* fractures. These combined patterns are more complex and more commonly result in articular incongruity and instability of the hip either anteriorly, centrally, or posteriorly. The both-column pattern differs from the basic transverse pattern in that no component of the articular surface of the acetabulum remains in continuity with the ilium, so the acetabulum is free floating in relation to the posterior sacroiliac complex for load transfer from the lower extremity.

Treatment

Once an acetabular fracture is defined radiographically, its effect on the function of the hip and lower extremity must be considered to determine the preferred treatment. The severity of acetabular fractures varies from nondisplaced fractures with no long-term effect on function to irreparable injury with functional salvage possible only with total hip arthroplasty or hip arthrodesis. There is no certain technique of predicting results of even the most perfect of surgical repairs, and each patient must be individually evaluated.

General treatment considerations include the patient's age and general health, the presence of osteopenia, stability of the hip, and congruency of the joint. In general, open reduction and internal fixation are not appropriate for elderly patients, especially those with osteopenia and limited preinjury ambula-

tion. An unstable hip that subluxes centrally, anteriorly, or posteriorly is a prime indication for open reduction and internal fixation. Articular incongruity of more than 3 to 5 mm, especially in the weight-bearing portions of the acetabulum, generally precludes good long-term results. Therefore this amount of incongruity is also an indication for open reduction and internal fixation.

Heterotopic ossification or periarticular calcification may interfere significantly with ROM after acetabular fracture. It is more common after posterior approaches to the hip, as well as in burn patients. Prophylaxis is usually offered in the form of indomethacin 25 mg orally three times a day or low-dose radiation, usually 1000 rads or less. Both treatments have associated risks. Excision of heterotopic ossification may be recommended if there is a significant loss of motion that does not respond to physical therapy.

Deep vein thrombosis and pulmonary embolus may result in chronic postphlebitic syndrome or death. There is no uniform successful treatment or preventative measure. Options include warfarin anticoagulation, mechanical measures such as compressive stockings, and venal caval filters. The patient must be informed of the risks and benefits of each option.

Postoperative treatment and rehabilitation are based on the amount of articular comminution and the amount of stability obtained by fixation.

REHABILITATION PROTOCOL

Stable Acetabular Fracture Treated Nonoperatively

INDICATIONS	• Stability • Less than 3 mm of articular incongruity
0 to 7 days	• In general, use Buck's traction (5 lbs) for comfort. When pain and spasm have decreased and the patient can perform straight leg raising, allow touchdown weight bearing using a heel-to-toe pattern with crutches.

• Begin active ROM exercises of the hip in the hospital.
• After discharge from the hospital, the follow-up protocol is the same as for operatively treated acetabular fractures (see below).

REHABILITATION PROTOCOL

Open Reduction and Internal Fixation of Acetabular Fracture
LETOURNEL

1 day	• Begin continuous passive motion (CPM) the day after surgery and continue for 18 to 21 days. The initial ROM is 0 to 40 degrees. The range of flexion is increased incrementally until 90 degrees of flexion is achieved at 5 to 6 days. • Use CPM initially 12 to 20 hours per day as tolerated.
4 to 5 days	• Perform active ROM exercises of all hip muscle groups twice daily under the supervision of the therapist.

10 to 14 days	• Begin ambulation with non–weight bearing or partial weight bearing (one fifth of body weight). • Continue active ROM exercises for hip, knee, and ankle.
10 to 12 weeks	• Begin full weight bearing when radiographic confirmation of healing is noted.

REHABILITATION PROTOCOL

Open Reduction and Internal Fixation of Acetabular Fracture
MATTA

1 day	• Begin CPM of the hip postoperatively with a flexion arc of 30 to 50 degrees at one cycle per minute. Increase the arc of flexion 5 to 10 degrees twice daily until 90 degrees is achieved. • Sit on side of bed.
2 to 7 days	• Transfer from bed to chair and begin physical therapy for active ROM exercises, including all ranges of motion for the hip. • Use a skateboard to encourage abduction and adduction.

• Initiate gait training as touchdown with 25 lbs of force applied to affected limb, if cleared by surgeon.
• Use radiographs to evaluate and confirm reduction.

7 to 14 days	• Begin progressive resistive exercises of the trunk and lower extremity. Emphasize abductors and quadriceps. • When the patient can perform independent transfers, attains 90 degrees of hip flexion, and can ambulate with two crutches, it is possible to discharge to home. *Continued*

REHABILITATION PROTOCOL—cont'd

Open Reduction and Internal Fixation of Acetabular Fracture

MATTA

2 to 6 weeks	• Begin outpatient physical therapy for active ROM exercises and progressive resistive exercises of the hip. • If other injuries do not preclude, begin swimming and riding a stationary bicycle.		• Begin a more vigorous program of progressive resistance exercises using weights or a Nautilus facility on a 3-times-a-week program. This may continue up to a year, until the patient has eliminated any Trendelenburg gait of abductor weakness. • Replace crutches with a cane when the patient walks without a limp.
6 to 12 weeks	• Take radiographs to document satisfactory maintenance of reduction and progressive healing. • Progress the weight-bearing program to 50 to 80 lbs using a bathroom scale and progress to full weight bearing with crutches over the next 4 to 6 weeks.	12 to 52 weeks	• Take radiographs at 12, 24, and 52 weeks to confirm healing and absence of avascular necrosis, heterotopic ossification, or posttraumatic arthropathy.

Hip Dislocation and Fracture-Dislocation

REHABILITATION RATIONALE

Injuries of the hip joint may include pure dislocation, dislocation with fracture of the femoral head, and dislocation with fracture of the acetabulum. The position of the femoral head in relation to the acetabulum at the time of injury and the mechanism of injury determine the type of injury produced. Because high-energy forces are required to cause these injuries, associated injuries to the pelvis or other systems are frequent.

Most hip dislocations can be reduced by closed manipulation, and this should be performed as soon as possible to decrease the risk of complications such as avascular necrosis of the femoral head. Reduction of the hip dislocation should take precedence over the treatment of any other skeletal injuries.

Posterior Dislocations

The femoral head is most often dislocated posteriorly; anterior dislocations occur in only about 12% of patients with traumatic hip dislocations. Thompson and Epstein classified posterior hip dislocations into the following five types according to the involvement of the acetabulum and/or femoral head fracture (Table 4-3):

Type I dislocations are treated with immediate closed reduction or with open reduction if closed manipulation does not obtain a concentric reduction. The treatment of types II through IV dislocations depends on the stability and congruency of the hip joint. Un-

TABLE 4-3 Thompson and Epstein Classification of Posterior Hip Dislocation

Type I	Dislocation without significant fracture of the acetabulum
Type II	Dislocation with a large single fracture of the posterior rim of the acetabulum (corresponds to posterior wall fracture in Judet classification of acetabular fractures)
Type III	Dislocation with comminution of the posterior acetabular rim with or without a major fragment
Type IV	Dislocation with fracture of the acetabular floor, which can be classified using Judet or Letournel classification
Type V	Dislocation with fracture of the femoral head

stable or incongruent types II, III and IV dislocations can be managed according to the Letournel or Matta protocols for acetabular fractures (pp. 149 and 150).

Type V dislocations, also known as Pipkin fracture-dislocations, are serious injuries when they involve the weight-bearing surface of the femoral head (Table 4-4). Most often the fracture of the femoral head is inferior and can be treated nonoperatively. Significant articular displacement may be an indication of the need for operative treatment, but the prognosis generally is poor. If acetabular fracture is present, open

TABLE 4-4 **Pipkin Subclassification of Type V Fracture-Dislocation**	
Type I	Posterior dislocation of the hip with fracture of the femoral head *caudad* to the fovea centralis
Type II	Posterior dislocation of the hip with fracture of the femoral head *cephalad* to the fovea centralis
Type III	Type I or II with associated fracture of the femoral neck
Type IV	Type I, II, or III with associated fracture of the acetabulum

TABLE 4-5 **Epstein Classification of Anterior Dislocation**	
Type I	Superior dislocations (includes pubic and subspinous dislocations)
Type IA	No associated fracture (simple dislocation)
Type IB	Associated fracture of the head of the femur (indentation type or transchondral type)
Type IC	Associated fracture of the acetabulum
Type II	Inferior dislocation
Type IIA	No associated fracture (simple dislocation)
Type IIB	Associated fracture of the head of the femur (indentation or transchondral type)
Type IIC	Associated fracture of the acetabulum

reduction and reconstruction usually are recommended. If the femoral head reduces concentrically into the acetabulum and the hip is stable, the limb is placed in skeletal traction through a Kirschner wire inserted near the tibial tuberosity. Traction is continued for 6 weeks, and then gradual weight bearing is allowed over the next 6 to 8 weeks. There have been no studies to date that document increased success with prolonged non–weight bearing. Partial weight bearing to fracture healing appears to be adequate.

Anterior Dislocations

Classifications are usually based on the position of the femoral head: pubic, obturator, or perineal (Table 4-5). After emergent closed reduction of the hip, the patient is placed in Buck's traction. If postreduction radiographs show a concentric reduction and no articular incongruity, progressive partial weight bearing is allowed. If closed reduction cannot be accomplished, the need for open reduction is indicated.

Anterior dislocations have a fairly high incidence of impaction of the femoral head, which may compromise long-term results. Patients should be monitored for the complications of late hip instability, posttraumatic arthropathy, heterotopic ossification, and avascular necrosis.

REHABILITATION PROTOCOL

Posterior Hip Dislocation

Thompson-Epstein Type I (without significant acetabular fracture)

1 day
- Begin quadriceps sets, gluteal sets, hamstring sets, and ankle pumps.
- Begin upper extremity exercises and bed mobility.
- Obtain occupational therapy consultation to help patient with activities of daily living (ADLs). (Include appropriate reaching devices for objects, utilizing shoe horn, etc.)
- Give patient an exercise sheet and review it with the patient, placing special emphasis on hip precautions to avoid recurrence of dislocation. (See Chapter 7.)

■ NOTE: *Hip precautions for anterior dislocation (external rotation and abduction) are opposite those for posterior hip dislocation (internal rotation and adduction).*

2 days
- Review exercise sheet, add new exercises, and clarify as needed.
- Initiate straight leg raises when tolerated.
- Initiate active-assisted ROM early for articular cartilage nutrition.
- Begin ambulation, weight bearing to tolerance with crutches.

3 to 7 days
- Allow progressive ambulation with partial weight bearing.

Continued

Posterior Hip Dislocation

Thompson-Epstein Type I (without significant acetabular fracture)—cont'd	**Thompson-Epstein Type II (with large single fracture of posterior acetabular rim)**
3 to 7 days —cont'd	• Perform ROM exercises of hip with a functional ROM. • Progress to full weight bearing at 6 to 12 weeks. • Follow rehabilitation protocols for acetabular fractures (pp. 149 and 150).	If the hip is stable within the range of 30 to 70 degrees of hip flexion, continue traction for 5 to 14 days, and then rehabilitation proceeds the same as for type I dislocation. If open reduction and internal fixation have been performed for instability or incongruous reduction, follow acetabular protocols (p. 150).

Pelvic Fracture

REHABILITATION RATIONALE

Pelvic fractures usually are caused by high-energy trauma in younger patients and by low-energy trauma only in elderly patients. Most patients have multiple associated injuries, and mortality rates of 10% to 20% have been reported in large series of pelvic fractures; open pelvic fractures have been reported to have mortality rates as high as 50%.

Young et al. developed a classification based on the mechanism of energy. *Anterior-posterior compression* forces result in diastasis of the symphysis pubis, with or without obvious diastasis of the sacroiliac joint or fracture of the iliac bone, with varying degrees of ligamentous disruption (sacrotuberous, sacrospinous, sacroiliac ligaments). *Lateral compression* forces result in rotation of the pelvis inward, leading to fracture in the sacroiliac area and fracture of the pelvic rami. *Vertical shear* forces disrupt the iliac or sacroiliac junction, causing upward displacement of the fracture component from the main pelvis. *Combined mechanical injuries* are caused by a combination of two forces, which results in a pattern of pelvic injuries that is a combination of two or more of the above types. The final category is *acetabular fractures*, in which the primary injury is acetabular and is produced by femoral loading with impaction of the femoral head.

Tile described another classification system, which has become the basis for the AO and the Orthopaedic Trauma Association classifications (Table 4-6).

Type A fractures are stable and can be treated nonoperatively. These include avulsion injuries of the anterior-superior iliac spine, anterior-inferior iliac spine, and ischial tuberosity, including "groin pulls" and isolated fractures of the pubic ramus.

Type B fractures (Fig. 4-2) are rotationally unstable and displaced, but are vertically stable. The sacrotuberous ligament and posterior sacroiliac complex are relatively intact. Variants consist of fractures of the pubis or ischium; and the sacrum, sacroiliac joint, or ilium may be involved. If no significant displacement or internal rotation of the lower extremities is present, type B fractures usually can be treated nonoperatively. For severe pain or significant narrowing of the pelvic outlet, external rotation reduction and application of an external fixator has been advocated.

Type C injuries (Fig. 4-3) are unstable vertically, posteriorly, and rotationally, with displacement either through the symphysis pubis or the pubic and ischial rami anteriorly and disruption of the sacrotuberous, sacrospinous, and posterior sacroiliac complex through the ilium, the sacroiliac joint, the sacrum, or a combined injury. Type C fractures are more likely

TABLE 4-6 Pelvic Fracture Classification

Type A	Rotationally and vertically stable A1—Fracture of the pelvis not involving the ring A2—Stable, minimally displaced fracture of the ring
Type B	Rotationally unstable, vertically stable B1—Open-book fracture B2—Lateral compression fracture: ipsilateral B3—Lateral compression fracture: contralateral (bucket handle)
Type C	Rotationally and vertically unstable C1—Unilateral C2—Bilateral C3—Associated with an acetabular fracture

From Tile M: *J Bone Joint Surg* 70(B):3, 1988.

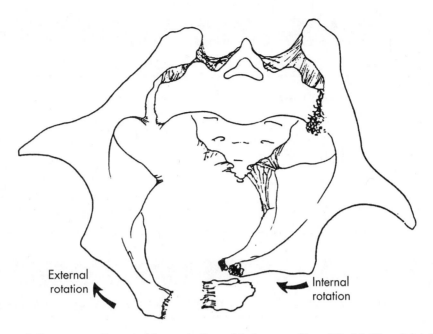

Figure 4-2 Rotationally unstable, vertically stable fracture. (From Tile M: *J Bone Joint Surg* 70B:1, 1988.)

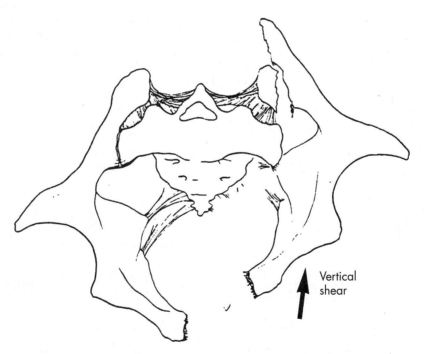

Figure 4-3 Rotationally and vertically unstable fracture. (From Tile M: *J Bone Joint Surg* 70B:1, 1988.)

to require open reduction and internal fixation. Most authors agree that, if operative intervention is required, both the anterior and posterior pelvic injuries must be treated. This usually requires a combination of open reduction and internal fixation or external fixation ofthe anterior ring injury combined with

posterior transiliac or posterior sacroiliac stabilization.

No currently used surgical procedure allows immediate full weight bearing after surgical stabilization. A partial weight-bearing program generally is recommended for up to 12 weeks.

REHABILITATION PROTOCOL

Stable Pelvic Fracture Treated Nonoperatively

0 to 7 days	• Allow partial weight bearing with crutches or walker.
7 to 14 days	• Begin progressive resistive exercise. • Begin closed- and open-chain exercises. (See box p. 147.) • Perform isometric exercises, including hip abductors and extensors.
4 to 8 weeks	• Allow progressive weight bearing with crutches or walker. May use a cane when the patient can apply full, unsupported weight to the extremity.
6 to 12 weeks	• Progress full weight bearing. When no Trendelenburg gait is present and full hip and back ROM is obtained, allow full weight bearing.

REHABILITATION PROTOCOL

Tile Type B Pelvic Fracture Treated With External Fixation

0 to 6 weeks	• If external fixation frames have been applied anteriorly, instruct the patient in care of the pin sites while in the hospital. • Once leg control is satisfactory, allow touchdown weight bearing on the affected extremity with crutches or walker. • Monitor with radiographs the first 2 weeks to confirm that there is no loss of reduction in the external fixator. • Periodically check the external fixator frame to ensure that it is not loosening. • Continue partial weight-bearing program with isometric exercises of the lower extremity for 6 weeks. • Progress from AAROM to AROM in all planes (supine and standing).
6 to 8 weeks	• If radiographs confirm maintenance of satisfactory alignment and evidence of early callus at 6 weeks, start progressive resistive exercises of the lower extremities. • Continue partial weight bearing with crutches or walker. • Begin closed-chain exercises. (See box p. 147.)
8 to 12 weeks	• Frequently the external fixation frame becomes uncomfortable because of pin-site irritation in the iliac crest anteriorly. If the patient can bear full weight on the extremity, the frame may be loosened, and lateral compression may be applied to the pelvis. • If the patient is asymptomatic, the external fixator may be removed, usually on an outpatient basis. Pin sites are left open and allowed to granulate in.

REHABILITATION PROTOCOL

Tile Type C Pelvic Fracture

These fractures are associated with the greatest frequency of malunion and continued pain referrable to the posterior sacroiliac complex. If patients are treated nonoperatively or with simple external fixation frames anteriorly, continue non–weight bearing, usually with bed-to-wheelchair transfers, for 6 to 12 weeks. Mobilize the patient with crutches after bony union is evident radiographically, then follow standard hip rehabilitation. (See Chapter 7.) Rehabilitation after operative stablization of type C fractures is modified according to the type of internal or external fixation used.	
1 day	• Mobilize the patient from bed to chair. • Begin isometric exercises for the lower extremities and general conditioning of the upper extremities.
2 to 5 days	• The patient continues to sit up in chair and is allowed to stand. • Progress ambulation with walker or crutches with touchdown weight bearing (less than 5 lbs) on the heel on the affected side, if sufficient stability is present after surgical stabilization.

REHABILITATION PROTOCOL—cont'd

2 to 5 days —cont'd	• Mobilize patients with bilateral fractures from bed to chair for the first 6 weeks and delay ambulation. • Perform lower extremity ROM in all planes.

1 week	• Discharge patient from hospital if following criteria are met:
	  1. Can get out of bed independently
	  2. Is able to ambulate independently 50 feet in the hall with assistive device as necessary or can perform bed to wheelchair transfer if nonambulatory
	  3. Can maneuver in and out of the bathroom independently
	• If discharge criteria are not met or if patient is elderly and lives alone, extended rehabilitative facility may be appropriate.

2 to 6 weeks	• Follow rehabilitation after acetabular fracture (Letournel) (p. 149).
6 to 12 weeks	• If fixation is stable and callus is evident on radiographs, test the patient on weight bearing using a bathroom scale to determine the amount of weight that is comfortable, usually in the 50- to 70-lb range. Allow partial weight bearing in this range for the next 4 to 6 weeks. • Begin closed-chain exercises as tolerated.
12 weeks	• Schedule the patient for external fixator removal. • Begin progressive ambulation, as in protocol for rehabilitation after hip fracture (pp. 159 to 160).

Femoral Neck, Subtrochanteric, and Intertrochanteric Fractures

REHABILITATION RATIONALE

Femoral Neck Fractures

The most commonly used classification for femoral neck fractures is that of Garden, which is based on the amount of fracture displacement (Table 4-7).

For young patients with good bone stock in the femoral neck, head, and lateral shaft, femoral neck fractures can be treated with anatomic open reduction and, if required, internal fixation with three cancellous screws in a lag-screw fashion. In older patients with less structurally stable bone stock, especially if the lateral cortex is thinned and weak, simple screw fixation often does not provide sufficient stability, and a hip compression screw with an accessory screw or hemiarthroplasty may be more appropriate. Most authors recommend some type of hemiarthroplasty, with the femoral component cemented, for complete displacement of the femoral neck fragment in an ambulatory patient with osteopenic bone. The relative advantages of endoprostheses and bipolar prostheses are still controversial. Bipolar arthroplasty usually is recommended for patients with an expected life span of more than 5 years. For patients with less than 2 years expected life span who are household ambulators with insufficient bone quality for internal fixation, some type of hemiarthroplasty, such as the Austin Moore, probably is more appropriate.

General treatment considerations include the age and general health of the patient (Fig. 4-5). In patients aged 20 to 40 years, this injury usually is caused by high-energy trauma, and avascular necrosis is frequent. Patients aged 40 to 60 years may exhibit underlying pathologic states, such as renal dystrophy or other organ system disease, that may affect surgical outcome. In patients over 60 years of age, femoral neck fractures are caused by low-energy trauma and may be considered part of a developing multiple organ system failure, because they frequently are associated with other diseases that complicate recovery, such as diabetes, cardiac conditions, and renal disease. It also is important to establish the preoperative ambulatory status of the patient (community ambulator, house-

TABLE 4-7 Garden Classification of Femoral Neck Fractures (Fig. 4-4)

Grade 1	Incomplete, impacted fracture
Grade 2	Nondisplaced fracture
Grade 3	Incompletely displaced fracture in varus malalignment
Grade 4	Completely displaced fracture with no engagement of the two fragments

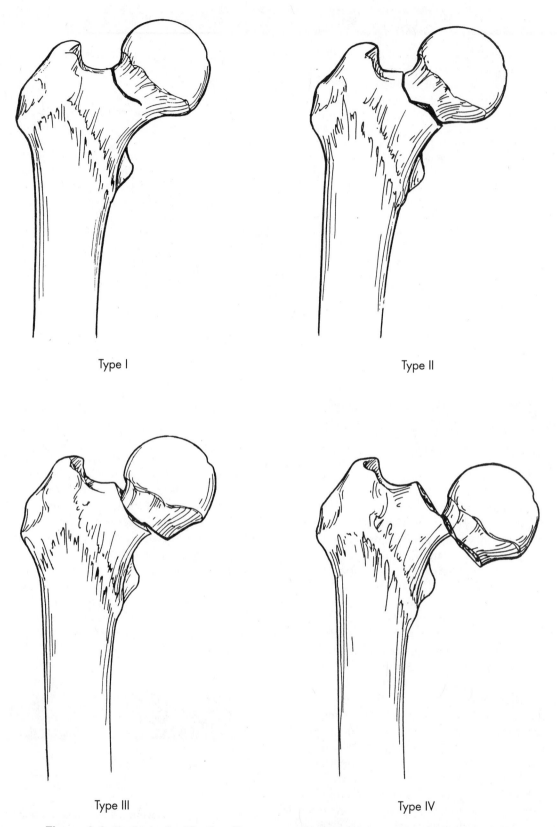

Type I

Type II

Type III

Type IV

Figure 4-4 Garden's classification. Treatment and avascular necrosis and union rates of femoral neck fractures are based on displacement. (From Kyle RF: *Fractures of the hip*. In Gustilo RB, Kyle RF, Templeman D, editors: *Fractures and dislocations*, St Louis, 1993, Mosby–Year Book.)

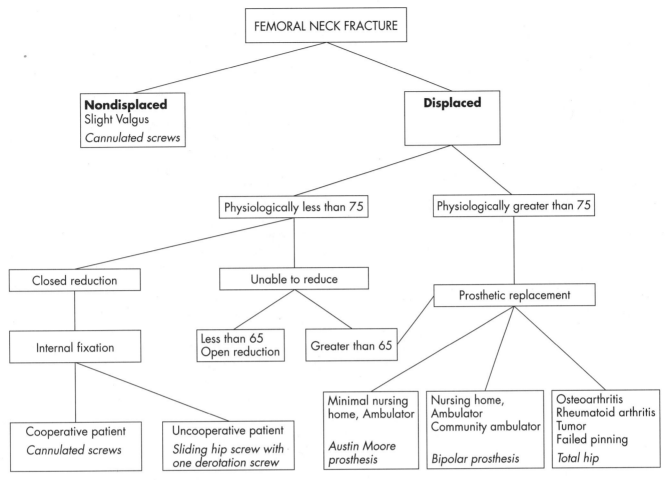

Figure 4-5 Flowchart for the treatment of femoral neck fractures. Treatment depends on the degree of displacement of the fracture and the age of the patient. Preexisting hip disease also dictates treatment. (From Kyle RF: *Fractures of the hip.* In Gustilo RB, Kyle RF, Templeman D, editors: *Fractures and dislocations,* St. Louis, 1993, Mosby–Year Book.)

hold ambulator, or essentially nonambulator), because this will affect treatment decisions.

Intertrochanteric Femoral Fractures

Intertrochanteric fractures of the femur occur most often in patients 66 to 76 years of age and affect more than 200,000 persons each year in the United States. Mortality for this fracture ranges from 15% to 20%, and frequently this injury is the start of multiple organ system failure in older patients. Most authors currently recommend a four-part classification, such as the Boyd, Evans, or Kyle classification, but alphanumeric classifications are gaining some advocates. The real question is whether the fracture is unstable because of loss of medial column support, or if it is stable with medial column support. The standard treatment at this time in the United States is fixation with a hip compression screw. Some authors have advocated intramedullary devices, but no studies have shown these implants to be superior to hip

compression screws. There has also been a tendency in the past few years to attempt a more anatomic reduction of the hip, with centralization of the compression hip screw in the center position of the femoral head on AP and lateral views for maximum stability and a decrease in the risk of cut-out. The prognosis for these fractures obviously is related to the degree of osteopenia and the comminution of the fracture. However, medial displacement osteotomies are rarely recommended.

It is important that once stabilization is obtained, these patients begin to get up, sit in a chair, and ambulate frequently, since many are borderline ambulators before injury. Early mobilization also helps to minimize the complications of prolonged bed rest. Thorough preoperative evaluation should determine the patient's preinjury mental status, independence at home, and especially ambulatory capabilities (nonambulator, household ambulator, or community ambulator).

Subtrochanteric Femoral Fractures

Boyd and Griffin, in their classification of peritrochanteric fractures of the femur, noted that fractures involving the subtrochanteric area had a much higher rate of failure with fixed implant designs. This fracture, indeed, has a reputation of nonunions and implant failures with the previous generation of implants. The key to stability of this fracture complex is very similar to that for intertrochanteric fracture: Is the medial column intact?

Russell and Taylor and others have noted the importance of supporting this fracture because of the high stresses across it. Russell and Taylor proposed a classification system (Fig. 4-6) that groups subtrochanteric fractures into four types to help determine the most appropriate type of operative stabilization. Fractures with stability of the lesser trochanter and an intact piriform fossa are similar to diaphyseal femoral fractures, and conventional interlocking nailing is advocated. In type IB fractures, the lesser trochanteric area and medial column are deficient, and there is no injury to the piriform fossa; for these fractures, a reconstruction-type intramedullary nail usually is recommended. In type IIA and IIB variants, the fracture extends from the subtrochanteric area up into the piriform fossa. If medial continuity is intact, as in type IA fractures, a standard hip compression screw can be used as for introchanteric fractures. Type IIB fractures, with comminution involving the piriformis fossa, medial comminution involving the lesser trochanter, and varying degrees of shaft comminution, frequently require indirect and open reduction techniques with hip compression screw fixation and autologous iliac bone grafting. If shaft comminution is extensive, occasionally open reduction and fixation with a reconstruction-type intramedullary nail are indicated because of the long diaphyseal fracture fragment.

Rehabilitation may include a hip exercise program for stable fixed fractures, with partial weight bearing until fracture healing is evident, whereas rehabilitation for patients with hemiarthroplasties follows the protocol for total hip arthroplasty, with emphasis on hip dislocation precautions. (See Chapter 7.) The surgeon should guide the rehabilitation team. Postoperative management must be individualized based on the patient's overall health and preinjury condition, the fracture characteristics, and the stability of the internal fixation.

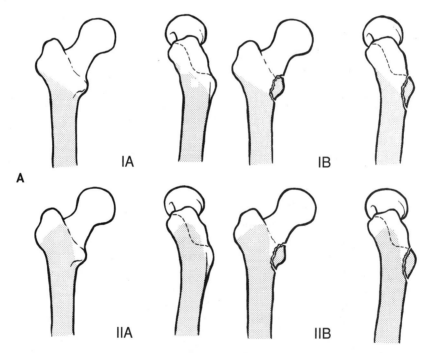

Figure 4-6 A, Russell-Taylor classification of subtrochantric fracture of femur based on involvement of piriformis fossa. Group 1 fractures do not extend into piriformis fossa: type IA—comminution and fracture lines extend from below lesser trochanter to femoral isthmus; type IB—fracture lines and comminution involve area of lesser trochanter to isthmus. Group 2 fractures extend proximally into greater trochanter and involve piriformis fossa: type IIA—without significant comminution or fracture of lesser trochanter; type IIB—with significant comminution of medial femoral cortex and loss of continuity of lesser trochanter. (From Russell TA: *Fractures of the hip and pelvis.* In Crenshaw AH, editor: *Campbell's operative orthopaedics,* St. Louis, 1993, Mosby–Year Book.)

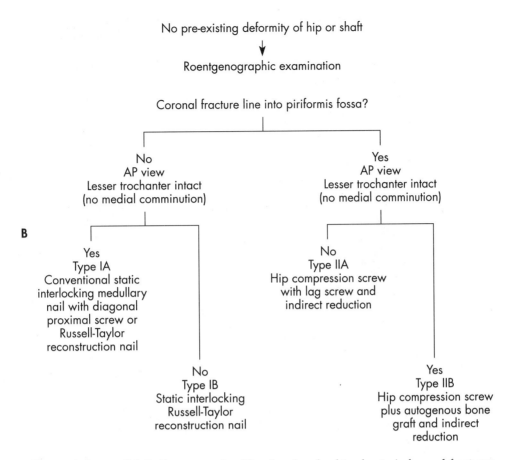

No pre-existing deformity of hip or shaft

Roentgenographic examination

Coronal fracture line into piriformis fossa?

B

No
AP view
Lesser trochanter intact
(no medial comminution)

Yes
Type IA
Conventional static
interlocking medullary
nail with diagonal
proximal screw or
Russell-Taylor
reconstruction nail

No
Type IB
Static interlocking
Russell-Taylor
reconstruction nail

Yes
AP view
Lesser trochanter intact
(no medial comminution)

No
Type IIA
Hip compression screw
with lag screw and
indirect reduction

Yes
Type IIB
Hip compression screw
plus autogenous bone
graft and indirect
reduction

Figure 4-6—cont'd B, Treatment algorithm for closed subtrochanteric femoral fractures based on the Russell-Taylor classification. (From Russell TA: *Fractures of hip and pelvis.* In Crenshaw AH: *Campbell's operative orthopaedics*, ed 8, 1992, Mosby–Year Book.)

REHABILITATION PROTOCOL

Femoral Neck Fractures, Intertrochanteric Fractures, and Subtrochanteric Fractures

1 day	• Begin quadriceps sets, hamstring sets, gluteal sets, and ankle pumps. • Perform gentle active-assisted abduction and adduction of the hip. • Perform supine leg slides for flexion of the hip and knee. • Institute bed mobility. • Provide an exercise sheet for the patient and family. Explain and demonstrate each exercise; the patient then performs the exercises with assistance of the therapist. • Provide occupational therapy to assist with ADLs. • Perform upper extremity exercises, especially if the patient is to be bedridden for any period. The use of Therabands for independent exercises can be helpful, with PNF patterns performed by the therapist with appropriate resistance.	2 days	• Review the exercise sheet with the patient and family. Answer any questions and add new exercises to achieve a complete home program. • Increase bed mobility (use of verbal cues more than assistance to get from supine to sitting will make the patient more independent). • Increase ambulation with appropriate weight-bearing status (e.g. TDWB with walker, then PWB with walker, etc.).
		3 to 7 days	• Encourage patient to be independent with exercises and assist in areas of difficulty. • Perform straight leg raises in all directions, lying position and standing (if the patient has good balance).

Continued

Femoral Neck Fractures, Intertrochanteric Fractures, and Subtrochanteric Fractures

3 to 7 days —cont'd	• If the patient is weight bearing to tolerance, start weight-shifting exercises and minisquats. • Begin gentle daily Thomas stretch of the anterior capsule and hip flexors. Pull the uninvolved knee to the chest while supine, simultaneously pushing the involved extremity against the bed. • Evaluate for assistive devices for the home (shower chair, elevated commode seat, etc.). • With a straight-back chair, work on sit/stand; increase repetitions as tolerated. • Continue ambulation 2 times a day with assistance.	• Perform quadriceps sets, gluteal sets, ankle pumps, hip and knee active ROM (hip slides in supine), supine abduction of the hip, progressive straight leg raises when tolerated by the patient. • Add standing hip abduction, adduction, extension, and flexion, with hip and knee flexion exercises. Include 4-point exercises. This involves flexing the knee while standing, then straightening the knee. Flex the knee again, then return the foot to the starting position. • Always reinforce good posture while exercising in the standing position.
1 to 2 weeks	• Discharge criteria: 1. Gets out of bed independently 2. Able to ambulate 50 feet in the hall independently with assistive device as necessary 3. In and out of the bathroom independently • If discharge criteria are not met or if patient is elderly and lives alone, an extended rehabilitative facility may be appropriate. • Institute home program with or without outpatient physical therapy (depending on the patient's preinjury activity level). Home exercise program should take the patient only 20 to 30 minutes 2 times per day to ensure compliance.	• Progress ambulation from use of a walker to use of a cane, but the walker should be used as long as the patient has a Trendelenburg lurch, which indicates continued gluteus medius weakness. • Emphasize gluteal strengthening, especially standing, to improve balance and proprioception. Do exercises on both legs to strengthen both concentric and eccentric components. • Stationary bicycle, pool exercises, treadmill may be of benefit.
Special Considerations		• Instruct patients with hemiarthroplasty in the use of adduction pillow, hip precautions (adduction, internal rotation, flexion), weight bearing to tolerance (WBTT). (See Chapter 7.)

Femoral Shaft Fractures

REHABILITATION RATIONALE

The most commonly used classification of femoral shaft fractures is that described by Winquist and Hansen (Fig. 4-7).

Currently, most femoral shaft fractures in adults, and many in adolescents, are treated with intramedullary nailing techniques. Fractures below the lesser trochanter to within 4 cm of the intercondylar notch can be stabilized with commercially available designs of intramedullary nails. Numerous studies have re-

ported union rates of 99%, infection rates of less than 1%, and overall complication rates of less than 5% with the use of intramedullary nails. Earlier mobilization and rehabilitation and improved care of polytrauma patients are advantages of intramedullary stabilization of femoral shaft fractures.

A contraindication to intramedullary nailing is contamination so severe that the open fracture wound cannot be converted to a clean contaminated wound, in which case traction or external fixation is used. External fixation may be converted to intramedullary fixation if wound stability is obtained within the first

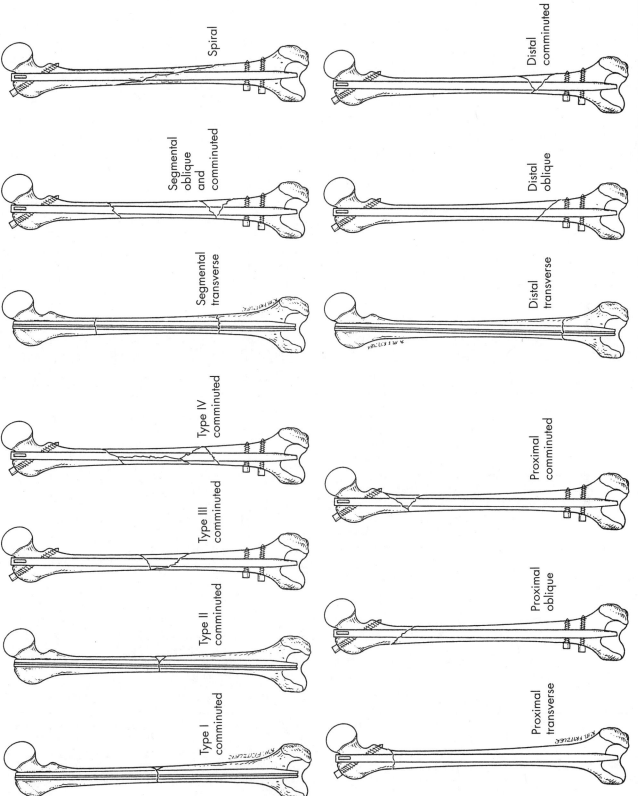

Figure 4-7 Winquist-Hansen classification of comminution (see text). (Redrawn from Winquist RA, Hansen RT, Clawson DK: *J Bone Joint Surg* 66A:529, 1984.) (From Kyle RF: *Fractures of the hip.* In Crenshaw AH, editor: *Campbell's operative orthopaedics,* St. Louis, 1993, Mosby–Year Book.)

2 weeks after injury; however, infection is much more likely when intramedullary nailing is performed after-prolonged external fixation or in patients with soft tissue envelopes with infection or drainage.

Plate-and-screw fixation is more appropriate for fractures with intraarticular extension into the hip or knee or in some patients with blunt chest trauma.

Traction rarely is used for adults with femoral shaft fractures, except for temporary stabilization until definitive stabilization can be obtained with external fixation or intramedullary nailing.

Technical aspects of intramedullary nailing that affect rehabilitation include the diameter of the nail used, the method of insertion, the mode of interlocking, the amount of fracture comminution, and the severity of soft tissue injuries.

Whether unreamed insertion techniques have any advantages over reamed insertion techniques is still controversial. However, nails inserted without reaming usually are of smaller diameter and have smaller screws than those inserted with reaming. Most au-

thors recommend a decrease in the amount of initial weight bearing when smaller diameter nails are used. Most static-locked 12-mm nails are sufficiently strong to permit unrestricted weight bearing if the fracture is stable with bone-on-bone contact. Partial weight bearing of 50 lbs usually is recommended during phase 1 (0 to 6 weeks) of rehabilitation if smaller diameter nails are used or if fracture comminution or bone loss prevents significant load sharing by the femur.

For transverse or short oblique fractures of the mid-shaft of the femur with good nail-to-bone fit, unlocked intramedullary nails can be used to control alignment. However, because the amount of fracture comminution often is underestimated and the amount of fracture stability often is overestimated, most authors currently recommend static locking (locking screws proximally and distally) of all intramedullary nails used for fixation of femoral shaft fractures to prevent late displacement and malunion. Dynamic locking (locking in only the proximal or distal fragment) rarely is indicated for femoral shaft fractures.

REHABILITATION PROTOCOL

Femoral Shaft Fracture Treated With Intramedullary Fixation

Phase 1
0 to 6 weeks

- If the fracture has bone-to-bone contact and a *stable* construct with a nail diameter of **12 mm** or more, allow weight bearing to tolerance, with progression to full weight bearing as tolerated, usually by 6 to 12 weeks. For patients with *unstable* fractures or fractures stabilized with **small-diameter nails**, begin with 25 kg ($\approx$ 50 lbs) weight bearing with crutches or walker as other injuries permit.
- Begin quadriceps sets, gluteal sets, hamstring sets, ankle pumps.
- Perform straight leg raising in all planes, supine and standing.
- Perform knee active ROM exercises (flexion and extension).
- Use stationary bicycle for ROM and strengthening.
- Instruct and observe crutch walking technique.
- Begin open- and closed-chain exercises as tolerated.

Phase 2
6 weeks to 3 months

- If full weight bearing is not possible, use a scale technique. The patient places the injured extremity on a scale to measure the amount of weight bearing that is comfortable. Instruct the patient to progress weight bearing in 5- to 10-kg

increments each week until full weight bearing is possible. Continue the crutches until the patient can bear full weight in the one-limb stance. Use a cane if necessary until gait is corrected with no lurch or Trendelenburg gait. Most patients regain 80% to 90% of full ROM during this phase. With smaller diameter nails (10 to 11 mm), achieve-full weight bearing incrementally using the scale technique for progression.
- Perform isokinetic exercises.
- Perform closed-chain exercises (p. 147).

Phase 3
3 to 6 months

- Most patients have progressed to full weight bearing and from crutches to a cane. If the patient is not full weight bearing and radiographic studies reveal lack of healing, consider either dynamization or bone augmentation (bone grafting, electrical stimulation).
- Continue closed-chain exercises until the patient obtains full knee and hip ROM, can perform a full squat, and can climb and descend stairs full weight bearing without an assistive device. Thigh circumference should be almost equal to the uninjured side before discontinuing rehabilitation.

REHABILITATION PROTOCOL—cont'd

Phase 4
>6 months
- Most patients have returned to athletic activities other than contact sports, which must be judged on an individual basis. If a plateau is reached with no improvement in the amount of weight bearing or evidence of nail loosening or screw breakage, and there are signs of radiographic nonunion, exchange nailing or autologous bone grafting may be considered.

CAUTION: If delayed healing is suspected, the patient should be evaluated to rule out occult infection, vascular insufficiency, or metabolic etiology for the nonunion.
- Resume full work and recreational activities as tolerated.

REHABILITATION PROTOCOL

Femoral Shaft Fracture Treated With Plate-and-Screw Fixation

Rehabilitation is the same as that following intramedullary nailing, with the exception that the patient is kept non–weight bearing with crutches for 8 to 12 weeks. Weight bearing is not progressed until evidence of consolidation of the fracture is visible on two radiographic views, usually at 3 to 6 months.

Phase 1
- Begin isometrics and upper extremity conditioning while in traction (preop).

Phase 2
- Apply cast brace or hinged, commercial rehabilitation brace.
- Ambulate with 20 kg weight bearing until evidence of bridging callus on two radiographic views.

- Begin open- and closed-chain exercises (p. 147).
- Perform ROM exercises for knee in cast brace.

Phase 3
- Remove brace.
- Ambulate with crutches until achieving full weight bearing in single leg stance.
- Progress open- and closed-chain exercises (p. 147).
- Stress active ROM and active-assisted ROM of the knee after cast removal.

Distal Femoral Metaphyseal and Epiphyseal Fractures

REHABILITATION RATIONALE

Because fractures in the distal femur frequently have intraarticular extension, they are more problematic than other fractures of the femoral shaft. The most commonly used classification of distal femoral fractures in adults is that of Müller et al. (Fig. 4-8). It is based on both the location and pattern of the fracture. In general, type A fractures involve only the metaphyseal area and have no intraarticular extension; type B fractures are medial, lateral, or posterior condylar fractures; and type C includes T and Y condylar fractures.

These fractures usually require open reduction and internal fixation for restoration of joint congruity. The type of internal fixation used varies with the type of fracture. Osteochondral blade plate-and-screw devices often are used for types A and C fractures, although more recently, intramedullary fixation techniques have been used successfully. Ganz described an indirect reduction and intramedullary fixation technique for type A fractures and nondisplaced type C1 fractures. This method maintains intraosseous blood supply by minimizing periosteal dissection. Maximum preservation of the soft tissue envelope results in less devascularization and earlier healing. Almost all type B fractures require fixation with lag screw techniques. Acute autologous bone grafting may be used in closed, severely comminuted (types A3 and C3) fractures.

Closed treatment with traction was advocated in the early part of the century, but currently this is used only for patients with osteopenic bone that is not suitable for stable internal fixation. External fixation rarely is indicated for these fractures.

■ *To avoid loss of reduction and malunion, weight bearing should be delayed for patients with distal femoral intraarticular fractures.*

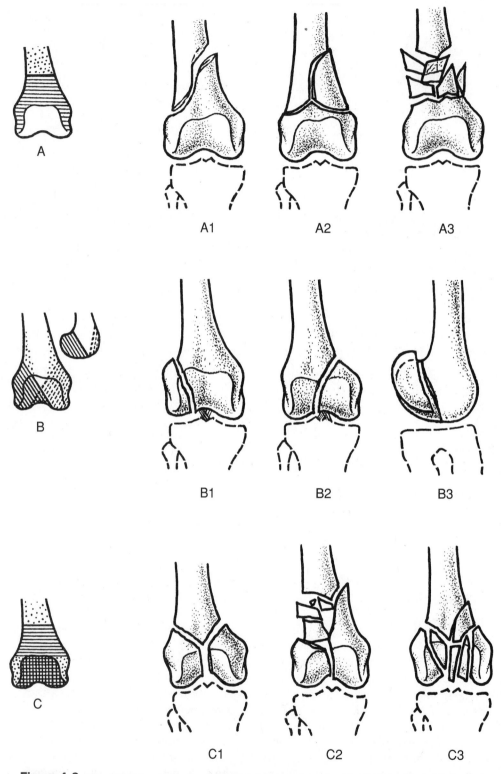

Figure 4-8 Classification of fractures of distal femur described by Müller et al. (Redrawn from Müller ME et al: *The comprehensive classification of fractures of long bones*, Berlin, 1990, Springer-Verlag.) (From Kyle RF: *Fractures of the hip*. In Crenshaw AH, editor: *Campbell's operative orthopaedics*, St Louis, 1993, Mosby–Year Book.)

REHABILITATION PROTOCOL

Distal Femoral Intraarticular Fracture With Plate-and-Screw or Intramedullary Fixation

Most patients do not regain full ROM after these injuries and should be advised of this early in the rehabilitation process.

Phase 1
0 to 6
weeks

- Begin active and active-assisted ROM exercises of the knee.
- May use CPM in the first 24 to 48 hours if fixation is sufficiently stable. In general, encourage 0 to 90 degrees of motion.
- Begin open-chain exercises (straight leg raises, quadriceps sets, and short arc quadriceps sets) and continue throughout rehabilitation.
- Allow only touchdown weight bearing.

Phase 2
6 to 12
weeks

- Begin stationary bicycling, minimal to no tension. Allow progression if fixation is stable and radiographs show callus and no fracture gap.
- Begin partial weight-bearing program with crutches or walker at 8 to 12 weeks, using the scale technique (p. 162).
- Begin closed-chain exercises and continue open-chain exercises (p. 147).

Phase 3
3 to 6
months

- Progress to full weight bearing.
- Perform closed- and open-chain exercises (p. 147).

■ *Delayed weight bearing, persistence of pain, and radiographic evidence of fracture gap at 3 to 6 months is an indication for cautious progression of weight bearing and the possibility of a delayed union or nonunion.*

Phase 4
>6 months

- Permit return to work and recreational activities, avoiding excessive squatting, climbing, and jumping. Avoid contact sports for 6 to 12 months, with evaluation of return to contact sports made on an individual basis.

Patellar Fractures

REHABILITATION RATIONALE

Patellar fractures are classified by several factors, including the amount of displacement, the severity of comminution, the amount of articular congruity, and the configuration of the fracture line. Patellar fractures in adults generally are classified as shown in the box.

Nondisplaced and stable fractures are treated nonoperatively. Functionally, this is indicated by the ability of the patient to extend the knee actively. An inability to extend the knee implies disruption of the extensor mechanism and functional loss, and is an indication for operative treatment. Other indications for operative treatment are comminution that requires total or partial patellectomy and an intraarticular fracture with more than 3 mm of displacement (step-off) of the articular surface. More than 3 mm of displacement or diastasis at the fracture site is a relative indication.

Most current fixation techniques for patellar fractures use a tension band concept that allows early, ac-

Classification of Patellar Fractures in Adults

Nondisplaced
Transverse
Vertical

Displaced
Transverse
Vertical

Comminuted
Entire patella (patellectomy)
Inferior pole (inferior pole patellectomy)
Superior pole (superior pole patellectomy)

Extraarticular

tive knee ROM after the soft tissues are stable. If patellectomy is performed, the retinaculum and extensor mechanism are repaired. Immobilization is continued for 6 to 8 weeks before ROM and closed-chain exercises are begun.

Patellar Fracture Treated Nonoperatively

0 to 6 weeks	• Wear long-leg cast for 2 to 3 weeks. • Allow weight bearing to tolerance with crutches. • Begin quadriceps sets, gluteal sets, hamstring sets, and straight leg raises in all planes (supine and standing) before discharge from the hospital (quadriceps sets help decrease adhesion formation during the healing process). • May begin open- and closed-chain exercises with the cast on, especially for hip strengthening. • Replace cast with controlled motion brace at 2 to 3 weeks. • Progress weight bearing to tolerance with crutches to weight bearing with the use of a cane. • In general, begin strengthening and ROM exercises at week 3 or 4 (open- and closed-chain exercises). • Begin gentle patellar mobilization; the patient should be independent with this exercise. • Begin scar mobilization to help desensitize the area. • Begin electrical muscle stimulation (EMS) for quadriceps reeducation. • Stationary bicycling with the seat elevated and no resistance is beneficial for ROM and strengthening. Initiate at approximately 6 weeks. • Begin isokinetic exercises at speeds of 60 to 120 degrees per second to strengthen the quadriceps musculature and decrease the forces on the patellofemoral joint that occur at lower speeds.

• Use stool scoots for hamstring strengthening (Fig. 4-9).
• Continue icing until effusion resolves.

6 to 12 weeks	• Begin and progress closed-chain exercises, such as minisquats and step-ups. • May use a Theraband for resistance in hip exercises and minisquats (Fig. 4-10). • Start BAPS board exercises. • Begin lunges. • Can use stationary bicycling with affected leg only to aid strengthening. • Since most patients with patellar fractures eventually develop some degree of chondromalacia, emphasize that restoration of quadriceps strength is essential to assist in the absorption of body-weight load that is transmitted up the kinetic chain. • The exercise program should emphasize restoration of lower extremity strength and flexibility. After this is achieved, implement a maintenance program with emphasis on closed-chain exercises. All exercises should be in a pain-free ROM. • Evaluate the entire lower extremity, especially for excessive pronation of the feet, which may add stresses to the knee and exacerbate patellofemoral-type symptoms. Use orthotics if excessive pronation is noted.

Patellar Fracture Treated With Open Reduction and Internal Fixation LOTKE AND ECKER

■ NOTE: *Rehabilitation protocols vary depending on the type of fracture, the surgical technique, and the rehabilitation philosophy of the surgeon. Gentle ROM intraoperatively after tension band wiring is often performed to observe the stability of the fracture and construct. This information is helpful for timing of postoperative ROM progression.*

1 to 2 days	• Permit weight bearing to tolerance in long-leg cast. • Ambulate and perform quadriceps sets. • Heel elevation for contralateral shoe is often used to help with ground clearance in straight leg cast during ambulation.
2 to 5 days	• Begin straight leg raises.
10 to 21 days	• Replace cast with controlled-motion brace. • Begin active ROM exercises (flexion and extension) of knee. Progress in controlled-motion brace by increasing locked setting on hinge.
6 weeks	• Begin passive ROM of knee.

REHABILITATION PROTOCOL—cont'd
Patellar Fracture Treated Nonoperatively

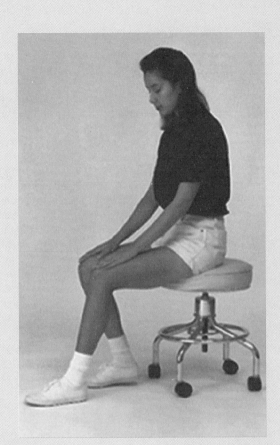

Figure 4-9 Stool scoots for hamstring strengthening.

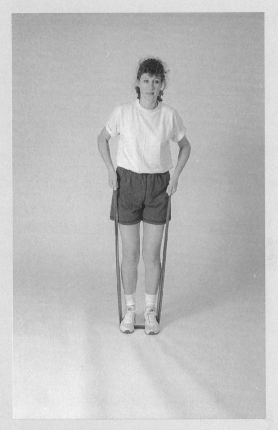

Figure 4-10 Theraband used for resistance during minisquats.

Acute Patellar Dislocation

REHABILITATION RATIONALE

Compared to recurrent patellar subluxation, acute patellar dislocation is rare. Almost all acute patellar dislocations are lateral, although intraarticular and superior dislocations have been reported. Because of the genu valgum of the normal knee, the quadriceps tendon tends to sublux the patella laterally, causing a tear in the medial retinaculum. The patella may dislocate over the edge of the lateral femoral condyle, and osteochondral fracture may occur. Patients with osteochondral fractures usually cannot flex the knee, have pain in the area of the medial retinaculum, and have severe hemarthrosis.

Most acute patellar dislocations are treated with closed reduction and immobilization in a cast or brace. Operative treatment may be necessary if an osteochondral fracture has occurred; any displaced osteochondral fragments are removed, and the disrupted medial tissues, including the vastus medialis muscle, are repaired.

Rehabilitation considerations include the mechanism of injury, the static patellar orientation (Q angle, patella baja or patella alta), and the dynamic patellar orientation (movement of the patella in functional movement patterns).

REHABILITATION PROTOCOL

Acute Patellar Dislocation

1 to 7 days	• Decrease edema with ice and elevation.
	• Begin isometric exercises, quadriceps sets, hamstring sets, gluteal sets, and adductor sets. (Because the vastus medialis obliquus [VMO] fibers originate from the adductor magnus, adductor strength is important in patellofemoral rehabilitation.)
	• Begin straight leg raises in all directions, with emphasis on adduction.
	• Evaluation of tight structures and stretching:
	  Iliotibial band may produce a lateral static force on the patella
	  Hamstrings, if tight, may increase the work of the quadriceps during knee extension
	  Gastrocnemius and soleus complex, if tight, may increase pronation during gait, which will increase the dynamic Q angle, causing the patella to track laterally
	• Perform manual resistive exercises (PNF for strengthening and to assess areas of weakness).
	• Perform short arc exercises to increase the amount of strength; use of EMS may be helpful.
	• Use stationary bicycle with the seat high and little to no resistance.
	• Use VMO biofeedback for VMO strengthening.

2 weeks	• Add weights to straight leg raises. If any pain, decrease the lever arm force by placing the weights around the proximal tibia or the distal thigh. • Increase VMO exercise range from 0 to 20 to 0 to 45 as tolerated and add resistance appropriately. • Continue stationary bicycle activity, progress to one-legged bicycling.

• Use standing hip machine or Theraband for resistance, again with emphasis on hip adduction.
• Pool exercises may be beneficial.
• Begin closed-chain exercises.
• Use BAPS board for ROM and proprioception.
• May use accessory weights to emphasize the concentric and the eccentric strength of the VMO.

3 to 6 weeks	• Begin isokinetics at a rate of 120 degrees per second in a pain-free ROM. • May use McConnell taping techniques (see Chapter 5) to assist with normalizing patellar alignment. Placing the patella in better alignment allows the VMO to fire at its optimal length, which increases its strength. • Progress closed-chain exercises. • Begin activities with both legs; progress to one-leg exercises, such as minisquats, stand-to-sit exercises, BAPS board, and wall sits. • Begin proprioceptive training with BAPS board and Fitter. • Use stair-climbing machine with short arcs and slow speeds.
6 to 12 weeks	• Continue closed-chain exercises. • Emphasize endurance with agility training as the patient returns to sports. • Consider placing a ¼-in wedge on the medial side under the shoe to decrease foot pronation and decrease stress on the knee while doing minisquats. • Evaluate for excessive pronation secondary to forefoot varus, rearfoot varus, or both. Make appropriate orthosis to correct the abnormalities.

Tibial Plateau Fractures

REHABILITATION RATIONALE

The most serious sequelae of tibial plateau fractures are articular incongruity and knee instability, which eventually lead to posttraumatic arthropathy and severe disability. Severe soft tissue injuries, including meniscal and ligamentous tears, often occur with tibial plateau fractures. Arterial and neurologic injuries also may occur with high-energy fractures.

Nondisplaced fractures with stable ligamentous structures may be treated with rest, immobilization and a cast-brace program with touchdown weight bearing. For displaced, depressed, or unstable frac-

tures, open reduction and internal fixation with a plate-and-screw device are indicated, except in patients with osteopenic bone, for stabilization of the epiphyseal, metaphyseal, and diaphyseal defects. Rasmussen listed as the primary indication for operative treatment varus/valgus instability of 10 degrees or more with the knee flexed less than 20 degrees. Because most of the tibia is subcutaneous, complications of wound dehiscence and infection are common with open reduction techniques. More recently, especially for severe fractures, limited internal fixation combined with external fixation of the metaphyseal component has proven successful.

The Schatzker classification of tibial plateau fractures (Fig. 4-11) has become the most widely used, replacing the earlier Hohl-Moore system. The Schatzker system aids in treatment decision making, as well as identifying the fracture type. **Type I** fractures are pure cleavage fractures for which screw fixation is adequate. **Type II** fractures are cleavage fractures, usually lateral, with depression. These require open reduction, elevation of the depressed fragment, fixation with a plate-and-screw device, and grafting with cancellous bone or a bone substitute. **Type III** fractures involve a central depression with no lateral wedge. They also require open reduction, internal fixation with buttress plating, and grafting. **Type IV** fractures are medial condylar fractures with either a split wedge or varying degrees of depression. These more severe injuries usually occur in younger patients, in whom ligamentous injuries should be suspected, and in patients with osteopenia. In addition to open reduction, internal fixa-

tion with a plate-and-screw device, and bone grafting, ligamentous repair often is required. Cruciate ligament avulsions with bony attachments are repaired at the time of fracture fixation. Repair of midsubstance cruciate ligament tears usually is delayed until active ROM knee is regained. **Type V** fractures are medial and lateral condylar fractures with a stable metaphyseal component. These usually are treated with open reduction and internal fixation with buttress plating or with external fixation supplemented by limited internal fixation of the intraarticular components. **Type VI** fractures are the most severe injuries, with condylar fractures and metaphyseal discontinuity; they require articular reconstruction and stabilization of the metaphyseal component. Recently, limited open reduction of the articular components and stabilization of the metaphyseal component with hybrid external fixation have been reported to give good results.

REHABILITATION PROTOCOL

Stable, Local Compression Fracture of the Tibial Plateau

LESS THAN 6-MM DEPRESSION, VARUS/ VALGUS STABILITY	• Begin early ROM (CPM, active assisted). • Keep non–weight bearing for 8 weeks, progressing to full weight bearing by 12 weeks.	**TIBIAL FRACTURES WITH LIGAMENTOUS INJURY**	• May limit ROM initially to allow healing of the ligamentous injury. • A motion control bracing system is preferable to a typical long-leg cast unless the patient is noncompliant.
GREATER THAN 6-MM DEPRESSION, VARUS/ VALGUS INSTABILITY MORE THAN 10 DEGREES	• Begin early ROM, use CPM. • Use touchdown to non–weight bearing for 8 weeks. Progress slowly to full weight bearing at 12 weeks. • Begin open-chain exercises. • Begin closed-chain exercises when weight bearing is allowed.		• Begin quadriceps sets, hamstring sets, gluteal sets, VMO strengthening, and straight leg raises with a stretching program that includes the hip, knee, and ankle. Tight hip flexors will shorten the involved leg, which is especially a problem if the patient already has decreased extension. • Begin patellar mobilization techniques (superior, inferior, medial, and lateral). • Delay full weight bearing for 8 to 12 weeks.
STABLE INTERNAL FIXATION POSSIBLE	• Begin CPM in recovery room. • The day after surgery, teach the patient quadriceps sets, hamstring sets, gluteal sets, and straight leg raises in all planes, supine and standing. • Delay weight bearing until healing is evident on radiographs, usually at 8 to 12 weeks. • When weight bearing is allowed, begin closed-chain exercises for the appropriate weight-bearing status of the patient (p. 147).		• May begin swimming and stationary bicycling at 8 weeks if clinical evidence of good healing is evident. • At 8 weeks, continue strength and ROM exercises. Begin a closed-chain exercise program and gradually progress. Begin PWB minisquats and gradually progress to stair-stepping.

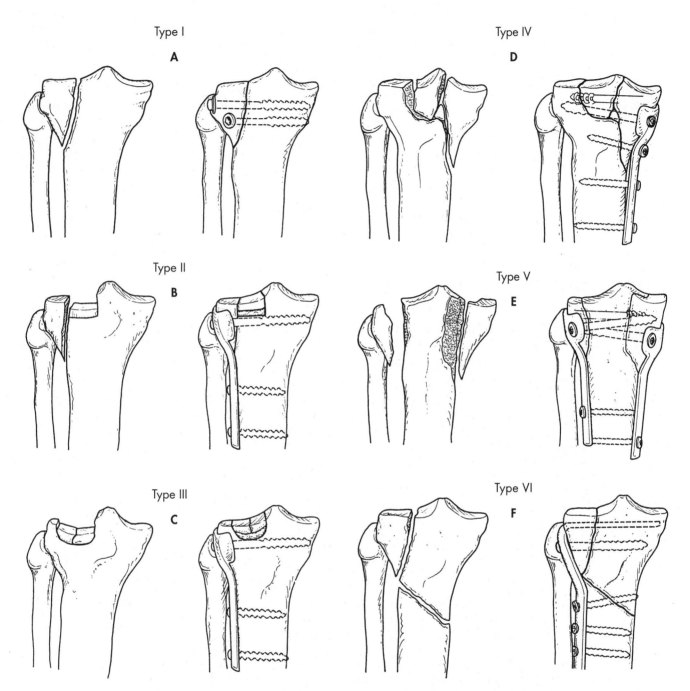

Figure 4-11 **A,** Type I, pure cleavage fracture. **B,** Type II, cleavage combined with depression. Reduction requires elevation of fragments with bone grafting of resultant hole in metaphysis. Lateral wedge is lagged on lateral cortex protected with buttress plate. **C,** Type III, pure central depression. There is no lateral wedge. Depression may also be anterior, posterior, or involve whole plateau. After elevation of depression and bone grafting, lateral cortex is best protected with buttress plate. **D,** Type IV. Medial condyle is either split off as wedge (type A) as illustrated, or it may be crumbled and depressed (type B), which is characteristic of older patients with osteoporosis (not illustrated). **E,** Type V. Note continuity of metaphysis and diaphysis. In internal fixation both sides must be protected with buttress plates. **F,** Type VI. Essence of this fracture is fracture line that dissociates metaphysis from diaphysis. Fracture pattern of condyles is variable and all types can occur. If both condyles are involved, proximal tibia should be buttressed on both sides. (Redrawn from Schatzker J, McBroom R, Bruce D: *Clin Orthop* 138:94, 1979).

REHABILITATION PROTOCOL

Stable Tibial Plateau Fracture or Operatively Stabilized Fracture

Phase 1
0 to 6 weeks

- Use CPM during hospitalization until obtaining 0 to 90 degrees of motion.
- Begin straight leg raises, quadriceps sets, and hamstring sets.
- Begin patellar mobilization techniques (medial, lateral, superior, and inferior).
- Begin active and active-assisted knee ROM exercises (**non**–weight bearing).
- Begin **gentle** passive ROM techniques for extension and flexion, including prone hangs, passive extension with roll under heel, and wall slides while lying supine.

Phase 2
6 to 12 weeks

- Begin progressive weight bearing, depending on fracture-fixation stability and radiographic findings of fracture repair.
- Allow stationary bicycling with minimal or no tension.

- Begin closed-chain exercises, initially with limited weight on affected extremity (8 to 12 weeks) (p. 147).

Phase 3
3 to 6 months

- Progress to full weight bearing and decrease dependence on ambulatory assistive devices in stepwise fashion (crutches-one crutch-cane).
- Continue open- and closed-chain exercises until thigh and calf circumferences are almost equal to opposite leg.
- Unaided stair climbing may be possible.
- Return to sedentary or light-duty work.

Phase 4
>6 months

- Progress work activities as tolerated. May require functional capacity evaluation for moderate to heavy work.
- Resume light recreation. No contact sports recommended for 1 year.

Tibial Shaft Fractures

REHABILITATION RATIONALE

Stable, Low-Energy Tibial Shaft Fractures

Closed reduction is preferred for stable, low-energy tibial shaft fractures. Exceptions include bilateral fractures, floating knee injuries, fractures with intraarticular extension, ipsilateral intraarticular fractures, and fractures in which closed reduction cannot be obtained or maintained. The patient is placed in a long, posterior splint with stirrup strap or a long-leg cast, and radiographs are obtained immediately to evaluate fracture alignment. No distraction of the fracture fragments should be accepted, because distraction of as little as 5 mm has been shown to increase healing time to as much as 8 to 12 months. Pins and plaster fixation of the tibial shaft fractures tends to distract the fracture and produces poorer results than do intramedullary nails and external fixators. Other criteria for an acceptable closed reduction are 10 degrees or less of angulation in any plane, 15 degrees or less of malrotation, and 1 cm or less of shortening.

The patient is admitted to the hospital for 24 to 36 hours to observe for possible compartment syndrome or tight cast. Immediate bivalving of the cast or measurement of compartment pressures should be performed if clinically indicated. During hospitalization, the leg should be iced at the fracture site and *maximally* elevated.

The average healing time of closed tibial shaft fractures treated with casting is 4 months. Sarmiento reported a 99.3% rate of union and no infections in his landmark article on the treatment of closed tibial fractures with a patellar-tendon bearing cast or functional brace. He observed that the initial shortening found on admission films was usually the maximum that would occur in closed treatment. Only 10% of his patients had shortening of 10 mm or more, and 3.9% had shortening of 1.5 cm or more (average shortening in all patients was 6.4 mm). There was a direct correlation of fracture healing to soft tissue injury, initial fracture displacement, comminution, an intact fibula, and time to bracing.

High-Energy, Unstable, or Open Tibial Shaft Fractures

Operative stabilization generally is required for high-energy tibial shaft fractures, many of which are open injuries. Relative indications for operative treatment include failure to obtain acceptable closed reduction, segmental fractures, displaced intraarticular fracture extension into the knee or ankle, bilateral shaft fractures, and fractures with compartment syndrome or vascular injury that requires arterial repair. Fixation may be obtained with plate-and-screw devices, intramedullary nails, or external fixators.

Gustilo-Anderson types (p. 144) I and II open tibial shaft fractures are treated with meticulous debridement and irrigation, removal of devitalized tissue and bone, and fixation with an unreamed, statically locked intramedullary nail. Proximal fractures (within 4 cm of the tibial plateau) or very distal fractures (within 5 cm of the ankle joint) may be treated with a biplanar external fixator. Type III open fractures are treated with meticulous sequential debridement and irrigation, removal of devitalized tissue and bone, soft tissue coverage as required, and fixation with a biplanar external fixator.

The likelihood of infection after open fracture can be decreased by meticulous debridement of devitalized or contaminated tissue and bone, combined with copious irrigation with 5000 to 10,000 cc of normal saline, followed by 2000 cc of bacitracin-polymixin solution. Early (5 to 7 days) soft tissue coverage is essential. Tissues are kept moist or provisional coverage, such as biologic dressing, is used until final coverage. Local or free-flap coverage of exposed bone should be done within 5 to 10 days to avoid bone devitalization.

Rehabilitation Principles

Postoperative rehabilitation of patients with operatively treated fractures depends on the following factors:

- Open or closed fracture. Open fractures have much higher incidences of delayed union and nonunion and have a poorer prognosis for healing than do closed fractures.
- Extent of injuries associated with open fracture, based on the Gustilo-Anderson classification (p. 144). This classification considers the mechanism of injury (high or low energy); the degree of soft tissue damage; the fracture configuration, comminution, and stability; the level of contamination; and concomitant neurovascular injuries.

- Stability of fracture fixation (strength and type of fixation used)
- Concomitant fractures of the ipsilateral or contralateral lower extremity. Other fractures may change the rate of rehabilitation and the progression of weight bearing.
- Overall medical condition of the patient. Some conditions are associated with delayed fracture healing, such as alcoholism, immunocompromise, and systemic diseases.
- Presence of superficial or deep infection.

Other Considerations

- **Bone graft by history.** If bone loss is more than 50% of cortical surface, early bone grafting is recommended at 6 to 8 weeks after the soft tissue environment has stabilized. Autogenous cancellous iliac bone is preferred.
- **Dynamization.** If bony consolidation is not progressing sequentially at approximately 6 weeks, options include removal of the screws from the longest fragment of the fracture to allow dynamization. This allows increased compression at the fracture, contact of the fracture ends, and improved healing. *Removing the screws from the longest fragment increases stability after removal.*
  If unacceptable shortening is anticipated because of bone loss, the implant should not be dynamized, but should be allowed to remain in static mode and a bone graft should be used.
- **Knee and foot ROM.** Active ROM exercises of the knee and foot should be continued whenever possible throughout the rehabilitation protocol to avoid knee flexion contracture or equinus deformity.
- **Early stabilization** of fractures in patients with multiple injuries reduces the incidence of pulmonary complications (adult respiratory distress syndrome, fat embolism, and pneumonia), decreases the number of days in the intensive care unit, and shortens the hospital stay (Bone et al.).
- The **rate of rehabilitation** may be slowed in type III wounds by soft tissue considerations. Anderson found that type III fractures averaged 3 months until soft tissue healing was complete. Soft tissue stability is aided by use of constructs such as foot mount on external fixators.

REHABILITATION PROTOCOL

Stable, Low-Energy Tibial Shaft Fracture Treated With Closed Reduction and Casting

0 to 3 weeks	• Begin quadriceps sets, hamstring sets, gluteal sets, and straight leg raises in all planes before discharge from the hospital. • Strongly encourage early weight bearing to tolerance on crutches. Use of a shoe lift for the contralateral extremity will aid in swing-through with a long, straight leg cast. • Make radiographs 7 to 10 days after reduction to check fracture alignment.
3 to 5 weeks	• Swelling should be diminished enough to allow careful fitting of a PTB cast or short leg cast. • Increase weight bearing as tolerated. • Begin active AROM exercises of the knee, 0 to 140 degrees. Perform straight leg raises and quadriceps sets several times a day, in addition to other open-chain exercises. • May use Theraband or ankle weights to add resistance. • Begin closed-chain exercises according to weight-bearing status.

6 to 8 weeks
• Patient should be ambulating weight bearing as tolerated in the PTB or short leg cast.
• Continue open- and closed-chain exercises for the hip and knee.
• Continue hip and knee ROM.

2 to 4 months
• Discontinue PTB or short leg cast when clinical evidence of complete healing is present (average healing time is 4 months). Determine healing with radiographic appearance and lack of tenderness on palpation and ambulation.
• Begin ankle stretching, ROM, and strengthening exercises.
• Continue progressive strengthening exercises, including leg presses, Stairmaster, lunges, toe raises, bicycling, and treadmill, until calf and thigh circumferences are equal to uninjured extremity.

■ *If fracture reduction is lost and alignment becomes unacceptable during weight bearing, the fracture probably should have been stabilized initially with an intramedullary nail. Treat loss of reduction with reduction and fixation with an intramedullary nail or biplanar external fixator.*

REHABILITATION PROTOCOL

Open Tibial Shaft Fracture Treated With Unreamed, Static Interlocked Intramedullary Nail

Phase 1
0 to 6 weeks
• Apply PTB or short leg cast.
• Patients with 8-mm or 9-mm nail begin touchdown weight bearing with crutches or walker.
• 10-mm nails or larger allow partial weight bearing with crutches.
• Begin active and passive knee ROM exercises.
• Begin quadriceps sets, VMO sets, short arc quadriceps exercises (open chain).
• Begin closed-chain exercises according to weight-bearing status (p. 147).

Phase 2
6 weeks to
3 months

STABLE FRACTURE
• Discontinue cast if early callus is present.
• Start ankle and subtalar ROM, continue knee therapy (active ROM plus towel stretches).
• Progress to weight bearing as tolerated with crutches.
• Progress closed-chain rehabilitation.

TYPE III OPEN FRACTURE
• Consider *"bone graft by history"* at 6 weeks, or eventual exchange nailing at 8 to 12 weeks, for 8- or 9-mm nail if no callus is visible or continued bone defect is present.

Continued

REHABILITATION PROTOCOL—cont'd

Open Tibial Shaft Fracture Treated With Unreamed, Static Interlocked Intramedullary Nail

Phase 3
3 to 6 months

- Progress to weight bearing as tolerated with crutches.
- Dynamize (remove distal or proximal screws) if minimal evidence of healing and gap present at fracture.
  NOTE: remove screws that are the greatest distance from fracture.
- Consider bone graft if no fracture gap and evidence of delayed healing in open fracture.
- If the fracture is united, progress to cane, then to independent ambulation.

- Resume functional activities and begin agility training; return to sports as tolerated.

Phase 4
>6 months

- If ununited, treat for **delayed union/ nonunion** with exchange nailing, bone graft, electrical stimulation, or fibular osteotomy.
- Rule out biologic problem, such as infection or vascular insufficiency.

REHABILITATION PROTOCOL

Tibial Shaft Fractures Treated With Biplanar Hexfix External Fixation

Stable Open Fractures

Phase 1
0 to 6 weeks

- Begin partial weight bearing with crutches (30 lbs).
- Begin knee and hip ROM exercises (open chain).
- Cover soft tissue at 5 to 7 days.
- Begin closed-chain rehabilitation according to weight-bearing status.

Phase 2
6 weeks to 3 months

- If soft tissues are stable, apply PTB cast or long-leg cast after fixator removal.
- If soft tissues are unstable, maintain and dynamize (see p. 172) external fixator; remove foot mount attachment when soft tissues are stable (Fig. 4-12).
- Continue with open-chain exercises and progress with closed-chain exercise.

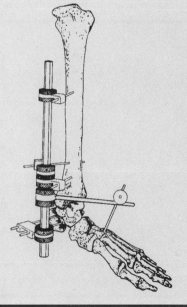

Figure 4-12 Immobilization of ankle and foot for fractures just proximal to ankle. Two pins are inserted into calcaneus, and one or more pins are placed in base of metatarsal. (Courtesy Smith & Nephew Richards, Inc, Memphis.)

REHABILITATION PROTOCOL—cont'd

Stable Open Fractures—cont'd

Phase 3
3 to 6 months
- If minimal callus, consider bone grafting.

Phase 4
6 months
- If healing is not progressing, treat as delayed union (see nonunion guidelines, p. 172).
- Do *not* use intramedullary nail fixation because of high incidence of infection with intramedullary nailing after external fixation.

Unstable Tibial Fractures (Closed and Open Types I and II)

Phase 1
0 to 6 weeks
- Begin touchdown weight bearing with crutches.
- Perform hip and knee ROM exercises (open chain).
- Stabilize foot with foot-mount attachment to control soft tissue motion in open fractures (especially distal third fractures).

Phase 2
6 weeks to 3 months
- Remove foot mount and dynamize frame (p. 172).
- Begin aggressive active and passive ROM of ankle and knee: SLRs, quadriceps sets, VMO exercises, short arc quadriceps sets.
- Progress weight bearing with crutches.
- Continue open-chain exercises and begin closed-chain rehabilitation.

Phase 3
3 to 6 months
- Begin weight bearing to tolerance with crutches.
- Perform bone graft if evidence of delayed healing.
- Ensure frame is properly dynamized.
- Progress closed-chain rehabilitation.

Phase 4
>6 months
- If no evidence of healing, treat for delayed union (p. 174).

Unstable Tibial Fracture (Open Type III)

Phase 1
0 to 6 weeks
- Begin touchdown weight bearing with crutches.
- Stabilize foot with foot-mount attachment on all frames for soft tissue stability.
- Begin hip and knee ROM exercises.

■ *Note: Be aware of the type of coverage used. For example, a free flap may not "take" if too much movement in the area decreases wound stability.*

Phase 2
6 weeks to 3 months)
- Bone graft by history at 6 weeks:
  Posterolateral—preferred because of good blood supply and better incorporation of bone graft; skin usually better.
  Posteromedial—often indicated in proximal fourth of tibia (where peroneal nerve makes posterolateral approach difficult).
  Anteromedial—skin must be in good condition.
- Slowly progress weight bearing over several weeks.
- If gap present at fracture, manually compress fracture in office or at time of surgery.
- Remove foot mount.
- Perform aggressive ankle and knee ROM exercises.
- Continue open-chain and begin closed-chain exercises.

Phase 3
3 to 6 months
- Begin weight bearing to tolerance with crutches.
- Dynamize fixator (see p. 174).
- Progress closed-chain rehabilitation.

Phase 4
>6 months
- If no evidence of healing, treat as delayed union or nonunion (p. 174).

Tibial Shaft Fracture Treated With Biplanar Ilizarov External Fixation

Phase 1
0 to 6 weeks
- Begin partial weight bearing as tolerated.
- In general, keep patients with intraarticular fractures at partial weight bearing at 30 to 50 lbs for 4 to 6 weeks (Fig. 4-13).
- Allow patients with nonarticular injuries to be weight bearing to tolerance.

■ *Patient must be at least partially weight bearing before discharge from hospital to avoid contracture.*

- Begin aggressive exercises for ankle and knee ROM: ankle pumps, ankle inversion and eversion exercises, SLRs, quadriceps sets, VMO exercises (open chain, p. 147).

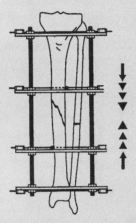

Figure 4-13 Ilizarov-type fixation of tibia and fibula.

- Retighten frame bolts before discharge from hospital.
- Use walking shoe and Theraband for dorsiflexion stretching to prevent equinus contracture if foot mount is not used.
- Use towel stretches for passive dorsiflexion of ankle.
- Begin closed-chain rehabilitation according to weight-bearing status.

Phase 2
6 weeks to 3 months
- Begin weight bearing to tolerance.
- Maintain wire tension and treat pin-tract infection aggressively.
- Evaluate for contractures and treat as necessary with passive ROM and active ROM exercises.
- Advance closed-chain rehabilitation.

Phase 3
3 to 6 months
- If evidence of delayed healing, compress fracture ¼ turn for 20 days.

Phase 4
>6 months
DELAYED UNION
- Ensure frame stability, revise and replace wires as necessary.
- Watch closely for pin-tract problems.
- Biologic treatment: bone graft or compression/distraction.
- Apply splint to avoid equinus contracture, if needed.

PREVENTION OF CONTRACTURES WITH THE USE OF ILIZAROV-TYPE EXTERNAL FIXATION

Ankle equinus and knee flexion contractures are the two most common deformities that occur with lower limb Ilizarov fixation. Hip flexion contractures may occur with femoral fixators. These may be avoided by stretching exercises, night positioning, splinting, and functional use of the extremity.

Passive stretching exercises for the calf and hamstring muscles should be done 2 to 3 hours each day. Calf stretching should include towel stretches, runners' stretch, use of an incline board, and use of rubberbands for dorsiflexion.

■ *Passive exercises are far more effective in preventing contractures than are active exercises.*

Night positioning is helpful in preventing contractures by changing the patient's usual sleeping posture. Most patients with an Ilizarov-type fixator choose a position that places the foot in plantar flexion and the knee in flexion. Patients are taught to place a pillow under the most distal ring of the fixator to keep the knee extended and to wear a shoe with the foot tied in dorsiflexion to the frame (Fig. 4-14).

Both static and dynamic splinting have a role in the management of patients with Ilizarov-type fixation. *Static splints* include fixed-position orthoses (AFO foot mount), straps, ropes, and other nonelastic devices to hold the foot out of equinus (in neutral). These devices are especially helpful at night, when the constant pressure of a dynamic splint may be too uncomfortable to allow sleep. *Dynamic splints* may be as simple as an elastic band from the shoe to the fixator. More elaborate devices include a spring-loaded, clamp-on dynamic extension splint.

Functional use of the extremity is important not only to prevent contractures, but also to encourage

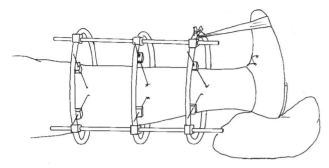

Figure 4-14 Ilizarov fixator. (Note that knee is straight and foot is in dorsiflexion.)

bone regeneration. Weight bearing is strongly encouraged. An obstacle course provides good motivation for younger patients. Retro walking on a treadmill decreases the amount of dorsiflexion needed in the gait. The amount of dorsiflexion needed can be controlled by increasing the incline of the treadmill. As ROM improves, the incline height can be gradually decreased until the patient is able to walk forward. This allows patients without full dorsiflexion to increase weight bearing on the involved leg and to ambulate without pain or limp.

Pilon Fractures of the Distal Tibia

REHABILITATION RATIONALE

Intraarticular fractures of the distal tibia are relatively uncommon, accounting for approximately 7% of all tibial fractures. They are caused either by axial compressive loads (e.g., a fall from a height) or from rotational forces, which usually are lower energy injuries. Pilon fractures can be severe injuries, with varying degrees of open fracture, soft tissue swelling, soft tissue loss, articular damage, bone loss, impaction, compromised circulation to bone fragments and soft tissues, and extension of the fracture into the tibial shaft. Rüedi and Allgöwer classified pilon fractures according to displacement and comminution, and Mast, Spiegel, and Pappas expanded this classification to include the mechanism of injury (Fig. 4-15).

Although restoration of articular congruity is of primary importance, severe soft tissue injuries can make both exposure and closure difficult, and severe comminution may make open reduction extremely difficult or impossible. Because of these difficulties, some authors prefer delayed internal fixation or limited open reduction and the use of either a circular external fixator that bridges the joint and foot or a hybrid half-pin fixator with a pin through the distal articular fragment to allow ankle motion. Operative treatment should include reduction and fixation of the fibula, anatomic reduction of the articular surface, bone grafting of the metaphyseal defect, and support of the fracture fragments medially with a buttress plate. In general, open reduction and internal fixation are recommended for patients with good soft tissue stability and minimal swelling; external fixation is recommended for patients with open wounds, severe swelling and contusion, and extremely comminuted fractures.

Early joint motion should be encouraged, but weight bearing should be delayed for 8 to 12 weeks after injury.

REHABILITATION PROTOCOL

Pilon Fractures of the Distal Tibia

0 to 6 weeks
- Use maximal elevation and icing for 7 to 10 days.
- Ensure non–weight bearing with crutches or wheelchair.
- Place compliant patients with stable fixation in removable commercial boot (e.g., 3-D boot).
- Continue straight leg raises and active ROM exercises for knee and hip throughout rehabilitation.

6 weeks to 3 months
- At surgeon's discretion, may begin swimming with continued non–weight bearing in pool.
- Partial weight bearing may be initiated at 8 to 12 weeks, depending on fracture stability, stability of fixation, and radiographic appearance of callus.

- At 8 to 12 weeks, begin passive towel stretches for ankle and gentle passive ROM exercises with therapist.

When full weight bearing is achieved:
- Progress bicycling with added tension and endurance, lowering the seat to increase ROM (avoid too low for anterior knee pain). Progress until only using involved leg.
- Initiate retro walking with incline, slowly decreasing the incline, and progress to forward walking.
- Toe raises, stair-stepper
- Vigorous passive stretching with focus on maximizing dorsiflexion
- Employ capsular stretching techniques with gentle joint manipulation to assist with joint ROM.

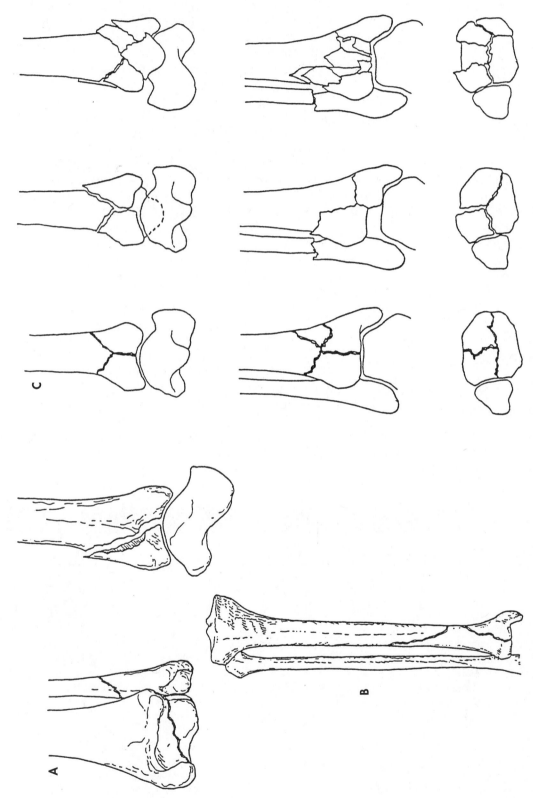

Figure 4-15 Classification of Mast, Spiegel, and Pappas for pilon fractures of tibia. **A,** Type I—supination–external rotation fracture with vertical loading at time of injury. **B,** Type II—spiral extension fracture. **C,** Type III—vertical compression fractures, graded according to displacement and comminution according to classification of Ruedi and Allgower. (Redrawn from Mast JW, Spiegel PG, Pappas JN: *Clin Orthop* 230:68, 1988.)

Bibliography

Alho A et al: Comparison of functional bracing and locked intramedullary nailing in the treatment of displaced tibial shaft fractures, *Clin Orthop* 227:243, 1992.

Alho A et al: Locked intramedullary nailing for displaced tibial shaft fractures, *J Bone Joint Surg* 72B(5):805, 1990.

Anderson LD et al: Fractures of the tibia and fibula treated by casts and transfixing pins, *Clin Orthop* 105:179, 1974.

Arnold WD: The effect of early weight-bearing on the stability of femoral neck fractures treated with Knowles pins, *J Bone Joint Surg* 66A:847, 1984.

Austin RT: The Sarmiento tibial plaster: a prospective study of 145 fractures, *Injury* 13:10, 1981.

Ayeni JP: Pilon fractures of the tibia: a study based on 19 cases, *Injury* 19:109, 1988.

Barrick EF, Jackson CB: Prophylactic intramedullary fixation of the tibia for stress fracture in a professional athlete, *J Orthop Trauma* 6(2):241, 1992.

Behrens F, Searles K: External fixation of the tibia: basic concepts and prospective evaluation, *J Bone Joint Surg* 68B:246, 1986.

Bennett FS et al: Ipsilateral hip and femoral shaft fractures, *Clin Orthop* 296:168, 1993.

Benirschke SK et al: Immediate internal fixation of open, complex tibial plateau fractures: treatment by a standard protocol, *J Orthop Trauma* 6(1):78, 1992.

Bergman GD et al: Subtrochanteric fracture of the femur, *J Bone Joint Surg* 69A:1032, 1987.

Blokker CP, Rorabeck CH, Bourne RB: Tibial plateau fractures: an analysis of the results of treatment in 60 patients, *Clin Orthop* 182:193, 1984.

Bogoch ER, Ouellette G, Hastings DE: Intertrochanteric fractures of the femur in rheumatoid arthritis patients, *Clin Orthop* 294:181, 1993.

Bone LB: Fractures of the tibial plafond: the pilon fracture, *Orthop Clin North Am* 18:95, 1987.

Bone LB, Johnson KD: Treatment of tibial fractures by reaming and intramedullary nailing, *J Bone Joint Surg Am* 68:877, 1986.

Bone LB et al: Early versus delayed stabilization of femoral fractures: a randomized study, *J Bone Joint Surg* 71A:336, 1989.

Bone LB et al: Prospective study of union rate of open tibial fractures treated with locked, unreamed intramedullary nails, *J Orthop Trauma* 8:45, 1994.

Bosse MJ et al: Heterotopic ossification as a complication of acetabular fracture: prophylaxis with low-dose irridation, *J Bone Joint Surg* 70A:1231, 1988.

Bourne RB, Rorabeck CH, Macnab J: Intra-articular fractures of the distal tibia: the pilon fracture, *J Trauma* 23:591, 1983.

Braten M et al: Bone loss after locked intramedullary nailing: computed tomography of the femur and tibia in 10 cases, *Acta Orthop Scan* 63(3):310, 1992.

Brien WW et al: Subtrochanteric femur fractures: a comparison of the Zickel nail, 95 degrees blade plate, and interlocking nail, *J Orthop Trauma* 5(4):458, 1991.

Briggs TW et al: Isolated tibial fractures in children, *Injury* 23(5):308, 1992.

Brumback RJ: Open tibial fractures: current orthopaedic management, *Instr Course Lect* 41:101, 1992.

Brumback RJ et al: Acetabular depression fracture accompanying posterior fracture dislocation of the hip, *J Orthop Trauma* 4:42, 1990.

Brumback RJ et al: Heterotopic ossification about the hip after intramedullary nailing for fractures of the femur, *J Bone Joint Surg* 72A:1067, 1990.

Burnett JW et al: Prophylactic antibiotics in hip fractures, *J Bone Joint Surg* 62A:457, 1980.

Carnesale PG, Anderson LD: Primary prosthetic replacement for femoral neck fractures, *Arch Surg* 110:27, 1975.

Carnesale PG, Stewart MJ, Barnes SN: Acetabular disruption and central fracture-dislocation of the hip: a long-term study, *J Bone Joint Surg* 57A:1054, 1975.

Cimino WG, Corbett ML, Leach RE: The role of closed reduction in tibial shaft fractures, *Orthop Rev* 19:233, 1990.

Connolly JF, Denhne E, Lafollette B: Closed reduction and early cast-brace ambulation in the treatment of femoral fractures, part II: results in one hundred and forty-three fractures, *J Bone Joint Surg* 55A:1581, 1973.

Cotler HB, LaMont JG, Hansen ST Jr: Immediate spica casting for pelvic fractures, *J Orthop Trauma* 2:222, 1988.

Cryer HM et al: Pelvic fracture classification: correlation with hemorrhage, *J Trauma* 28:973, 1988.

Court-Brown CM: Fractures of the tibial diaphysis. *Int J Orthop Trauma* 3(2):40, 1993.

Cuckler JM, Tamarapalli JR: An algorithm for the management of femoral neck fractures, *Orthopedics,* 17(9):789, 1994.

Dabezies EJ et al: Fractures of the femoral shaft treated by external fixation with the Wagner device, *J Bone Joint Surg* 66A:360, 1984.

DeLee JC, Clanton TO, Rockwood CA Jr: Closed treatment of subtrochanteric fractures of the femur in a modified cast-brace, *J Bone Joint Surg* 63A:772, 1981.

DeLee JC, Evans JA, Thomas J: Anterior dislocation of the hip and associated femoral-head fractures, *J Bone Joint Surg* 62A:960, 1980.

Den Outer AJ et al: Conservative vs operative treatment of displaced noncomminuted tibial shaft fractures: a retrospective comparative study, *Clin Orthop* 252:231, 1990.

Drennan DB, Locher FG, Maylahn DJ: Fractures of the tibial plateau: treatment by closed reduction and spica cast, *J Bone Joint Surg* 61A:989, 1979.

Edeiken-Monroe BW, Browner BD, Jackson H: The role of standard roentgenograms in the evaluation of instability of pelvic ring disruption, *Clin Orthop* 240:63, 1989.

Edwards CC: Staged reconstruction of complex open tibial fractures using Hoffmann external fixation: clinical decisions and dilemmas, *Clin Orthop* 178:130, 1983.

Ekeland A et al: Interlocking intramedullary nailing in the treatment of tibial fractures: a report of 45 cases, *Clin Orthop* 231:205, 1988.

Epstein HC, Wiss DA, Cozen L: Posterior fracture dislocation of the hip with fractures of the femoral head, *Clin Orthop* 201:9, 1985.

Fischer MD, Gustilo RB, Varecka TF: The timing of flap coverage, bone-grafting, and intramedullary nailing in patients who have a fracture of the tibial shaft with extensive soft-tissue injury, *J Bone Joint Surg* 73A(9):1316, 1991.

Fishmann AJ et al: Prevention of deep vein thrombosis and pulmonary embolism in acetabular and pelvic fracture surgery, *Clin Orthop* 305:133, 1994.

Frederick D, Seligson D: Developments in locked femoral nailing, *Orthopedics* 13:1141, 1990.

Ganz R, Thomas RJ, Hammerle CP: Trochanteric fractures of the femur: treatment and results, *Clin Orthop* 138:30, 1979.

Garden RS: Reduction and fixation of subcapital fractures of the femur, *Orthop Clin North Am* 5:683, 1974.

Gerber C, Strehle J, Ganz R: The treatment of fractures of the femoral neck. *Clin Orthop* 292:77, 1993.

Ghalambor N, Matta JM, Bernstein L: Heterotopic ossification following operative treatment of acetabular fracture: an analysis of risk factors, *Clin Orthop* 305:96, 1994.

Gill SS, Nagi ON, Dhillon MS: Ipsilateral fractures of femoral neck and shaft, *J Orthop Trauma* 4:293, 1990.

Goldhill VB et al: Bipolar hemiarthroplasty for fracture of the femoral neck, *J Orthop Trauma* 5(3):318, 1991.

Gray G: *Chain reaction*, Kirkland, Wash, 1989, Wynn Marketing.

Green A, Trafton PG: Early complications in the management of open femur fractures: a retrospective study, *J Orthop Trauma* 5:51, 1991.

Gustilo RB: *Management of open fractures and their complications*, Philadelphia, 1982, WB Saunders.

Gustilo RB, Gruninger RP, Davis T: Classification of type III (severe) open fractures relative to treatment and results, *Orthopedics* 10:1781, 1987.

Gustilo RB, Mendoza RM, Williams DN: Problems in the management of type III (severe) open fractures: a new classification of type III open fractures, *J Trauma* 24:742, 1984.

Hammer R: Team approach to tibial fracture: 37 consecutive type III cases reviewed after 2-10 years, *Acta Orthop Scand* 63(5):471, 1992.

Heckman JD et al: Acceleration of tibial fracture-healing by non-invasive, low-intensity pulsed ultrasound, *J Bone Joint Surg* 76A:26, 1994.

Henderson RC et al: Residual bone-mineral density and muscle strength after fractures of the tibia or femur in children. *J Bone Joint Surg Am* 74(2):211, 1992.

Henley MB, Meier M, Tencer AF: Influences of some design parameters on the biomechanics of the unreamed tibial intramedullary nail, *J Orthop Trauma* 7(4):311, 1993.

Hohl M: Tibial condylar fractures: an instructional course lecture, the American Academy of Orthopaedic Surgeons, *J Bone Joint Surg* 49A:1455, 1967.

Holmes CA et al: Biomechanics of pin and screw fixation of femoral neck fractures, *J Orthop Trauma* 7(3):242, 1993.

Holt EM et al: 1000 femoral neck fractures: the effect of pre-injury mobility and surgical experience on outcome, *Injury* 25(2):91, 1994.

Hooper GJ, Keddell RG, Penny ID: Conservative management or closed nailing for tibial shaft fractures: a randomized prospective trial, *J Bone Joint Surg* 73B(1):83, 1991.

Horne G et al: Disability following fractures of the tibial shaft, *Orthopedics* 13:423, 1990.

Hougaard K, Thomsen PB: Traumatic posterior fracture-dislocation of the hip with fracture of the femoral head or neck, or both, *J Bone Joint Surg* 70A:233, 1988.

Jalovaara P, Virkkunen H: Quality of life after primary hemiarthroplasty for femoral neck fracture: 6-year follow-up of 185 patients, *Acta Orthop Scan* 62(3):208, 1991.

Jensen DB et al: Tibial plateau fractures: a comparison of conservative and surgical treatment, *J Bone Joint Surg* 72B:49, 1990.

Johnson EE, Kay RM, Dorey FJ: Heterotopic ossification prophylaxis following operative treatment of acetabular fracture, *Clin Orthop* 305:88, 1994.

Johnson EE et al: Delayed reconstruction of acetabular fractures 21-120 days following injury, *Clin Orthop* 305:20, 1994.

Judet R, Judet J, Letournel E: Fractures of the acetabulum: classification and surgical approaches for open reduction: preliminary report, *J Bone Joint Surg* 46A:1615, 1964.

Kaempffe FA, Bone LB, Border JR: Open reduction and internal fixation of acetabular fractures: heterotopic ossification and other complications of treatment, *J Orthop Trauma* 5(4):439, 1991.

Kaufer H, Matthews LS, Sonstegard D: Stable fixation of intertrochanteric fractures: a biomechanical evaluation, *J Bone Joint Surg* 56A:899, 1974.

Kebaish AS, Roy A, Rennie W: Displaced acetabular fractures: long-term follow-up, *J Trauma* 31(11):1539, 1991.

Keller CS, Laros GS: Indications for open reduction of femoral neck fractures, *Clin Orthop* 152:131, 1980.

Koval KJ et al: Complications of reamed intramedullary nailing of the tibia, *J Orthop Trauma* 5:184, 1991.

Koval KJ et al: Indirect reduction and percutaneous screw fixation of displaced tibial plateau fractures, *J Orthop Trauma* 6(3):340, 1992.

Leenen LP et al: Internal fixation of open unstable pelvic fractures. *J Trauma* 35(2):220, 1993.

Letournel E: Acetabulum fractures: classification and management, *Clin Orthop* 151:81, 1980.

Letournel E, Judet R: *Fractures of the acetabulum*, New York, 1981, Springer-Verlag.

Leung KS et al: Operative treatment of unstable pelvic fractures, *Injury* 23(1):31, 1992.

Lu-Yao GL et al: Outcomes after displaced fractures of the femoral neck: a meta-analysis of one hundred and six published reports, *J Bone Joint Surg* 76(1):15, 1994.

Marya SKS, Bhan S, Dave PK: Comparative study of knee function after patellectomy and osteosynthesis with a tension band wire following patellar fractures, *Int Surg* 72:211, 1987.

Matta JM: Operative indications and choice of surgical approach for fractures of the acetabulum, *Techniques Orthop* 1:13, 1986.

Matta JM: Operative treatment of acetabular fractures through the ilioinguinal approach: a 10-year perspective, *Clin Orthop* 305:10, 1994.

Matta JM et al: Fractures of the acetabulum: a retrospective analysis, *Clin Orthop* 205:230, 1986.

Matta JM, Saucedo T: Internal fixation of pelvic ring fractures, *Clin Orthop* 242:83, 1989.

Mauer DJ, Merkow RL, Gustilo, RB: Infection after intramedullary nailing of severe open tibial fractures initially treated with external fixation, *J Bone Joint Surg Am* 71:835, 1989.

Mawhinney IN, Maginn P, McCoy GF: Tibial compartment syndromes after tibial nailing, *J Ortho Trauma* 8(3):212, 1994.

Mayo KA: Open reduction and internal fixation of fractures

of the acetabulum: results in 163 fractures, *Clin Orthop* 305:31-7, 1994.

McConnell J: The management of chondromalacia patellae: a long-term solution, *Aust J Physiother* 32:215, 1986.

McKellor H et al: Control of motion of tibial fracture with use of a functional brace or an external fixator, *J Bone Joint Surg* 75A:1019, 1993.

Mendez AA, Joseph J, Kaufman EE: Stress fractures of the femoral neck following hardware removal from healed intertrochanteric fractures, *Orthopedics* 16(7):822, 1993.

Merchant TC, Dietz FR: Long-term follow-up after fracture of the tibial and fibular shafts, *J Bone Joint Surg* 71A:599, 1989.

Moed BR, Watson JT: Intramedullary nailing of fractures of the tibial shaft utilizing an intraoperative two-pin external fixator, *J Bone Joint Surg* 17(3), 1993-1994.

Moore TM: Fracture-dislocation of the knee, *Clin Orthop* 156:128, 1981.

Müller ME et al: *The comprehensive classification of fractures of long bones,* Berlin, 1990, Springer-Verlag.

Nielsen JO, Dons-Jensen H, Sørensen HT: Lauge-Hansen classification of malleolar fractures: an assessment of the reproducibility in 118 cases, *Acta Orthop Scand* 61:385, 1990.

Nilsson LT et al: Function of the hip after femoral neck fractures treated by fixation or secondary total hip replacement, *Int Orthop* 15(4):315, 1991.

Nilsson LT, Johansson A, Stromqvist B: Factors predicting healing complications in femoral neck fractures: 138 patients followed for 2 years, *Acta Orthop Scan* 64(2):175, 1993.

Pantazopoulos T et al: Surgical treatment of acetabular posterior wall fractures, *Injury* 24(5):319, 1993.

Pitsaer E, Samuel AW: Functional outcome after intertrochanteric fractures of the femur: does the implant matter? a prospective study of 100 consecutive cases, *Injury* 24(1):35, 1993.

Quan-yi L, Jia-Wen W: Fracture of the patella treated by open reduction and external compressive skeletal fixation, *J Bone Joint Surg* 69A:83, 1987.

Rae PS, Khasawneh ZM: Herbert screw fixation of osteochondral fractures of the patella, *Injury* 19:116, 1988.

Richardson JB et al: Measuring stiffness can define healing of tibial fractures, *J Bone Joint Surg* 76B(3):389, 1994.

Routt MLC Jr, Swiontkowski MF: Operative treatment of complex acetabular fractures: combined anterior and posterior exposures during the same procedure, *J Bone Joint Surg* 72A:897, 1990.

Rüedi T, Allgöwer M: Fractures of the lower end of the tibia into the ankle joint: results 9 years after open reduction and internal fixation, *Injury* 5:130, 1973.

Rüedi TP, Allöwer M: The operative treatment of intraarticular fractures of the lower end of the tibia, *Clin Orthop* 138:105, 1979.

Sanders R et al: Retrograde reamed femoral nailing, *J Orthop Trauma* 7(4):293, 1993.

Sarmiento A: A functional below-the-knee cast for tibial fractures, *J Bone Joint Surg* 49A:855, 1967.

Sarmiento A: A functional below-the-knee brace for tibial fractures: a report on its use in one hundred thirty-five cases, *J Bone Joint Surg* 52A:295, 1970.

Sarmiento A et al: Factors influencing the outcome of closed tibial fractures treated with functional bracing, *Clin Orthop* 315:8, 1995.

Sarmiento A et al: Prefabricated functional braces for the treatment of fractures of the tibial diaphysis, *J Bone Joint Surg* 66A:1328, 1984.

Schatzker J: Compression in surgical treatment of fractures of the tibia, *Clin Orthop* 105:220, 1974.

Schatzker J, McBroom R, Bruce D: The tibial plateau fracture: the Toronto experience 1968-1975, *Clin Orthop* 138:94, 1979.

Schatzker J, Waddell JP: Subtrochanteric fractures of the femur, *Orthop Clin North Am* 11:539, 1980.

Shih CH, Wang KC: Femoral neck fractures: 121 cases treated by Knowles pinning, *Clin Orthop* 271:195, 1991.

Sikorski JM, Barrington R: Internal fixation versus hemiarthroplasty for the displaced subcapital fracture of the femur: a prospective randomised study, *J Bone Joint Surg* 63B:357, 1981.

Simpson LA, Kellam JF, Tile M: The surgical management of femoral head fractures occurring with anterior dislocation of the hip, *Techniques Orthop* 1:23, 1986.

Tile M: Pelvic ring fractures: Should they be fixed? *J Bone Joint Surg* 70B:1, 1988.

Trafton PG: Subtrochanteric-intertrochanteric femoral fractures, *Orthop Clin North Am* 18:59, 1987.

Triffitt PD et al: Cast immobilization and tibial diaphyseal blood flow: an initial study, *J Orthop Res* 10(6):784, 1992.

Triffitt PD et al: Compartment pressures after closed tibial shaft fracture: their relation to functional outcome, *J Bone Joint Surg Br* 74(2):195, 1992.

Trunkey DD, Hapman MW, Lim RC: Management of pelvic fractures and blunt traumatic injury, *J Trauma* 14:912, 1974.

van Veen IH et al: Unstable pelvic fractures: a retrospective analysis, *Injury* 26(2):81, 1995.

Watson JT: Current concepts review: treatment of unstable fracture of the shaft of the tibia, *J Bone Joint Surg* 76A:1575, 1994.

Whittle AP et al: Treatment of open fracture of the tibial shaft with the use of interlocking nailing without reaming, *J Bone Joint Surg* 74A:1162, 1992.

Whittle AP, Wester W, Russell TA: Fatigue failure in small diameter interlocking tibial nails: implications for postoperative care, *Clin Orthop* 136, 1995.

Wickstrom J, Corban MS: Intramedullary fixation for fractures of the femoral shaft: a study of complications in 298 operations, *J Trauma* 7:551, 1967.

Winquist RA, Hansen ST Jr: Comminuted fractures of the femoral shaft treated by intramedullary nailing, *Orthop Clin North Am* 11:633, 1980.

Wiss DA, Brien WW: Subtrochanteric fractures of the femur: results of treatment by interlocking nailing. *Clin Orthop* (283):231, 1992.

Wiss DA, Brien WW, Stetson WB: Interlocked nailing for treatment of segmental fractures of the femur, *J Bone Joint Surg* 72A:724, 1990.

Wu C, Shih C: Complicated open fractures of the distal tibia treated by secondary interlocking nailing, *J Trauma* (6):792, 1993.

Wu CC, Shih CH: Femoral shaft fractures associated with unstable pelvic fractures. *J Trauma* 34(1):76, 1993.

Ylinen P, Santavirta S, Slätis P: Outcome of acetabular fractures: a 7-year follow-up, *J Trauma* 29:19, 1989.

CHAPTER FIVE

The Knee

S. BRENT BROTZMAN, MD
PENNY HEAD, PT

Anterior Cruciate Ligament Reconstruction

REHABILITATION RATIONALE

Rehabilitation after reconstruction of the anterior cruciate ligament (ACL) has changed significantly in recent years, with protocols becoming increasingly aggressive. Despite changes in protocol design, however, the goal of rehabilitation has remained the same: to return the patient to a preinjury level of activity. This involves restoration of normal range of motion (ROM), strength, and stability of the knee to allow return to functional activities. In athletes, the rehabilitation program must also strive to restore agility, skill, and speed, as well as a functionally stable knee that can withstand all rigors of sports-related activities.

After ACL reconstruction, the proper balance between protection of the reconstructed ligament and prevention of disuse sequelae may be difficult. The reconstructed ligament must be properly protected to allow healing and to prevent excessive strain on the graft; however, prolonged immobilization is not desirable because of the numerous detrimental effects associated with this form of treatment, including disuse atrophy of muscle tissue, severe changes in articular cartilage and ligaments, and the loss of joint ROM from the formation of intraarticular adhesions.

Although numerous rehabilitation protocols have been based on clinical observations of ACL patients, a relative paucity of research exists to provide basic scientific information on how rehabilitation affects the reconstructed ligament *in vivo*. "Accelerated" rehabilitation programs have recently become widely used, despite their apparent divergence from accepted biomechanical and histologic principles. These accelerated protocols are based on the observation that patients who did not comply with the restrictions imposed by a traditional protocol had better ROM, strength, and function without compromising joint stability than did those who complied.

Rehabilitation programs continue to progress as new information becomes available about factors affecting the reconstructed ligament. Although no definitive ACL protocol has been universally agreed on as the most effective, most current protocols stress the following principles:

- Initiation of early ROM and weight bearing
- Early edema control techniques
- Avoidance of excessive stress to the graft (avoiding excessive *early* open-chain exercises)
- Early hamstring strengthening to provide dynamic joint stability and to decrease strain on the graft
- Proprioceptive retraining and neuromuscular reeducation.
- Muscle strengthening and conditioning
- Incorporation of closed kinetic chain exercises

- Sports-specific agility training
- Aerobic cardiovascular training
- A bracing algorithm
- Criteria-based progression from one level to the next
- Criteria-based return to athletic activity

BASIC SCIENCE AND BIOMECHANICS

■ *In early stages of healing, failure of the ACL graft usually occurs at the site of fixation, rather than in the graft itself.*

Central third patellar tendon graft (bone-patellar tendon-bone graft)

According to Huegel and Indelicato, the central third patellar tendon graft is fixed in position through bony or fibrous union within 6 to 8 weeks postoperatively. Lambert suggests that union may occur as early as 3 weeks, while Kurosaka et al. report that 3 to 4 months may be necessary to achieve stable, solid graft incorporation.

Noyes et al. demonstrated that a 14- to 15-mm patellar tendon graft has 175% of the tensile strength of the normal ACL. This figure is somewhat deceiving, however, because most ACL grafts used today are 10 mm wide. The 10-mm patellar tendon graft is believed to be 107% as strong as the normal ACL at the time of implantation. Extrapolation of Clancy et al.'s original data predicts that the 10-mm graft is 57% as strong as the original ACL at 3 months after surgery, 56% at 6 months, and 87% at 9 and 12 months.

Andrews and Wilk developed a theoretic graft strength model in humans, based on extrapolation of the collective work of Clancy, Noyes, and Warren. The extrapolated values point out two principles: (1) the clinically used 10-mm patellar tendon graft has significantly less strength than the 14-mm graft, and (2) significant loading and stress during the weakened periods of graft necrosis, synovial envelopment, remodeling, and revascularization should be minimized to avoid possible graft elongation or failure.

Arnoczky et al. report that although revascularization may be complete at 5 months after surgery, the graft does not resemble the normal ACL in structural, vascular, and histologic appearance until 1 year; therefore, the graft has not developed the strength to oppose normal ACL forces at the time of complete revascularization.

Noyes et al. suggest that most strenuous activities seldom expose the ACL to more than 50% of its maximum load. Therefore, according to the extrapolated values, the ACL graft should be capable of tolerating an intense weight program at 3 months after reconstruction and jogging on level surfaces at 5 months. O'Meara et al. suggests that by 9 months after reconstruction, the ACL has attained its maximum level of tensile strength.

Histologic studies of ACL graft tissue from 6 weeks to 4.75 years after implantation by Amiel et al. and Clancy et al. showed that the transplanted tissue remained consistently viable, attaining maximum fibroblast size and number by 6 months after surgery and proceeding in maturation to "ligamentization." Shelbourne et al. suggest that accelerated rehabilitation may actually speed the process of ligamentization by guiding the graft to a more functional cellularity; that is, accelerated rehabilitation may actually strengthen the graft rather than stretch it.

Hamstring Grafts

Hamstring grafts (semitendinosus and gracilis) provide weaker initial fixation and have a more prolonged and variable rate of fixation into bone than do central third patellar tendon grafts. Hamstring grafts also have the disadvantage of bone-to-tendon healing rather than the more stable bone-to-bone healing. For these reasons, hamstring grafts have not been recommended for ACL reconstruction unless the patellar tendon graft is contraindicated or not possible. Recently there has been some return to the use of hamstring grafts because of a fairly significant incidence of patellofemoral/anterior knee pain associated with harvesting the patellar tendon graft.

Allografts

The morbidity to the extensor mechanism (donor site) in autologous patellar tendon grafting has resulted in an increased use of allografts for ACL reconstruction. Current indications for the use of allograft tissue are previous failure of autograft surgery, significant patellofemoral arthrosis, a narrow patellar tendon, and patients who do not want to sacrifice their own tissue.

Four areas of concern must be carefully considered before deciding to use allograft tissue for ACL reconstruction: (1) immunogenicity of the allograft, (2) preservation and secondary sterilization of the graft tissue, (3) remodeling and its effects on mechanical properties, and (4) potential disease transmission. Several methods of graft preparation have been studied, including freeze-drying, ethylene oxide, fresh-freezing, irradiation, and various combinations of these. Some authors currently recommend high-dose radiation (up to 4 megarads) to sterilize the graft, despite studies that show a decrease in structural strength with irradiation. These authors suggest that sterilization is inadequate with 2 megarads of radiation. The maturation process of allografts appears comparable to that of autologous grafts, but may be slower. Current data suggest minimal differences between the ultimate biomechanical properties of allografts and autografts. Autologous central third patellar tendon graft failure rates range from 10% to 17%, whereas allograft failure rates range from 10% to 16%. We seldom employ allografts except in cases of failed autograft surgery. This avoidance is based on the catastrophic consequence of transmission of the HIV virus.

REHABILITATION CONSIDERATIONS

Preoperative Rehabilitation

Preoperative rehabilitation of acute ACL injury should focus on the following:

- Decreasing joint effusion
- Restoring full ROM
- Strengthening the quadriceps and hamstrings
- Restoring a normal gait pattern

Joint effusion usually can be controlled with limb elevation, cryotherapy, compression, and modalities such as high-voltage galvanic stimulation (HVGS); however, aspiration also may be required. It is extremely important to diminish joint effusion because of its neuromuscular inhibitory effects on the quadriceps, which result in rapid atrophy of the quadriceps muscles.

Several studies report an increased incidence of *arthrofibrosis* after reconstruction of an **acutely** injured ACL. Shelbourne et al. noted a decreased incidence of arthrofibrosis by delaying surgery at least 3 weeks. We delay ACL reconstruction until the patient has regained full ROM with minimal to no pain. This avoids the risk of loss of motion associated with attempting to rehabilitate a swollen knee with an acutely inflamed, painful synovium.

Graft Fixation

The type of fixation used to secure the graft is an important consideration in determining the rehabilitation program. The advent of stronger initial fixation, such as interference Kurosaka screws, and stronger graft tissue (central third patellar tendon grafts) has allowed successful implementation of earlier ROM and weight bearing after ACL reconstruction, which avoids many of the complications associated with prolonged immobilization. With a bone-patellar tendon-bone graft, union of the osseous tunnels may occur as early as 3 weeks or as long as 3 to 4 months after surgery (Fig. 5-1). Until union occurs, the fixation site is the weakest link in resisting tensile forces, not the graft itself.

Early Motion in an "Accelerated" Protocol

Historically, patients with ACL reconstructions were treated with prolonged immobilization to protect the graft tissue. This conservative form of treatment resulted in numerous complications, such as intraarticular adhesions, joint stiffness, patellofemoral crepitus and pain, and profound quadriceps weakness. Eriksson and Haggmark demonstrated 40% quadriceps atrophy after just 5 weeks of immobilization. In addi-

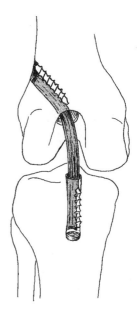

Figure 5-1 Central third patellar tendon ACL graft with interference screw fixation.

tion, the rate of atrophy was increased with immobilization in a shortened position (such as joint flexion). A rapid decline in the biomechanical and histologic properties of bone, ligament, and articular cartilage with prolonged immobilization has been well documented in the literature. Because of these proven effects of immobilization, rehabilitation has become increasingly focused on obtaining early motion of the knee.

■ *The hallmark of accelerated rehabilitation protocols is an emphasis on aggressive, early accomplishment and long-term maintenance of full knee extension.*

Clancy et al. reported a decrease in knee flexion contractures from more than 10 degrees at 8 weeks after surgery with traditional rehabilitation, to an incidence of 1.7% using an accelerated protocol. Shelbourne and Nitz also reported a decreased incidence of arthrofibrosis from 12% with traditional ACL rehabilitation to 4% using the accelerated protocol.

The goals for ROM in an accelerated protocol, according to Fu et al., are full knee extension (equal to the uninvolved knee) within 2 to 3 weeks after surgery and full flexion within 8 weeks.

Reducing Stress on the ACL Graft

The current trend of accelerated ACL rehabilitation appears to diverge somewhat from the established basis of science and rehabilitation principles. To minimize postoperative complications, such as arthrofibrosis and quadriceps atrophy, ACL rehabilitation has become more aggressive; however, this aggressive rehabilitation must be performed in a manner that minimizes inflammation and avoids excessive loading on the reconstructed ligament.

Closed Kinetic Chain (CKC) Exercises Versus Open Kinetic Chain (OKC) Exercises

Knee exercises for rehabilitation after ACL reconstruction are divided into two broad categories: open kinetic chain and closed kinetic chain.

Closed kinetic chain (CKC) exercises are those in which motion at the knee is accompanied by motion at the hip and ankle. The distal segment of the extremity (foot) is in contact with a pedal, platform, or ground surface. Examples of CKC exercises include minisquats, cycling, and leg presses (Fig. 5-2).

CKC exercises promote cocontraction and increase stability through increased joint compressive loads. Cocontraction minimizes the anterior translation of the tibia on the femur that occurs with increased compressive loads, thus reducing shear forces on the joint and strain on the ACL. Because of reduced strain on the ACL, CKC exercises can be incorporated early in

the rehabilitation program to strengthen the quadriceps.

In addition to developing muscle strength, CKC exercises optimize functional capacity by reeducating proprioceptors in a manner that stimulates functional and sports-related activity. Because CKC exercises use the body's natural movements and planes, all proprioceptors are stimulated to some extent. The use of multiplanar movements, acceleration, and deceleration allows a much more sport-specific form of rehabilitation. This form of exercise strengthens both the agonist and the antagonist muscles, thus enhancing neuromuscular coordination and proprioception required during functional activities.

Open kinetic chain (OKC) exercises are those in which motion at the knee is independent of motion at the hip and ankle. The distal segment of the extremity (foot) is free to move. Examples of OKC exercise include leg extensions and leg curls.

OKC quadriceps exercise, e.g., Kin-Com quadriceps strengthening, often is avoided early in ACL rehabilitation because of the significant stress it places on the reconstructed ligament. Numerous studies have demonstrated that OKC quadriceps exercises through a full ROM may damage the graft. This form of exercise isolates quadriceps activity, thus increasing anterior translation of the tibia and placing excessive strain on the ACL graft from 30 degrees flexion to full extension.

OKC quadriceps exercise can be used in a restricted ROM, avoiding the last 30 to 45 degrees of knee extension, to allow the isolated quadriceps strengthening that is necessary to restore normal strength and muscle girth.

Quadriceps setting is a form of OKC exercise that is used early in many ACL protocols. Early use of this isometric exercise improves neuromuscular control of the quadriceps and reduces the risk of quadriceps shutdown. It also aids in the resorption of joint effusion and provides superior mobilization of the patella, thus helping to prevent infrapatellar contracture syndrome and knee flexion contracture.

Straight leg raising is another OKC exercise that can be used early in ACL protocols. This exercise involves isometric contracture of the quadriceps with simultaneous isotonic contraction of hip musculature (adductors, abductors, flexors, or extensors). Straight leg raises initiated early in the rehabilitation program help reduce atrophy and weakness of the quadriceps and hip musculature. The patient should be able to perform a quadriceps set sufficiently to prevent an extensor lag before beginning straight leg raising exercises.

OKC hamstring curls can be performed early in the rehabilitation program because they decrease the level of strain on the ACL throughout the entire ROM. Because the hamstrings are the primary dynamic stabi-

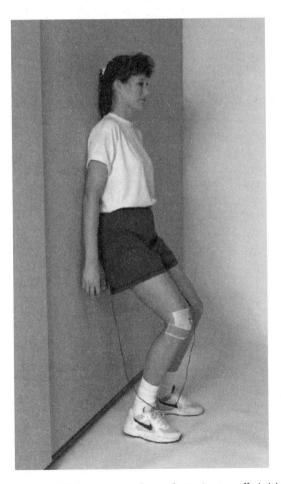

Figure 5-2 Minisquats performed against wall initially (wall sits). Patient does not flex beyond 30 degrees. These are later performed without a wall.

lizers of the knee, early initiation of hamstring strengthening should be emphasized.

Active, isolated quadriceps contraction in a non–weight-bearing position (OKC), places undesirable shearing stress on the reconstructed ligament by increasing anterior translation of the tibia on the femur. When external resistance as low as 7 lbs. is applied to the distal tibia, the quadriceps force required to extend the leg is almost 2 times the force required with no resistance. This significantly increases the stress on the reconstructed ACL.

■ *Shearing stress on the ACL is greatest from 30 degrees of flexion to full extension.*

This stress can be neutralized either by simultaneous, isometric contraction of the hamstrings with the quadriceps (cocontraction), in either an open- or closed-chain fashion, or by avoiding open-chain quadriceps exercises between 0 to 45 degrees of flexion. This restriction of ROM avoids isolated quadriceps contraction in the zone of greatest ACL stress.

Cocontraction of the hamstrings with the quadriceps (such as in minisquats or leg presses) adds a posterior translatory force to counteract anterior translation induced by the quadriceps; therefore, cocontraction is thought to stabilize the knee during the strengthening process. Many ACL protocols avoid active-resisted isolated quadriceps strengthening for several months after ACL reconstruction because of the potential stress on the graft. Instead, they incorporate CKC exercises to promote cocontraction of the hamstrings and quadriceps to protect the graft during strength training. The hamstrings are the primary dynamic stabilizers of the knee, acting synergistically with the ACL, as well as protecting it from excessive stress. Reestablishing a hamstring/quadriceps strength ratio that is equivalent to or higher than that of the unoperated limb has produced better functional outcomes after ACL reconstruction.

Another advantage of CKC exercises is the significant decrease in patellofemoral joint forces compared with those generated by OKC quadriceps exercises in the range of 60 to 90 degrees of knee flexion. CKC quadriceps exercises generally are performed with the knee in nearly full extension, thus avoiding one of the most common pitfalls of ACL rehabilitation: the patellofemoral pain syndrome. Paulos' "paradox of exercise" is successfully avoided by using CKC quadriceps strengthening instead of OKC exercises from 60 to 90 degrees.

Timing of Rehabilitation Progression

The exact time constraints for healing and maturation of ACL grafts, as well as the loads that they can withstand at specific points of time, are not entirely understood.

After carefully studying ACL stresses and elongation involved in functional and rehabilitative activi-

ties, Henning et al. concluded that the proper order of a rehabilitation program, with regard to ACL stress, should be the following:

1. Crutch walking
2. Stationary cycling
3. Walking
4. Slow running on level surface
5. Faster running on level surface

They also determined that CKC exercises, such as minisquats, could be incorporated early in the rehabilitation progression because of the minimal amount of ACL elongation produced with these exercises. They caution patients to avoid downhill running, because running down a 4.5-degree decline at 5 mph produces ACL elongation twice as great as running on a level treadmill. OKC knee extension exercises through a full ROM also are avoided because they cause significant elongation of the ACL.

Rubenstein and Shelbourne base their postoperative program on rehabilitation of the donor site rather than on protection of the ACL graft, and they stress early motion (including full extension) and quadriceps strengthening. Their guidelines include the following:

- Careful selection of patients with consideration of age and activity demands and desires
- Preoperative rehabilitation to attain ROM and quadriceps strength
- Delay of surgery until the patient is physically and mentally ready
- Regular visits to monitor rehabilitation after surgery so that developing problems can be recognized and corrected
- Long-term follow-up.

Rubenstein and Shelbourne believe that common postoperative complications are largely avoided if the following goals are attained by 2 weeks after surgery:

- Full knee extension
- Minimal swelling
- Leg control (active control by quadriceps)
- 90 degrees of flexion

Neuromuscular Retraining

The intact ACL has been demonstrated to have an important sensory function in the normal knee. Studies indicate that the normal ACL has mechanoreceptors that may be able to detect joint position, as well as sudden or slow joint position changes. Disruption of the ACL destroys the mechanoreceptors, thus eliminating normal joint proprioception. Reconstruction of the ligament does not restore these mechanoreceptors. In addition, immobilization after ACL reconstruction decreases proprioception in the muscles, tendons, and other ligaments around the knee joint, causing the mechanoreceptors to "forget" their role in controlling acceleration and deceleration of the lower extremity.

Developing proprioception and incorporating intricate timing with muscular strength and power are essential to performing functional activities. More traditional rehabilitation protocols emphasize the concepts of strength and motion; accelerated protocols incorporate the concepts of proprioception and agility, making these protocols more functional.

Through preathletic-training exercise, increasingly complex knee-joint activities are gradually introduced. With this progression of exercise, the patient may be able to learn to rely more heavily on the knee's remaining proprioceptive structures, thus compensating for the loss of the ACL mechanoreceptors.

Proprioceptive retraining involves sensory activation of the tendons, ligaments, capsules, and muscles. This process begins early in accelerated rehabilitation protocols. Early, controlled weight bearing and CKC exercises help to reeducate proprioceptors in the lower extremity. Passive cycling is an example of proprioceptive retraining that can be initiated relatively early. More complex proprioceptive activities, such as agility training, are typically introduced later in the rehabilitation progression.

Joint Effusion

Joint effusion is a secondary effect of any operative procedure. Persistent joint effusion occurs in approximately 12% of patients with ACL reconstructions. The primary complication of joint effusion is its inhibitory effect on the quadriceps muscles. Patients with joint effusions typically experience significant quadriceps atrophy because of neuromuscular inhibition. Studies demonstrated that a 60-cc infusion of normal saline into a knee joint results in a 30% to 50% inhibition of voluntary quadriceps contraction. As joint pressure increases, stimulation of types I and II mechanoreceptors increases the threshold of the spinal reflex arc by Hoffmann's reflex, resulting in neuromuscular inhibition.

Because of its inhibitory effect, it is important to diminish joint effusion as early as possible after ACL reconstruction. Typically, the patient is instructed in edema control techniques, such as ice, compression, limb elevation, and active quadriceps setting and ankle pumps. Many clinicians also use commercially available cooling/compression devices, such as the CryoCuff (Aircast Inc., Summit, NJ), immediately after surgery to minimize joint effusion.

Loss of Motion

Loss of motion (LOM) is one of the most common complications after ACL reconstruction. Sachs et al. reported a 24% incidence of knee flexion contracture of more than 5 degrees after ACL reconstruction, and Harner et al. reported an 11.1% incidence.

Fu et al. define LOM as knee flexion contracture of more than 10 degrees and/or knee flexion ROM of less than 125 degrees. Functionally, loss of knee extension appears to be more serious than loss of knee flexion.

Loss of knee extension after ACL surgery may lead to an abnormal gait, quadriceps weakness, and patellofemoral pain.

Arthrofibrosis

Several studies report a frequent occurrence of arthrofibrosis after reconstruction of an acutely injured ACL. Shelbourne et al. suggest that delaying surgery at least 3 weeks from the time of injury significantly decreases the incidence of arthrofibrosis. ACL reconstruction should be delayed until the patient has regained full ROM of the knee with only minimal pain. Postoperative rehabilitation of a knee with an acutely inflamed, painful synovium may increase the risk of LOM.

Cross-Over Effect

The cross-over effect is a neurophysiologic concept in which exercise in one extremity causes strengthening in the opposite extremity. This concept can be used early in the rehabilitation program with isometric quadriceps setting bilaterally to induce a stronger quadriceps contraction in the involved extremity. Some clinicians also have patients continue with exercises on both the operated and nonoperated knees to increase this cross-over effect. It has been reported that strength in the involved extremity may be increased as much as 30% through this effect.

Continuous Passive Motion (CPM)

Continuous passive motion (CPM) is a gentle method of promoting and advancing knee ROM. It was introduced by Salter et al. in 1970, and its use has been shown to have distinct physiologic effects on soft tissue and joint surfaces. Numerous studies have reported the benefits of initiating early motion, including nutrition of the articular cartilage, retarding intraarticular adhesions and joint stiffness, and providing early controlled forces acting on collagenous tissues. The literature suggests, however, that there are also dangers in the use of CPM.

Studies that advocate the judicious use of CPM after ACL reconstruction include those of Noyes and Mangine, who demonstrated increased knee ROM with no increase in joint effusion and no increase in joint laxity in their patients; O'Driscoll et al., who reported accelerated clearance of blood and fluid from the joint, which may facilitate mobility of the joint; and Salter et al., who concluded that CPM can counter the deleterious effects of immobilization by inhibiting intraarticular adhesions, improving articular cartilage nutrition, accelerating the clearance of hemarthrosis, and improving matrix formation by stimulation of the chondrocytes.

Many clinicians prefer to involve patients actively in their own rehabilitation as early as possible. This can be done by using active, active-assisted, and passive ROM initiated by the patient, rather than by a

CPM device. Other concerns regarding the use of CPM include danger to the reconstruction if the ROM settings are inappropriate or if the unit is incorrectly placed on the patient, potential damage to the graft through cyclic fatigue at the notch margins, and development of knee flexion contracture or extensor lag because the CPM does not always permit terminal knee extension. Rosen et al. found no beneficial or detrimental effects with CPM use, but did note its significant financial cost.

Electromyogram (EMG) Biofeedback

The use of electromyogram (EMG) biofeedback can be a valuable tool in neuromuscular reeducation of the quadriceps. This modality provides visual and/or auditory feedback when a preset goal has been obtained with muscle contraction; stronger contractions elicit stronger feedback. This form of treatment requires active participation by the patient, and "rewards" the patient when the goal of muscle contraction is reached. EMG biofeedback can be used with both OKC and CKC exercises.

EMG biofeedback transforms myoelectric signals produced by the muscle into visual and/or auditory signals for the patient. A threshold or goal is set by the therapist for the patient to try to obtain. Once the patient produces a strong enough muscle contraction to exceed the threshold level, the visual and/or auditory signals occur. The threshold can then be raised to elicit a stronger contraction by the patient.

A common use for EMG biofeedback is to improve contraction of the vastus medialis obliqus (VMO) (Fig. 5-3). When joint effusion inhibits quadriceps activity, research indicates that the VMO "wastes first and wastes most." Because it is the only medial dynamic stabilizer of the patella, weakness of the VMO results in patellar maltracking, which may lead to patellofemoral pain syndrome.

Electrical Muscle Stimulation

The use of electrical muscle stimulation (EMS) after ACL reconstruction remains controversial. The primary goal of EMS for these patients is to minimize postoperative quadriceps atrophy and weakness. Results in the literature vary widely regarding the benefits of EMS. Some studies describe significant clinical benefits, such as decreased strength loss in the early postoperative period, more rapid gains in ROM, and increased overall rate of return to athletic activity; other studies report less optimistic results, stating that EMS is no more effective than volitional exercise in maintaining quadriceps strength.

A more recent study by Snyder-Mackler et al. reported that the use of a high-intensity electrical stimulation regimen, in conjunction with an aggressive postoperative training program, resulted in at least

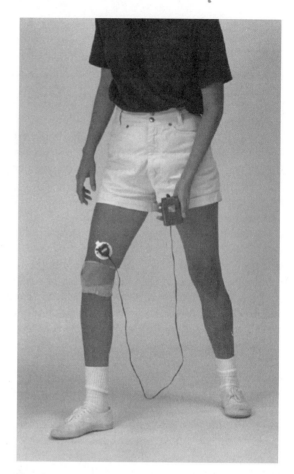

Figure 5-3 EMG biofeedback of vastus medialis oblique (VMO) muscle to improve quality of contraction.

70% quadriceps strength recovery by 6 weeks after surgery. This was compared with 51% strength recovery using low-intensity electrical stimulation (portable muscle stimulation) and 57% strength recovery with volitional training alone. Snyder-Mackler et al. report that although low cost and ease of use may tempt clinicians to use portable electrical stimulators after ACL reconstruction, results do not support their effectiveness in improving quadriceps strength recovery. They recommend the use of high-intensity electrical stimulation in addition to an aggressive rehabilitation program for promoting quadriceps recovery and improving functional outcome.

ACL BRACING

Knee braces are classified into four categories: prophylactic, rehabilitative, functional and transitional.

Prophylactic Braces

Prophylactic braces attempt to prevent or reduce the severity of knee ligament injuries. These braces are designed to protect the medial collateral ligament by resisting medial joint opening. Theoretically, this brace should also prevent injury to the anterior and posterior cruciate ligaments from a valgus-producing force. At present there is no convincing clinical or biomechanical evidence to support the routine use of prophylactic braces to reduce the number or severity of knee injuries.

Rehabilitative Braces

Rehabilitative braces are designed to allow protected, controlled motion of injured knees treated operatively or nonoperatively. Many surgeons use a rehabilitative brace immediately after ACL reconstruction to permit a limited amount of motion, thus avoiding the complications of total immobilization. The ROM prescribed by the brace varies among protocols, depending on the surgeon's preference, graft selection, graft fixation, and concomitant surgical procedures.

Rehabilitative braces provide a compromise between motion and protection by restricting knee flexion and extension; however, they provide little, if any, anterior/posterior stability and may allow more extension than expected to occur with the adjusted settings. Several studies indicate that these braces allow as much as 15 to 20 degrees past the set extension stop. Some authors recommend setting the extension stop at least 10 to 20 degrees greater than the desired limit to avoid this problem. Because many patients demonstrate a different degree of knee flexion than the preset stop on the brace, it is important to measure the knee ROM in comparison with the brace and to allow for any differences.

Hoffmann et al. tested six rehabilitative braces on fresh cadaver specimens and concluded that braces with medial and lateral plastic shells and offset hinges provided more stability. The main criticism of this study is the lack of control over how tightly the brace was applied.

Rehabilitative braces should have the ability to adjust to any patient. A close fit to the leg minimizes slipping and aids in the comfort of the patient. These braces should be easily applied and removed and should provide ready access to incisions around the knee.

Functional Braces

Functional braces are designed to assist or provide functional stability for the unstable knee and to provide prophylactic support during exercise and strenuous activity in the stable reconstructed knee. The efficacy of functional knee braces is still controversial. Most biomechanical studies indicate that these braces may restore knee laxity to normal levels under low-load conditions, but are minimally effective when subjected to the higher forces associated with functional and athletic activities.

Under low-load conditions, 50% to 80% of patients have significantly decreased anterior translation of the tibia and improved rotatory stability with the use of a functional brace. However, at higher loads the brace may not significantly decrease tibial translation.

Functional knee braces have been demonstrated to provide support during side-cutting activity. The brace appears to work either by reducing the need for muscle activity during a cut or by altering limb position during a cut, thus reducing the need for muscle stabilization. Furthermore, 90% of patients claim subjective feelings of support, and 70% claim improved performance when wearing a brace. For these reasons, many surgeons opt to use a functional knee brace during the rehabilitative period and with sporting activity for up to 1 year after reconstruction.

Two basic types of functional knee braces are available, both using hinges and posts. The primary difference between the two is whether they employ thigh and calf enclosures or use straps for suspension.

Transitional Braces

Transitional braces may be used during the time between postoperative rehabilitative bracing and functional bracing. During the rehabilitation process, patients work on increasing muscle strength and girth. The lack of muscle girth sometimes poses a problem when fitting the patient for a functional brace. Most insurance companies allow reimbursement for only one brace, not a series of braces, causing a financial burden for the patient. To bridge the gap between rehabilitative bracing and functional bracing, many manufacturers have designed conversion systems for their rehabilitative braces. These braces continue to provide controlled ROM in an overall shortened brace. Typically, these braces are easily converted and provide adequate support for the knee. The transitional brace should allow for increasing girth and adjustments to limb alignment. The use of such a brace allows added safe rehabilitation time before the patient is fitted with a functional knee brace. According to Nelson, this type of brace is used from the twelfth through the twenty-sixth postoperative weeks. Many clinicians prefer an early fit of the functional brace and do not use transitional braces.

FUNCTIONAL TESTING

Functional testing after ACL rehabilitation attempts to evaluate the functional stability of the knee joint. This stability is provided by passive restraints of the knee ligaments, active restraints generated by the muscles, and joint geometry. Functional testing attempts to simulate, in a controlled environment, the forces experienced during common activities such as running, hopping, or cutting.

Traditionally, variables such as thigh musculature

TABLE 5-1 Function Testing After Anterior Cruciate Ligament Rupture

Rationale: Ruptures of the ACL result in varying amounts of functional limitations of the lower extremity. In order to assess these limitations quantitatively, objective testing under simulated activity conditions is required. Four one-legged hop function tests were devised; their effectiveness and sensitivity in detecting limitations was assessed in two studies. These tests should be used with other clinical measuring tools (isokinetic testing, questionnaires) to verify functional limitations.

	One-Legged Single Hop for Distance	One-Legged Timed Hop	One-Legged Triple Hop for Distance	One-Legged Cross-Over Hop for Distance
Methods	The patient stands on one limb, hops as far as possible, and lands on the same limb. The total distance hopped is measured. Each limb is tested twice; the means of each are calculated and used to determine limb symmetry.	The patient hops on one limb a distance of 6 m as fast as possible. The total time to cover the distance is recorded. Each limb is tested twice; the times are calculated to the nearest one-hundredth of a second with a stop watch. The means of each limb are calculated and used to determine limb symmetry.	The patient stands on one limb, performs three consecutive hops as far as possible, and lands on the same limb. The total distance hopped is measured; each limb is tested twice. The means of each limb are calculated and used to determine limb symmetry.	A distance of 6 m in length, with a 15-cm long strip marked in the center of the floor, is designated. The patient hops three consecutive times on one limb, crossing over the center strip on each hop. The total distance hopped is measured; each limb is tested twice. The means of each limb are calculated and used to determine limb symmetry.
Calculation	Limb symmetry = mean score of the involved limb divided by mean score of the noninvolved limb; result is multiplied by 100. $\dfrac{\text{involved}}{\text{noninvolved}} \times 100$	Limb symmetry = mean time of the noninvolved limb divided by mean time of the involved limb; result is multiplied by 100. $\dfrac{\text{noninvolved}}{\text{involved}} \times 100$	Limb symmetry = $\dfrac{\text{involved}}{\text{noninvolved}} \times 100$	Limb symmetry = $\dfrac{\text{involved}}{\text{noninvolved}} \times 100$

Study Results	Normal limb symmetry was determined to be 85%. Approximately one-half of ACL-deficient knees demonstrated abnormal test scores. Results of normals and ACL-deficient knees showed low false-positive and high specificity rates, indicating test is of value in confirming lower limb limitations. The low sensitivity rates found exclude the use of this test as a screening tool.	Normal limb symmetry was determined to be 85%. Approximately 42% to 49% of ACL-deficient knees had abnormal test scores. Low false-positive and high specificity rates allow test to be used to confirm lower limb limitations. Low sensitivity rates exclude its effectiveness in screening for limitations.	Data available for 26 ACL-deficient knees only. One-half of the patients had abnormal symmetry scores. The low sensitivity rate excludes the test as a screening tool.	Data available for 26 ACL-deficient knees only. Fifty-eight percent of the patients had abnormal symmetry scores. Test showed highest percentage of abnormal symmetry scores compared to the other three; however, the low sensitivity rate does not allow it to be used as a screening test.

Conclusion/Summary

The tests designed and the statistical analyses performed in these two studies attempted to correct deficiencies found in previous reports. The data collected on 93 normal knees showed no effect of gender, sports-activity level, or dominance on limb symmetry. This allowed an overall normal symmetry limb score to be determined from the population as a whole, which was 85%, and simplified analysis of test scores of ACL-deficient knees. The percentage of ACL-deficient knees that had abnormal symmetry scores increased when the results of two tests were analyzed versus just one test. Any two tests can be used; an analysis of the six possible two-test combinations did not reveal any one combination that had a higher sensitivity rate. These tests should be used with other clinical measuring tools (isokinetic testing, questionnaires) to confirm abnormal lower limb symmetry. Patients with normal symmetry scores should still be considered at risk for giving way during sports activities.

From Barber SD et al: Rehabilitation after ACL reconstruction: functional testing, *Sports Med Rehab Series* 15:969, 1992.

strength, hamstring to quadriceps strength ratios, static laxity testing, ROM, and muscle girth have been used to evaluate the functional capacity of an athlete after ACL reconstruction. Lephart et al. demonstrated that athletes who returned to preinjury levels of sport activity performed functional tests significantly faster than athletes who were unable to return to preinjury levels of sport activity after ACL reconstruction. Based on their findings, Lephart et al. suggest that functional testing be included in the battery of assessments used to determine when an athlete can return to functional activity.

Several functional knee tests are described in the literature; however, many of these testing procedures have been poorly evaluated and do not provide reliable results. The most commonly used functional tests include the four one-legged hop tests and the vertical jump test. The one-legged hop tests include the following:

- One-legged single hop for distance
- One-legged timed hop
- One-legged triple hop for distance
- One-legged cross-over hop for distance

Barber et al. demonstrated that the one-legged single hop test and the one-legged timed hop test had low sensitivity rates, low false-positive rates, and high specificity rates (Table 5-1, pp. 192-193). The authors indicate that these tests should be used to confirm lower limb limitations; however, they cannot be used alone to detect such limitations, since a high sensitivity rate must be present to be considered a screening test. Barber et al. also recommend the use of the one-legged triple hop and the one-legged cross-over hop for distance to confirm lower limb limitations; however, they cannot be used alone, either.

The vertical jump test is another commonly used functional test. In this test, the patient stands with the uninvolved leg positioned closest to the wall, at a distance of 1 foot. The patient then performs a one-legged vertical jump and is given three trials. The average of the three trials is the score. The test is then repeated on the involved leg and limb symmetry is calculated by dividing the involved score by the uninvolved score and multiplying by 100. Although commonly used to determine function, research does not indicate a high reliability factor for this test.

Risberg and Ekeland suggest that functional tests can be categorized into two different functions: daily life function and strength/stability function. Their study indicates that after 3 months the figure eight test and the stair-running test (two-legged tests) provide a quantitative assessment of daily life function. After 6 months the patient should be able to perform the triple-jump test (one-legged test) to assess strength/stability function.

Functional testing plays an important role in deter-

mining whether an athlete can return to sports-related activity and should be used in conjunction with other diagnostic evaluation methods, such as isokinetic strength testing and KT-1000 laxity testing, to assess lower limb limitation.

CRITERIA FOR RETURN TO SPORTS

Return to sports activity is the usual goal after ACL reconstruction. Several different guidelines have been established to help determine when an athlete may safely return to sports; these guidelines vary among rehabilitation protocols.

Paulos and Stern

Paulos and Stern recommend a return to sports when the following criteria are met:

- Minimum of 9 months after surgery
- No swelling
- Completed jog/run program
- Isokinetic testing of the quadriceps indicates 85% strength compared with uninvolved leg
- Isokinetic testing of the hamstrings indicates 90% strength compared with uninvolved leg
- Single leg hop for distance test 85% of uninvolved leg
- Full ROM (0 to 140 degrees)

Although recognizing that the efficacy of bracing for graft protection is questionable, Paulos and Stern use a functional ACL brace during sporting activities for 1 year after surgery. They use a 20-degree extension stop in the brace to limit the limb to 7 to 10 degrees of extension.

Andrews and Wilk

Andrews and Wilk recommend a return to sports at 5 to 6 months after surgery if the following criteria are met:

- Isokinetic testing of quadriceps and hamstrings fulfills criteria
- KT-1000 test unchanged from initial test
- Functional test 80% or greater compared with contralateral leg
- Proprioceptive test 100% of contralateral leg
- Satisfactory clinical exam

The criteria for isokinetic test results, as well as what types of functional and proprioceptive tests are used, are not given by the authors.

Shelbourne and Nitz

Shelbourne and Nitz recommend a return to sports at 4 to 6 months after surgery if the following criteria are met:

- Isokinetic test indicates quadriceps strength is greater than 80% of the contralateral leg at 60, 180, and 240 degrees per second

- Full ROM
- No joint effusion
- Satisfactory ligament stability test using the KT-1000
- Successful completion of functional progression

Shelbourne and Nitz recommend the use of a functional ACL brace up to 1 year after reconstruction.

Frndak and Berasi

Frndak and Berasi recommend a return to sports when the following criteria are met:
- Minimum of 9 months after surgery
- Full ROM
- Isokinetic test indicates quad strength at least 90% of uninvolved leg
- No pain or swelling
- Successful completion of preathletic agility training

Campbell Clinic

At the Campbell Clinic, therapists use the following guidelines to determine when an athlete can return to sport:
- Full ROM
- No joint effusion
- Isokinetic test indicates quadriceps strength is 80% or more than uninvolved leg
- Isokinetic test indicates hamstring strength is 85% or more than uninvolved leg
- One-legged hop for distance test is 85% compared with uninvolved leg
- Successful completion of running program
- Successful completion of sports-specific agility program
- Satisfactory clinical exam

Return to sport varies between 6 and 12 months, depending on the surgeon's preference. The use of an ACL functional brace also depends on the surgeon's preference.

Rehabilitation After Central Third Patellar Tendon ACL Reconstruction

The following section provides descriptions of several established ACL protocols. Both traditional and accelerated protocols are presented.

REHABILITATION PROTOCOL

ACL Reconstruction CAMPBELL CLINIC

The Campbell Clinic protocol (Table 5-2) emphasizes early ROM, weight bearing, and functional rehabilitation similar to the Shelbourne protocol; however, it is not considered to be as aggressive in terms of the timing of certain activities and return to sporting activity.

0 to 2 weeks	• During the initial postoperative period, emphasize decreasing joint effusion, improving quadriceps control, and obtaining full knee extension (Fig. 5-4).

- Initiate quadriceps setting (QS) in full knee extension (Fig. 5-5) on the first postoperative day to prevent neurophysiologic shutdown of the quadriceps muscles; continue until 3 to 4 weeks.
- Initiate straight leg raises in all planes when the patient can perform a QS sufficient to prevent an extensor lag (Fig. 5-6). Add ankle weights when the patient can correctly perform 3 sets of 10 to 15 repetitions with ease. Progress the weights according to patient's tolerance. Begin active hamstring curls, prone and standing, early in the rehabilitation progression.
- Perform passive ROM exercises, such as towel extensions (Fig. 5-7), on postoperative day 1 to obtain full knee extension.
- As pain subsides, use prone leg hangs to promote or maintain full extension (Fig. 5-8). Perform passive ROM for knee flexion to 90 degrees by sitting on the edge of the bed and lowering the involved extremity with the uninvolved extremity (Fig. 5-9).
- When the patient is able to achieve 80 to 90 degrees of flexion, initiate wall slides (Fig. 5-10).
- Begin patellar mobilizations (Figs. 5-11 and 5-12), especially superior gliding, during this initial postoperative period.
- Use electrical stimulation for neuromuscular reeducation if the patient demonstrates a poor QS on initial evaluation by the physical therapist.
- Bracing and weight bearing depend on the surgeon's preference and the surgical procedure performed. Typically, the patient is placed in a straight leg immobilizer or a rehabilitative brace, allowing 0 to 90 degrees of motion. The brace or immobilizer may be removed to perform ROM exercises several times throughout the day. The brace can also be removed for showering or bathing once the incisions have healed.

Text continued on p. 199.

REHABILITATION PROTOCOL—cont'd

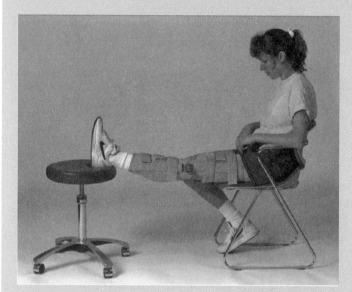

Figure 5-4 Extension of knee on stool.

Figure 5-5 Quadriceps sets.

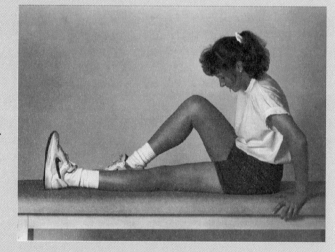

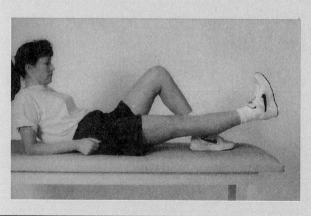

Figure 5-6 Straight leg raise.

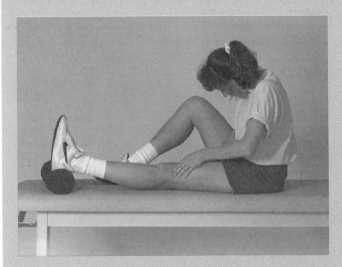

Figure 5-7 Patient places heel on rolled towel to aid in knee extension. Patient may be instructed to push downward on quadriceps with the hands to passively increase extension.

Figure 5-8 Prone leg hangs to increase knee extension.

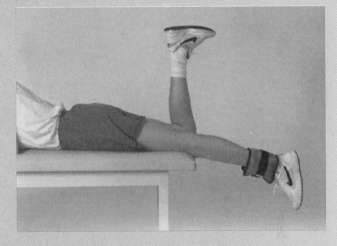

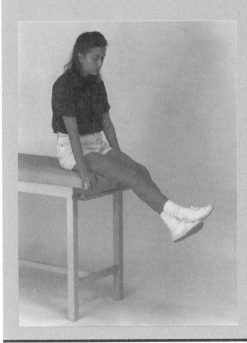

Figure 5-9 Passive flexion of the knee.

Continued

ACL Reconstruction   CAMPBELL CLINIC

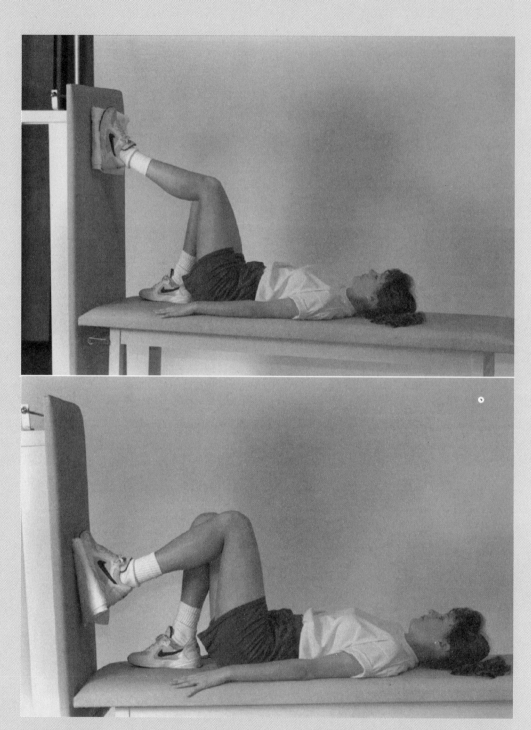

Figure 5-10 Wall slides aid with knee flexion by utilizing gravity to assist flexion. The patient slowly slides the foot down the wall until a sustained stretch is felt in the knee.

REHABILITATION PROTOCOL—cont'd

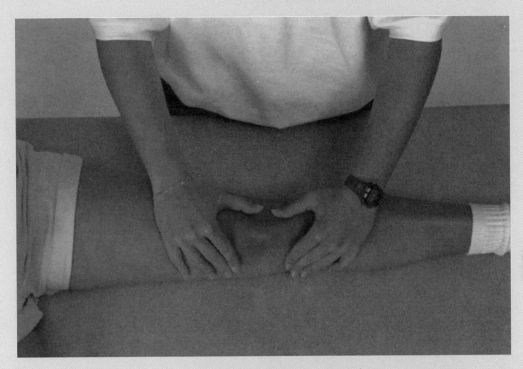

Figure 5-11 Patellar mobilization to avoid contractures (e.g., patella infera).

0 to 2 weeks —cont'd	• Allow weight bearing to tolerance with crutches if the brace is locked in full extension; the patient remains non–weight bearing if concomitant meniscal repair is performed. Encourage a normal, symmetric gait.
2 to 4 weeks	• Open the brace to allow full ROM. • Continue to emphasize maintenance of extension using prone leg hangs, towel extensions, and passive ROM by the therapist if indicated. • Knee flexion should progress to 120 degrees by the end of 4 weeks. • Add weights to prone and standing hamstring curls as tolerated.

• Also progress weights with the SLR program. Once the patient can lift 10 lbs in each direction, use the multihip machine for hip strengthening.
• Initiate the stationary bicycle during week 2 if knee flexion ROM is adequate. Use minimal resistance early in the bicycling program.
• Initiate closed kinetic chain (CKC) exercises at 2 weeks after surgery, unless concomitant meniscal repair is performed. These exercises include minisquats and leg presses, beginning with both legs and progressing to a single leg as tolerated (Fig. 5-13).

Continued

ACL Reconstruction CAMPBELL CLINIC

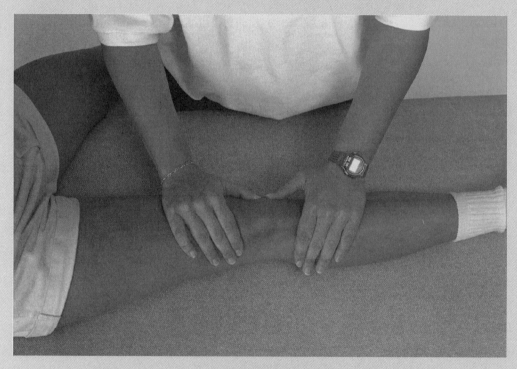

Figure 5-12 The patella is mobilized medially, laterally, and especially superiorly.

2 to 4 weeks —cont'd	• Initiate wall sits, another form of CKC exercise, at a 45-degree angle (see Fig. 5-2). It is important to make sure the patient's tibia remains vertical during this exercise to prevent excessive stress to the graft. The patient progresses the exercise by increasing the sitting time.

• Begin proprioceptive training early with the BAPS board, starting with two legs and progressing to one; and progress weight-shifting activities to one-legged stance (Fig. 5-14).

• Begin lateral step-ups on a 2- to 4-inch step when the patient can perform single leg minisquats. Progress this exercise by increasing the height of the step as strength improves (Fig. 5-15).

• Begin ambulation on the treadmill (forward and retro) between 2 and 3 weeks with emphasis on a normal gait. A mirror may be used to provide visual feedback during ambulation.

• Perform submaximal active knee extension in the 90- to 60-degree range, with manual resistance by the therapist.

• Progress to full weight bearing without crutches when patient can ambulate without a limp. This usually occurs by the third or fourth postoperative week.

4 to 6 weeks	• Full ROM should be achieved by 6 weeks. • Continue to emphasize full knee extension.

REHABILITATION PROTOCOL—cont'd

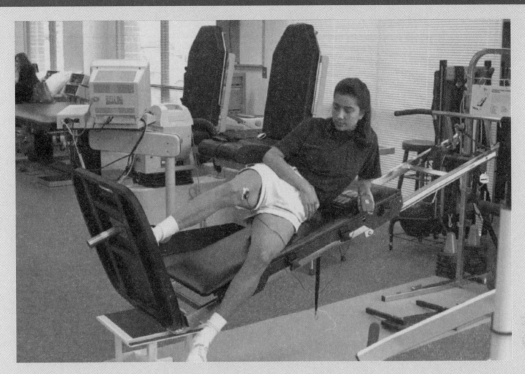

Figure 5-13 Leg press.

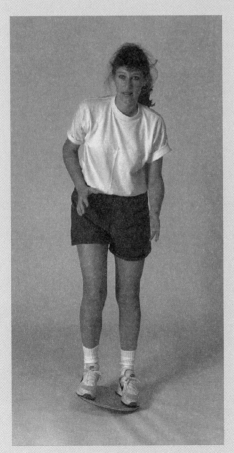

Figure 5-14 Proprioception with BAPS board.

Continued

REHABILITATION PROTOCOL—cont'd

ACL Reconstruction   CAMPBELL CLINIC

4 to 6 weeks —cont'd	• May begin use of Stairmaster or Nordic-Track cross-country ski machine (Fig. 5-16). • Continue to progress strengthening program according to patient's tolerance. • Begin hamstring progression from isotonics to isokinetics on the Kin-Com. • Also use the Kin-Com for quadriceps strengthening in the isotonic mode from 90 to 40 degrees, with the tibial pad placed proximally. At 6 weeks, employ higher speed isokinetic quadriceps work in conjunction with the isotonic training; the range is still limited to 90 to 40 degrees, and the pad is still proximal. • The typical procedure is to fit the patient for an ACL functional brace at 6 weeks postoperatively, depending on the surgeon's preference.

8 to 10 weeks	• Progress all of the above exercises, and add lunges (Fig. 5-17). • Initiate slow-form running with the Sport-Cord (forward and retro). • Continue isokinetic quadriceps work at various speeds. • Begin lateral strengthening and agility at 10 weeks using the Fitter and the slide board (Fig. 5-18).
12 weeks	• Allow full-range isotonics for the quadriceps on the Kin-Com; move the tibial pad to midrange. Progress isokinetic quadriceps work to full extension by 16 weeks postoperatively. • Begin the knee extension machine with emphasis on low weight and high repetitions.

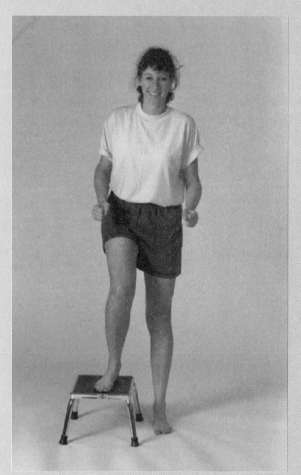

Figure 5-15 Lateral step-ups. Patient stands on a stable stair step. The operated leg is bent slowly, lowering the opposite foot to the floor. Return to the starting position.

REHABILITATION PROTOCOL—cont'd

12 weeks —cont'd
- Initiate slow, controlled lateral SportCord drills.
- Continue progression of the strength program.
- Perform an isokinetic evaluation of hamstring strength.
  If the test indicates hamstring strength is 85% or better, discontinue isokinetic hamstring workouts; however, encourage the patient to continue hamstring workouts on the machines.

16 to 18 weeks
- Evaluate quadriceps strength isokinetically; retest the hamstrings if necessary.
- Institute a jogging program and a plyometric program if quadriceps strength is at least 65% of the uninvolved extremity, no effusion is present, the patient has full ROM, and the knee is stable.

5 to 6 months
- Begin agility training and sports-specific drills if the above criteria have been met.
- Perform retesting of the quadriceps if necessary.
- Return to sport depends on the surgeon's preference; however, the patient must exhibit at least 80% quadriceps strength and 85% hamstring strength (see p. 195).
- If a functional brace was prescribed by the surgeon, it is usually recommended that it be worn for sporting activity for at least 1 year after surgery.

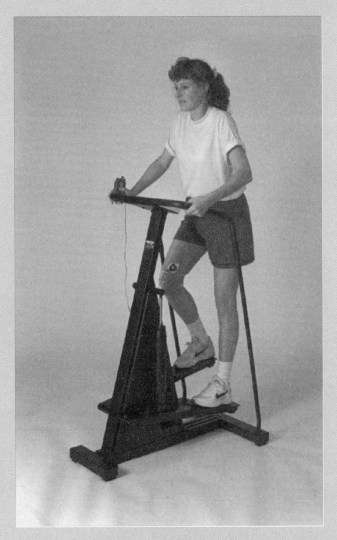

Figure 5-16 Stairmaster exercises.

Continued

ACL Reconstruction   CAMPBELL CLINIC

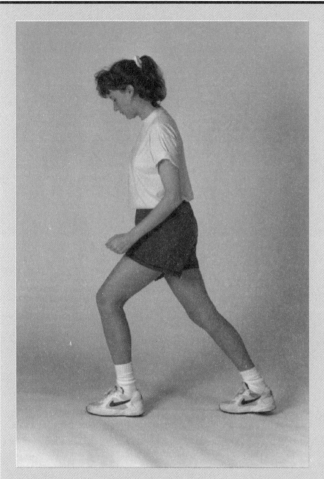

Figure 5-17 Lunges.

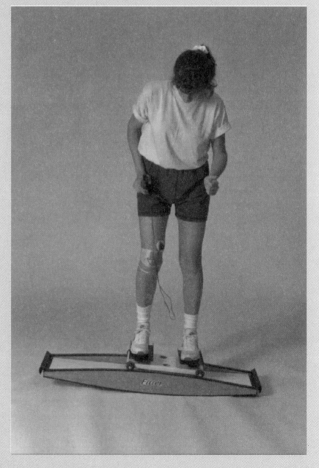

Figure 5-18 Fitter for lateral agility.

REHABILITATION PROTOCOL—cont'd

TABLE 5-2 **Campbell Clinic ACL Rehabilitation Protocol—ACL Reconstruction**

	Weeks					Months			
	1-2	3-4	5-6	7-8	9-12	4	5	6	7-12
Bracing									
Straight leg immobilizer/motion control brace (MCB) at 0 degrees	X	X							
Functional brace with exercise/sport			X	X	X	X	X	X	X
Range of Motion									
Braced in extension except with exercise	X	X							
Prone hangs/towel extension	X	X	X	X	X				
Knee flexion out of brace									
90 degrees	X								
120 degrees		X							
Full flexion (135 to 140 degrees)			X						
Weight Bearing									
50% weight bearing	X								
75% to 100% weight bearing			X						
Discontinue crutches			X						
Delay weight bearing with meniscal repair			X						
Strengthening									
Quad sets/SLR (all planes)	X	X	X						
Stool scoots	X	X							
Wall sits			X	X	X	X	X	X	
Hamstring curls (prone/standing)	X	X	X	X	X	X	X	X	X
Multihip machine			X	X	X	X			
Progressive closed-chain activities			X	X	X	X	X	X	X
Knee extension (90 to 60 degrees)/proximal resistance	X	X							
Knee extension (90 to 40 degrees)/proximal resistance				X	X	X			
Knee extension (full range)						X	X	X	X
Conditioning									
Stationary bike—low resistance	X	X							
Stationary bike—progress resistance			X	X	X	X	X	X	X
Outdoor bike					X	X	X	X	X
Treadmill (forward/retro)		X	X	X	X	X			
Stairmaster/cross-country ski machine			X	X	X	X	X	X	X
Jogging/running						X	X	X	X
Agility/Sport-Specific Training									
Fitter/slide board					X	X	X	X	
Resisted running with SportCord					X	X	X	X	
Plyometric training						X	X	X	X
Carioca, cutting, figure 8's, etc.						X	X	X	X

ACCELERATED REHABILITATION PROTOCOL

ACL Reconstruction   SHELBOURNE AND NITZ

This four-phase rehabilitative protocol emphasizes early restoration of full knee extension (equal to the uninvolved knee), immediate weight bearing, and closed-chain exercises (Table 5-3). Although the protocol is accelerated in terms of early full extension, quadriceps activity, and early return to athletic play, the term accelerated does *not* apply to the initial 2 weeks after surgery.

During the first 14 days of postoperative rehabilitation, the patient focuses on five goals: full extension, wound healing, good quadriceps leg control, minimal swelling, and flexion to 90 degrees. Allow weight bearing to tolerance with the assistance of crutches, but encourage the patient to be up and about only for bathroom privileges

and meals. During the remainder of this time, encourage the patient to limit walking and to elevate the limb. Shelbourne and Nitz believe that this initial 2 weeks of rest greatly decreases postoperative swelling, therefore allowing faster advancement toward normal activities of daily living and earlier return to sports activity.

Phase 1   This phase actually begins shortly after the acute knee injury and weeks before the reconstructive surgery. The initial focus is on regaining ROM and decreasing joint effusion. A CryoCuff (Aircast, Summit, NJ) is used to provide both cooling and compression in the attempt to decrease swelling. Patients also work

TABLE 5-3   Shelbourne and Nitz Accelerated ACL Rehabilitation Protocol

	Weeks					Months			
	1-2	3-4	5-6	7-8	9-12	4	5	6	7-12
Bracing									
Straight leg immobilizer/MCB at 0 degrees	X								
Functional brace with exercise/sport		X	X	X	X	X	X	X	X
Range of Motion									
Braced in extension except with exercise	X								
Passive range of motion (PROM) for full knee extension	X	X	X						
CPM	X								
Knee flexion ROM	X	X	X						
Weight Bearing									
Weight bearing to tolerance with crutches	X								
Full weight bearing without crutches		X							
Strengthening									
Quadriceps sets/SLR (all planes)	X	X							
Active knee extension (90 to 30 degrees)	X	X	X	X	X				
Calf raises		X	X	X	X	X	X	X	X
Minisquats/step-ups		X	X	X	X	X	X	X	X
Progressive closed-chain activities		X	X	X	X	X	X	X	X
Conditioning									
Biking		X	X	X	X	X	X	X	X
Swimming		X	X	X	X	X	X	X	X
Stairmaster		X	X	X	X	X	X	X	X
Running (if strength test 70%)			X	X	X	X	X	X	X
Agility/Sport-Specific Training									
Lateral shuffles			X	X	X	X	X	X	X
Cariocas			X	X	X	X	X	X	X
Jumping rope			X	X	X	X	X	X	X

ACCELERATED REHABILITATION PROTOCOL—cont'd

Phase 1 —cont'd
on restoring a normal gait pattern during this phase. Once swelling and pain are decreased and full ROM is restored, begin strengthening exercises.

Phase 2
The second phase of the accelerated protocol encompasses the initial 2 weeks after surgery. Place the patient in a straight leg immobilizer immediately after surgery; also apply the CryoCuff. Begin the use of CPM once the patient returns to the hospital room on postoperative day 1 and continue until discharge from the hospital, on the second or third postoperative day. Use the CPM for 10 minutes every hour with the heel of the operative extremity propped on pillows to allow full knee extension. Place a 2.5-lb ankle weight on the proximal tibia to help promote full knee extension. Also begin PROM for terminal knee extension and for knee flexion to 90 degrees out of the CPM.

The patient begins working on leg control on the first postoperative day. This is done by using active quadriceps setting and straight leg raising. Perform the above exercises for knee flexion/extension PROM and leg control 3 times a day during the initial 2 weeks. Also perform active quadriceps contractions in the range of 90 to 30 degrees.

Allow weight bearing to tolerance with crutches immediately after surgery; however, as mentioned above, encourage patients to limit activity to meals and bathroom privileges during the first 2 weeks.

After discharge from the hospital, usually on postoperative day 2, patients continue with PROM, leg control exercises, and active knee extension 90 to 30 degrees. Initiate prone leg hangs and towel extensions (see Fig. 5-8) at week 1 to maintain or promote full knee extension. Begin wall slides (see Fig. 5-10), heel slides (Fig. 5-19), and active-assisted flexion to promote knee flexion ROM.

During the second week after surgery, it is permissible for patients to return to classes or light office work on a part-time basis, depending on the amount of swelling in the knee.

Use the straight leg immobilizer during the initial 2 weeks after surgery when the patient is out of the house. It is not required when ambulating around the house. At follow-up evaluation by the surgeon at 7 days postoperatively, measure the patient for a functional brace without blocks to extension or flexion. This brace replaces the immobilizer after the initial 2 weeks and works as a protective device during inclement weather and when the patient is returning to athletic activity.

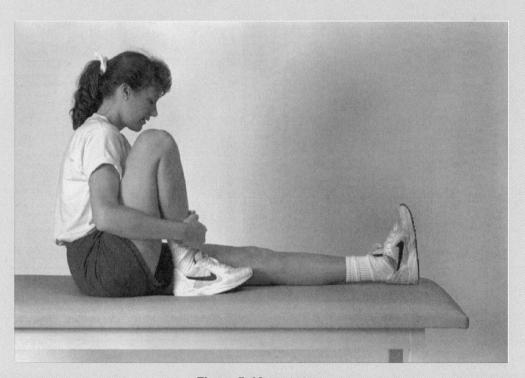

Figure 5-19 Heel slides.

Continued

ACL Reconstruction SHELBOURNE AND NITZ

Phase 3 This phase of rehabilitation usually encompasses 3 to 5 weeks postoperatively. Emphasize a normal gait pattern without the use of crutches, as well as a gradual return to normal activities of daily living. Full knee extension with minimal swelling continues to be a primary focus. Encourage the restoration of normal knee flexion; patients typically achieve full flexion (135 degrees) 5 weeks postoperatively.

May initiate strengthening exercises, such as calf raises, minisquats, leg presses, and step-ups (see p. 206), between 2 and 3 weeks postoperatively. Patients may also begin using the Stairmaster, bicycling, and swimming.

Phase 4 The final phase of the accelerated protocol begins at 5 weeks after surgery. Perform an isokinetic strength evaluation with a 20-degree extension block at 180 and 240 degrees per second. If strength testing shows that the involved extremity has reached at least 70% of the strength of the uninvolved extremity, institute a running program. The patient may also begin lateral shuffles, cariocas (Fig. 5-20), and jumping rope. It is also permissible to implement sports-specific agility training. Continue strength training, as well as bicycling, swimming, and/or using the Stairmaster.

Throughout this phase, temper aggressive activity by the control of swelling and the maintenance of ROM. It is noted by Shelbourne et al. that if the patient does not desire a rapid return to sport, a near-normal level of strength will be restored through normal activities of daily living over 1 to 2 years. If the patient does desire a rapid return to sport, intensify strength training in this final phase.

At 10 weeks, perform another isokinetic evaluation at 60, 180, and 240 degrees per second. Perform a KT-1000 to assess ligament stability. Increase agility workouts.

At 16 to 24 weeks, repeat the isokinetic evaluation; allow return to sports if strength is greater than 80% and functional progression has been successfully completed.

Patients can perform most of the rehabilitation on their own. Patients are followed at 1, 2, 5, 9, and 15 weeks postoperatively by both the physician and the physical therapist. During these visits, the therapist guides the patient in progression of exercises and activity. Perform additional follow-up at 6 and 12 months.

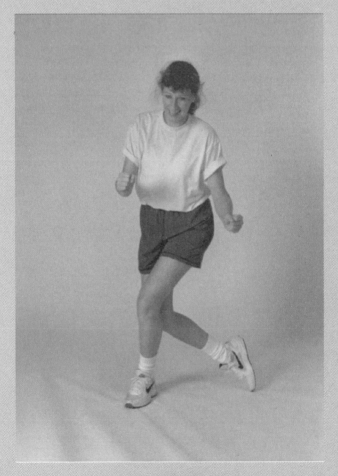

Figure 5-20 Carioca.

ACL Reconstruction

KERLAN-JOBE CLINIC, SETO, BREWSTER, LOMBARDO, AND TIBONE

1 to 10 days
- The patient remains in the hospital for 2 to 4 days. Immediately after surgery, use CPM (see Table 5-4 for CPM protocol) to promote knee ROM and continue for 2 to 4 weeks after surgery.
- Straight leg raises are discouraged during the early stages of rehabilitation because of the stresses placed on the patellar tendon and the reconstructed ligament through isolated quadriceps contraction. Instead, instruct the patient to use either the uninvolved leg or the hands to help lift the involved leg when necessary. By internally or externally rotating the leg, the patient can also recruit the hip abductors or adductors to help raise the involved leg.

10 to 14 days
- Initiate supervised passive ROM, such as wall slides, and isometric hamstring and quadriceps exercises with the knee slightly flexed, using a towel roll or small bolster under the knee at 10 days postoperatively.
- Perform quadriceps setting with simultaneous hamstring cocontraction to reduce the amount of anterior tibial translation.
- Initiate isometric hip adduction to strengthen the adductor muscles and keep the adductor tendon taut.

2 to 6 weeks
- Continue ROM and isometric exercises.
- Discontinue CPM when passive flexion reaches 125 to 130 degrees.
- Use heel slides to increase knee flexion when the patient reaches 110 degrees.
- Initiate hamstring curls when the patient has at least 80 to 90 degrees of passive knee flexion; 2 to 3 sets of 10 repetitions beginning with 5 lbs or more, according to the patient's ability; progress weight as tolerated.
- Initiate active-resistive hip adduction, abduction, and extension in the form of multiplanar straight leg raises.
- Can also initiate calf raises once patient is full weight bearing.
- Begin weight bearing to tolerance at 2 to 3 weeks postoperatively, with the brace locked at 0 degrees extension so that negligible shear force is produced. This allows the patient to perform more functional activities without jeopardizing the graft. Maintain the brace in extension for ambulation until 7 to 8 weeks postoperatively, then allow full flexion in the brace.

- Begin stationary bicycling when passive knee flexion is at least 110 degrees. The bicycle seat should be adjusted to 15 to 20 degrees extension to avoid terminal knee extension on the downstroke.
- Begin short-arc quadriceps (SAQ) exercises in the 40- to 0-degree range, with simultaneous hamstring cocontraction (Fig. 5-21). Maintain the cocontraction of the hamstrings by performing hip extension into the bolster while the knee is extended. If pain in the area of the patellar tendon occurs, these exercises may be postponed until 6 to 8 weeks.

6 weeks to 3 months
- Exercises continued during this stage of rehabilitation are primarily to emphasize the hamstrings.
- Progress progressive resistance exercises (PREs) as tolerated.
- Allow ambulation without the extension lock.

3 to 4 months
- May discontinue the brace with activities of daily living.
- Continue progression with all resistive exercises and gradually increase the duration and tension during bicycling.
- Initiate eccentric quadriceps exercises with weights to enhance quadriceps strength. For example, with the SAQ exercise, emphasis is on slowly lowering the weight. Continue to encourage a cocontraction of the quadriceps and hamstrings.
- If there is anteromedial rotatory instability, perform strengthening of the pes anserinus muscles group to enhance dynamic stability.

4 to 5 months
- Initiate step-ups to train the quadriceps specifically to resist eccentric loading. Step-ups simulate activities of daily living and help to strengthen various muscle groups, especially the quadriceps. Begin this exercise by using a 4- to 5-inch step and progressively increasing to an 8-inch step height as strength improves.
- Initiate jogging in place on a trampoline if the patient can lift 15 lbs during the SAQ exercise. This is the first stage in the running protocol. Progress gradually until patient can tolerate jogging 10 to 15 minutes without complications.

Continued

REHABILITATION PROTOCOL—cont'd

ACL Reconstruction
KERLAN-JOBE CLINIC, SETO, BREWSTER, LOMBARDO, AND TIBONE

TABLE 5-4 Kerlan-Jobe Clinic ACL Rehabilitation Protocol
Seto, Brewster, Lombardo, and Tibone

	Weeks					Months			
	1-2	3-4	5-6	7-8	9-12	4	5	6	7-12
Bracing									
Brace locked in full extension with ambulation	X	X	X	X					
Brace unlocked for ambulation				X	X	X			
Discontinue brace with activities of daily living						X			
Range of Motion									
CPM	X	X							
Passive ROM knee flexion	X	X	X						
Weight Bearing									
Weight bearing to tolerance—full extension with crutches		X							
Progress to partial weight bearing/full weight bearing		X	X						
Brace unlocked for ambulation					X				
Strengthening									
Isometric QS with ham cocontraction and knee flexed slightly	X								
Isometric hamstring sets	X								
Isometric hip adduction	X								
SLR for hip adduction, abduction, and extension		X	X	X	X	X			
Resisted ankle plantar flexion/calf raises		X	X	X	X	X			
Hamstring curls		X	X	X	X	X	X	X	X
Short arc quadriceps (40 to 0 degrees) with ham cocontraction			X	X	X	X	X	X	
Eccentric quadriceps work						X	X	X	
Step-ups						X	X	X	
Conditioning									
Stationary bike		X	X	X	X	X	X	X	
Jogging on trampoline						X	X		
Jog/run on treadmill if strength sufficient								X	X
Agility/Sport-Specific Training									
Lateral/backward running									X
Vertical jumping									X
Jumping rope									X
Carioca, high knee drill, Figure-eight's									X
Practice sport-specific drills if hamstring/quadriceps ratio is 80%									X

REHABILITATION PROTOCOL—cont'd

4 to 5
months
—cont'd

- Begin isokinetic strengthening. Perform ten repetitions at 240, 180, and 120 degrees per second in descending order. Also perform a 30- to 45-second endurance at 300 degrees per second.

5 to 6
months

- At the end of 5 months, perform an isokinetic strength test of the quadriceps and hamstrings. Sufficient muscle strength and an average hamstring/quadriceps strength ratio of 60% to 70% should be present before the patient begins jogging and running.
- Once this has been accomplished, the patient begins running on the treadmill and discontinues jogging on the trampoline.
- When the patient is able to run 10 to 15 minutes at a 7- to 8-mph pace, progress to running on a track or on grass.
- Emphasize endurance before proceeding to agility drills.

7 to 8
months

- Initiate agility drills. Once the patient is able to run 2 to 3 miles, institute drills such as lateral and backward running, vertical jumping, rope jumping, carioca, and high knee drills.

- Once these skills are mastered, add figure-eight running to the program. As with running, these drills should not cause pain or swelling. If a specific maneuver results in pain, it should be temporarily discontinued until the symptoms subside.

8 to 9
months

- At the end of 8 months, a second isokinetic test may be performed. Because of the role the hamstrings play in dynamic stability of the knee, the goal at this stage of rehabilitation is for the hamstrings to be within 80% of the quadriceps strength value. Also examine the quadriceps strength ratio of the uninvolved versus the involved leg. If this ratio shows a 20% or greater strength deficit, this will affect the hamstring:quadriceps ratio of the involved leg.
- If the patient is able to complete the agility exercises without complications and has a hamstring/quadriceps ratio of at least 80%, it is permissible to begin to practice the drills of the specific sport. Emphasize technique, endurance, and accuracy.
- Once the athlete has successfully performed these drills and practiced with the team for 2 to 3 weeks, allow a return to full athletic participation.

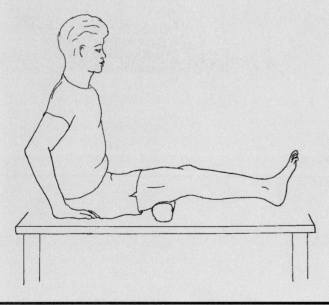

Figure 5-21 Short arc quadriceps (SAQ) exercises with simultaneous hamstring contraction.

REHABILITATION PROTOCOL

ACL Reconstruction PAULOS AND STERN

Paulos and Stern developed three procedure-based ACL protocols to meet the needs of their patients. The *standard ACL protocol* (Table 5-5) leaves the weight-bearing and brace settings blank; this allows the surgeon to individualize the protocol according to the specific surgical procedure and the patient's situation. Use this protocol for patients with special requirements or with concomitant surgical procedures. Use the *accelerated ACL protocol* (Table 5-6) for patients with isolated ACL reconstructions or with ACL reconstructions and partial meniscectomies only. This protocol allows earlier functional weight-bearing exercises. The *semitendinosus tendon protocol* (Table 5-7) is progressed slower in consideration of the weaker initial fixation, greater graft compliance, and slower soft tissue–to–bone healing after the use of these grafts.

BRACING
- Place all patients in a postoperative rehabilitative brace.
- For patellar tendon grafts or Achilles tendon allografts with interference screw fixation, allow immediate motion from 0 to 90 degrees passively and 40 to 90 degrees actively.
- Allow hamstring grafts 10 to 70 degrees passively and 30 to 60 degrees actively due to weaker initial fixation.
- Begin passive ROM on the first postoperative day with wall slides (see p. 200) for knee flexion and prone leg hangs (see p. 198) for knee extension.

WEIGHT BEARING
- For the accelerated protocol, allow 50% weight bearing at 2 weeks after surgery. Begin full weight bearing when the patient demonstrates no more than 5 degrees extension loss, no extensor lag, minimal swelling, and enough quadriceps strength to allow nearly normal gait; this generally occurs by the end of the third postoperative week.
- Patients with concomitant meniscal repairs may proceed more slowly with weight bearing, depending on the surgeon's preference.
- Patients treated for full-thickness chondral defects remain non–weight bearing for 6 weeks to avoid damaging the developing neocartilage by shear stress or axial loading.

- Delay weight bearing for patients with hamstring grafts until the beginning of the sixth postoperative week, then allow 50% weight bearing, and progress to full weight bearing over 2 weeks.

STRENGTHENING
- The first strengthening exercises allowed are QS and straight leg raising (see p. 197). These exercises begin on the first postoperative day and continue through 8 weeks. They are performed with the brace locked at 30 to 40 degrees to prevent inadvertent active knee extension.

PREs
- The first progressive resistance exercises (PREs) initiated are those that isolate the agonist muscles, predominantly the hamstrings.
- Perform hamstring curls in either a seated or prone position, beginning the second week.
- Continue hamstring strengthening throughout the rehabilitation program.
- Also initiate PREs for hip musculature in the second postoperative week by using a total hip machine or by performing multiplanar straight leg raises with ankle weights.
- Continue hip strengthening through 8 weeks postoperatively.
- Closed-chain exercises, such as leg press and minisquats, train both the agonist and antagonist muscles using cocontraction. These exercises begin when 50% weight bearing is allowed, typically by 3 weeks for those with patellar tendon and Achilles grafts, and 6 weeks for those with meniscal repairs and hamstring grafts. Continue these exercises through the rehabilitation program. As a starting point, allow 10% of the patient's body weight for both quadriceps and hamstring exercises, with increases according to the patient's tolerance. The use of a brace is preferred during these exercises.

REHABILITATION PROTOCOL—cont'd

PREs—cont'd

- Begin bicycling with the well leg in week 1 and continue until week 3.
- Begin stationary bicycling in the third week for the accelerated protocol if knee flexion is at least 105 degrees, and in the fifth week for the standard and hamstring graft protocols. Continue this form of exercise throughout the rehabilitation program.
- Allow outdoor bicycling in the seventh week on level ground only; the patient may progress to seated hill climbing at 4 months and to standing hill climbing at 6 months.

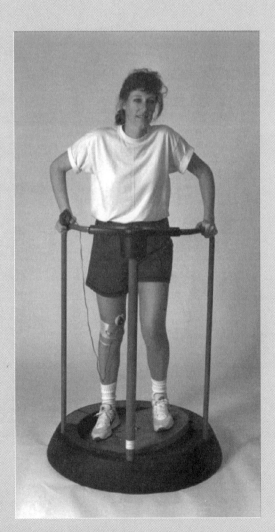

Figure 5-22 KAT (R) machine for proprioception and balance.

BALANCE ACTIVITIES

- Delay BAPS, KAT (Fig. 5-22), and balance board until 6 weeks in the accelerated protocol, and 8 weeks in the standard and hamstring graft protocols. These activities are to increase proprioception and coordination; continue throughout the rehabilitation program.
- The Fitter helps to promote balance, coordination, and lateral strengthening and agility (see p. 205).
- May also use lateral movements with SportCord resistance to promote lateral strengthening and agility. Do not initiate these exercises until 3 months and continue throughout the rehabilitation program.

CARDIOVASCULAR CONDITIONING

- May initiate the upper body ergometer (UBE) during 1 week postoperatively and continue throughout the rehabilitation program.
- Initiate walking when full weight bearing is allowed; use the rehabilitative brace with a 20-degree extension stop until 12 weeks, then discontinue the brace for walking.
- Initiate the Stairmaster and cross-country ski machine during week 7 in the accelerated protocol, and month 3 in the standard hamstring graft protocols. Use a 20-degree extension stop in the brace for these activities.
- May begin running/jogging at 6 months, using a functional brace with a 20-degree extension stop.
- Continue all cardiovascular conditioning exercises throughout the rehabilitation program.

ISOKINETIC STRENGTHENING

- These activities are generally the last to be introduced (see p. 214).

RETURN TO SPORT

- See p. 194.

Continued

REHABILITATION PROTOCOL—cont'd

ACL Reconstruction   PAULOS AND STERN

TABLE 5-5 Standard ACL Protocol   (LONNIE PAULOS, MD)

Activities/Daily Living	Week								Month					
	1	2	3	4	5	6	7	8	3	4	5	6	9	12
Shower without brace				➤➤➤➤➤➤➤➤➤➤➤➤➤➤➤➤➤										
Sleep without brace						➤➤➤➤➤➤➤➤➤➤➤➤➤								
Break down brace						➤➤➤➤➤➤➤➤➤➤➤➤➤								

Range of Motion	Week								*Extension*
	1	2	3	4	5	6	7	8	• Lie on stomach and lower leg into extension
Passive									• Sit on firm surface and place 5 to 10 lbs above knee
Extension/flexion	0/90	0/90	0/100	0/110	0/120	0/130	0/140	Full	*Flexion*
Active									• Lie on back; use gravity to slide foot down wall
Extension/flexion	40/90	40/90	30/100	20/110	10/120	0/130	0/140	Full	• While sitting use gravity and opposite leg to bend knee

Brace Settings	Week								Month					
	1	2	3	4	5	6	7	8	3	4	5	6	9	12
Weight bearing									Full ➤➤➤➤➤➤➤➤➤➤					
Knee-brace ROM setting	• Brace locked at 30 degrees for first 2 weeks postoperatively													
For exercise	• Unlock brace to exercise angles after 2 weeks postoperatively													
Extension/flexion	40/90	40/90	30/100	20/110	20/120	20/open	➤➤➤➤➤➤➤➤➤➤➤➤➤➤							
For ambulation														
Extension/flexion									D/C'd for walking at 12th week					

Strength Training	Week								Month					
	1	2	3	4	5	6	7	8	3	4	5	6	9	12
Quad sets, SLRs (brace locked at 40 degrees)	➤➤➤➤➤➤➤➤➤➤➤➤➤➤➤➤													
Electrical stimulation (brace locked at 40 degrees)	➤➤➤➤➤➤➤➤➤➤➤➤➤➤➤➤													
Hamcurls		➤➤➤➤➤➤➤➤➤➤➤➤➤➤➤➤➤➤➤➤➤➤➤➤➤➤➤➤➤												
Total hip		➤➤➤➤➤➤➤➤➤➤➤➤➤➤➤												
Minisquat/leg press/toe rise						➤➤➤➤➤➤➤➤➤➤➤➤➤➤➤➤➤➤➤➤➤								
Cycling—stationary					➤➤➤➤➤➤➤➤➤➤➤➤➤➤➤➤➤➤➤➤➤➤➤									
Cycling—outdoor								Level ground only		Seated hill climb		Standing hill climbs		

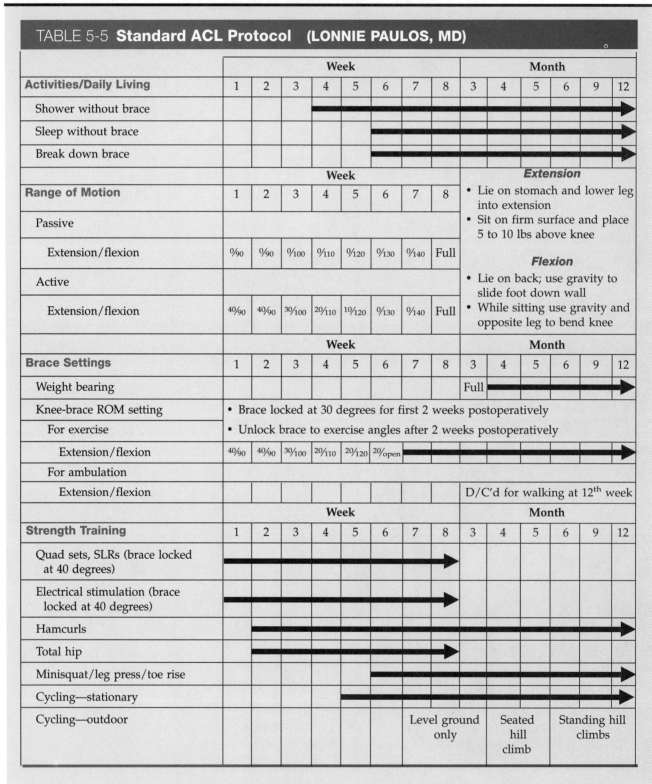

REHABILITATION PROTOCOL—cont'd

TABLE 5-5—cont'd

	Week								Month					
Balance/Coordination	1	2	3	4	5	6	7	8	3	4	5	6	9	12
Baps/KAT/Sandunes/Rhomberg/ tape touch									■■■■■■■■■■■■■■■■■■■►					
Profitter									■■■■■■■■■►					
SportCord lateral agility									■■■■■■■■■►					

	Week								Month					
Conditioning	1	2	3	4	5	6	7	8	3	4	5	6	9	12
Cycle with well leg	■■■■■■►													
UBE (upper body ergonometer)	■■■■■■■■■■■■■■■■■■►													
Swimming (refer to pool protocol)					20° ■■■■■■■■■■►									
Walking (100% weight)								10° ■■■■►						
Stairmaster									20° ■■■►					
Cross-country ski machine									20° ■■■►					
Rowing									30°/90° ■■►					
Run/jog (sports brace must be worn)												20° ■►		

	Week								Month					
Power Training	1	2	3	4	5	6	7	8	3	4	5	6	9	12
Low repetitions—leg press/ squats/hamcurls								20°/90° ■■■►						
Isokinetics (refer to protocol)											■■►			

To Return to Sports:
- Minimum of 9 months postoperatively
- No swelling
- Complete jog/run program
- Quadriceps strength 85% of opposite knee
- Hamstring strength 90% of opposite knee
- Hop distance 85% of opposite knee
- ROM 0 to 140 degrees

Modified from Jackson DW: *The anterior cruciate ligament: current and future concepts,* New York, 1993, Raven Press.

Continued

REHABILITATION PROTOCOL—cont'd

ACL Reconstruction PAULOS AND STERN

TABLE 5-6 Accelerated ACL Protocol   (LONNIE PAULOS, MD)

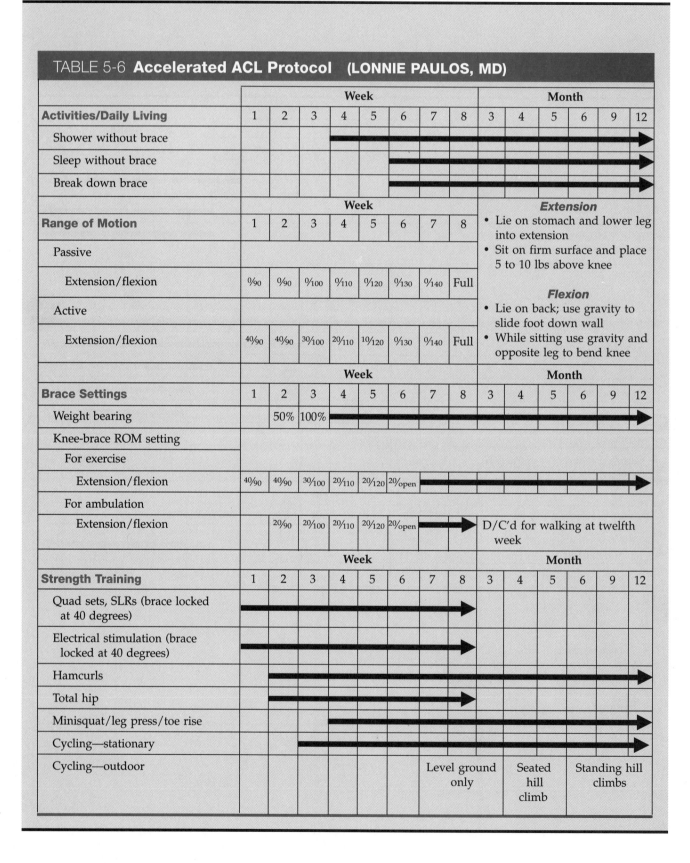

Activities/Daily Living	Week								Month					
	1	2	3	4	5	6	7	8	3	4	5	6	9	12
Shower without brace				████████████████████████████████████▶										
Sleep without brace						████████████████████████████████▶								
Break down brace						████████████████████████████████▶								

Range of Motion	Week								**Extension**
	1	2	3	4	5	6	7	8	• Lie on stomach and lower leg into extension
Passive									• Sit on firm surface and place 5 to 10 lbs above knee
Extension/flexion	$^0/_{90}$	$^0/_{90}$	$^0/_{100}$	$^0/_{110}$	$^0/_{120}$	$^0/_{130}$	$^0/_{140}$	Full	**Flexion**
Active									• Lie on back; use gravity to slide foot down wall
Extension/flexion	$^{40}/_{90}$	$^{40}/_{90}$	$^{30}/_{100}$	$^{20}/_{110}$	$^{10}/_{120}$	$^0/_{130}$	$^0/_{140}$	Full	• While sitting use gravity and opposite leg to bend knee

Brace Settings	Week								Month					
	1	2	3	4	5	6	7	8	3	4	5	6	9	12
Weight bearing		50%	100%	████████████████████████████████████▶										
Knee-brace ROM setting														
For exercise														
Extension/flexion	$^{40}/_{90}$	$^{40}/_{90}$	$^{30}/_{100}$	$^{20}/_{110}$	$^{20}/_{120}$	$^{20}/_{open}$	████████████████████████████▶							
For ambulation														
Extension/flexion		$^{20}/_{90}$	$^{20}/_{100}$	$^{20}/_{110}$	$^{20}/_{120}$	$^{20}/_{open}$	██████▶	D/C'd for walking at twelfth week						

Strength Training	Week								Month					
	1	2	3	4	5	6	7	8	3	4	5	6	9	12
Quad sets, SLRs (brace locked at 40 degrees)	████████████████████████████████▶													
Electrical stimulation (brace locked at 40 degrees)	████████████████████████████████▶													
Hamcurls		██▶												
Total hip		████████████████████████████▶												
Minisquat/leg press/toe rise				████████████████████████████████████▶										
Cycling—stationary			████████████████████████████████████▶											
Cycling—outdoor								Level ground only		Seated hill climb		Standing hill climbs		

REHABILITATION PROTOCOL—cont'd

TABLE 5-6—cont'd

	Week								Month					
Balance/Coordination	1	2	3	4	5	6	7	8	3	4	5	6	9	12
Baps/KAT/Sandunes/Rhomberg/tape touch						➞								→
Profitter									➞					→
SportCord lateral agility									➞					→

	Week								Month					
Conditioning	1	2	3	4	5	6	7	8	3	4	5	6	9	12
Cycle with well leg	➞	➞												
UBE (upper body ergonometer)	➞													→
Walking (100% weight)			10°											→
Swimming (refer to pool protocol)					20°									→
Stairmaster							20°							→
Cross-country ski machine							20°							→
Rowing								20°						→
Run/jog (sports brace must be worn)												20°		→

	Week								Month					
Power Training	1	2	3	4	5	6	7	8	3	4	5	6	9	12
Low repetitions—leg press/squats/hamcurls									20°/90°					→
Isokinetics (refer to protocol)											➞			→

To Return to Sports:
- Minimum of 9 months postoperatively
- No swelling
- Complete jog/run program
- Quadriceps strength 85% of opposite knee
- Hamstring strength 90% of opposite knee
- Hop distance 85% of opposite knee
- ROM 0 to 140 degrees

Modified from Jackson DW: *The anterior cruciate ligament: current and future concepts*, New York, 1993, Raven Press.

Continued

REHABILITATION PROTOCOL—cont'd

ACL Reconstruction PAULOS AND STERN

TABLE 5-7 Semitendinosus Protocol (LONNIE PAULOS, MD)

Activities/Daily Living	Week								Month					
	1	2	3	4	5	6	7	8	3	4	5	6	9	12
Shower without brace				➤➤➤➤➤➤➤➤➤➤➤➤➤➤➤										➤
Sleep without brace						➤➤➤➤➤➤➤➤➤➤➤➤➤								➤
Break down brace						➤➤➤➤➤➤➤➤➤➤➤➤➤								➤

Range of Motion	Week								Extension
	1	2	3	4	5	6	7	8	• Lie on stomach and lower leg into extension • Sit on firm surface and place 5 to 10 lbs above knee
Passive									
Extension/flexion	10/70	10/70	10/70	0/90	0/100	0/110	0/120	Full	**Flexion**
Active									• Lie on back; use gravity to slide foot down wall
Extension/flexion	30/60	30/60	25/70	20/80	15/90	10/100	5/110	0/120	• While sitting use gravity and opposite leg to bend knee

Brace Settings	Week								Month					
	1	2	3	4	5	6	7	8	3	4	5	6	9	12
Weight bearing						50%	75%	100%	Full ➤➤➤➤➤➤➤➤➤➤➤➤					➤
Knee-brace ROM setting	• Brace locked at 30 degrees for first 2 weeks postoperatively													
For exercise	• Unlock brace to exercise angles after 2 weeks postoperatively													
Extension/flexion	30/60	30/60	25/70	20/80	15/90	10/100	5/110	0/120	Open ➤➤➤➤➤➤➤➤➤					➤
For ambulation														
Extension/flexion						20/100	20/110	20/120	D/C'd for walking at twelfth week					

Strength Training	Week								Month					
	1	2	3	4	5	6	7	8	3	4	5	6	9	12
Quad sets, SLRs (brace locked at 40 degrees)	➤➤➤➤➤➤➤➤➤➤➤➤➤➤➤➤							➤						
Electrical stimulation (brace locked at 40 degrees)	➤➤➤➤➤➤➤➤➤➤➤➤➤➤➤➤							➤						
Hamcurls		➤➤➤➤➤➤➤➤➤➤➤➤➤➤➤												➤
Total hip		➤➤➤➤➤➤➤➤➤➤➤➤➤						➤						
Minisquat/leg press/toe rise						➤➤➤➤➤➤➤➤➤➤➤								➤
Cycling—stationary					➤➤➤➤➤➤➤➤➤➤➤➤									➤
Cycling—outdoor								Level ground only		Seated hill climb	Standing hill climbs			

REHABILITATION PROTOCOL—cont'd

TABLE 5-7—cont'd

	Week								Month					
Balance/Coordination	1	2	3	4	5	6	7	8	3	4	5	6	9	12
Baps/KAT/Sandunes/Rhomberg/ tape touch									███████████████→					
Profitter									███████████████→					
SportCord lateral agility									███████████████→					
	Week								**Month**					
Conditioning	1	2	3	4	5	6	7	8	3	4	5	6	9	12
Cycle with well leg	████████→													
UBE (upper body ergonometer)		████████████████████→												
Swimming (refer to pool protocol)					20°███████→									
Walking (100% weight)								10°████→						
Stairmaster									20°████→					
Cross-country ski machine									20°████→					
Rowing									30°/90°███→					
Run/jog (sports brace must be worn)												20°████→		
	Week								**Month**					
Power Training	1	2	3	4	5	6	7	8	3	4	5	6	9	12
Low repetitions—leg press/ squats/hamcurls								20°/90°████→						
Isokinetics (refer to protocol)												████→		

To Return to Sports:
- Minimum of 9 months postoperatively
- No swelling
- Complete jog/run program
- Quadriceps strength 85% of opposite knee
- Hamstring strength 90% of opposite knee
- Hop distance 85% of opposite knee
- ROM 0 to 140 degrees

Modified from Jackson DW: *The anterior cruciate ligament: current and future concepts*, New York, 1993, Raven Press.

COMPLICATIONS/TROUBLESHOOTING

Loss of Motion

Loss of motion, or arthrofibrosis, is recognized as one of the most common postoperative complications following ACL reconstruction. As stated earlier, loss of motion is defined by Fu et al. as a knee flexion contracture of more than 10 degrees and/or knee flexion ROM less than 125 degrees.

It is important to begin passive full knee extension exercises early in the rehabilitation program to prevent scar tissue formation in the intercondylar notch. These exercises, such as prone leg hangs and towel extensions, should be performed until maintenance of full knee extension is assured.

Patellar mobilization, especially superior gliding, should be initiated immediately to prevent shortening of the patellar tendon and decreased patellar mobility.

Mobilization of the tibiofemoral joint may also be necessary to promote knee flexion and extension ROM. Early edema control is important to prevent induration of the peripatellar soft tissues. Induration of these tissues may lead to decreased patellar mobility with resulting loss of motion. Joint effusion may also be exacerbated by an aggressive strengthening program. Nonsteroidal antiinflammatory medication (NSAIDs), as well as modification of the rehabilitation program, may be necessary until the effusion can be controlled.

Infrapatellar contracture syndrome may develop if a fibrous hyperplasia of the anterior soft tissues of the knee occurs. The fibrous hyperplasia entraps the patella and limits knee motion. Early detection of this condition is necessary to prevent significant complications. Signs and symptoms include induration of the peripatellar tissues, painful ROM, restricted patellar mobility, extensor lag, and a "shelf sign."

Patients with unacceptable motion, defined by Graf and Uhr as a flexion contracture of 10 degrees or more or a limitation of flexion of less than 130 degrees, are treated initially with aggressive physical therapy. The use of a Dynasplint (Dynasplint Systems) may be considered; this device produces a low-load prolonged force on restricted soft tissues to restore ROM. If conservative measures fail, patients are treated surgically. At less than 6 months postoperatively, Graf and Uhr and Paulos et al. recommend closed manipulation of the knee, with arthroscopic lysis of adhesions and debridement of the intercondylar notch as necessary. At more than 6 months after surgery, open debridement is recommended.

Patellofemoral Pain

Patellofemoral pain may be caused by flexion contracture, prolonged immobilization, quadriceps weakness, or aggressive open-chain (OKC) quadriceps exercises.

Shelbourne and Nitz found fewer problems with patellofemoral pain symptoms in patients undergoing accelerated ACL rehabilitation, probably because of the initiation of early ROM and CKC quadriceps exercise.

OKC quadriceps strengthening should be performed in a pain-free ROM to prevent exacerbation of patellofemoral pain. Generally, OKC quadriceps exercises in the 90- to 60-degree range produce the highest forces on the patellofemoral joint. A low-weight/high-repetition program should be emphasized with quadriceps exercise if the patient complains of patellofemoral pain.

The use of CKC strengthening decreases the amount of force at the patellofemoral joint. CKC exercises are generally performed near full extension, thus avoiding the increased compressive forces generated from 90 to 60 degrees.

Patellar Tendonitis

Wilk et al. reported that patellar tendonitis is not caused by harvest of the patellar tendon graft. They suggest that if meticulous procurement of the graft is performed, followed by immediate motion and weight bearing, patellar mobilization, and quadriceps strengthening, complications such as patellar tendonitis can be avoided.

Patients often develop symptoms of patellar tendonitis with the initiation of aggressive quadriceps strengthening. It is important to monitor patients for such symptoms, so that a chronic inflammatory process does not ensue. If treated in the acute phase with NSAIDs, ice-cup massage, flexibility exercises, and a reduction or modification of the quadriceps strengthening program, patellar tendonitis generally can be reversed. Some clinicians advocate eccentric quadriceps strengthening in the treatment of patellar tendonitis. Once in the chronic phase, patellar tendonitis becomes harder to treat and can hinder the patient's progress with rehabilitation.

ACL RECONSTRUCTION WITH CONCOMITANT MENISCAL REPAIR

Rehabilitation protocols for the ACL reconstructed knee with concomitant meniscal repair vary according to surgeons' preferences and surgical consideration (see box).

Medial and Lateral Collateral Ligament Injury of the Knee

REHABILITATION RATIONALE

Medial collateral ligament (MCL) injuries usually are caused by a valgus stress. The most common mecha-

Variables Affecting Rehabilitation After ACL Reconstruction and Meniscal Repair

- Type of surgical procedure
  Arthrotomy
  Arthroscopic assisted
  Endoscopy
- Graft type
  Patellar tendon
  Semitendinosus
  Iliotibial band
- Graft fixation
  Screw
  Button
  Staple
  Suture
- Graft placement
  Isometricity
  Nonisometricity
- Graft tensioning
- Tourniquet time
- Concomitant surgeries
  Menisci lesion
  Capsular deficiencies
  Collateral ligament injuries
  Posterior cruciate ligament injuries
  Chondral lesions
  Surgical notchplasty
- Patient variables
  Size
  Alignment
  Activity level
  Compliance

nism is a blow to the lateral aspect of the knee. The examiner must make sure, by examination or magnetic resonance imaging (MRI), that concomitant injuries of the knee are not present. The classic O'Donoghue triad of injury is MCL, ACL, and peripheral medial meniscus, but more recent reports indicate that the most common triad is MCL, ACL, and lateral meniscal tear. Isolated MCL injury should be treated nonoperatively, but concomitant intraarticular ligament injuries (ACL) typically require surgical reconstruction. Meniscal pathology also requires surgical intervention. Seventy percent to 80% of patients with acute ACL disruptions present with significant traumatic effusion. The incidence of significant knee effusion with isolated MCL tears is significantly lower (usually 1+ rather than 4+).

Examination

To test for MCL injury, a valgus stress is applied with the knee in full extension and then with the knee in 30 degrees of flexion (Fig. 5-23). As the knee moves into extension, the role of secondary restraints other than the MCL increases. Isolated MCL tear is indicated by instability only at 30 degrees of flexion. Instability in full extension indicates that secondary restraints are disrupted in addition to the MCL. Tenderness to palpation usually is present over the tibial or femoral attachment. The severity of MCL and lateral collateral ligament (LCL) tears is based on a standard system (Table 5-8 and Fig. 5-24).

Treatment

Isolated MCL tests are treated nonoperatively with protective bracing, early ROM, and physical therapy. Grades 1 and 2 injuries are treated with immediate

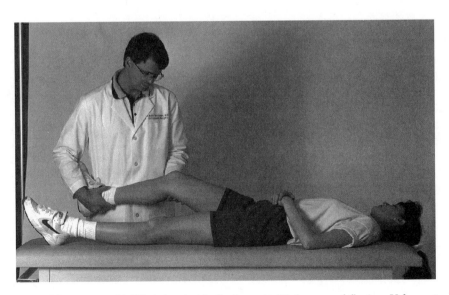

Figure 5-23 Testing of MCL injury with the knee in 30 degrees of flexion. Valgus stress is placed across the knee.

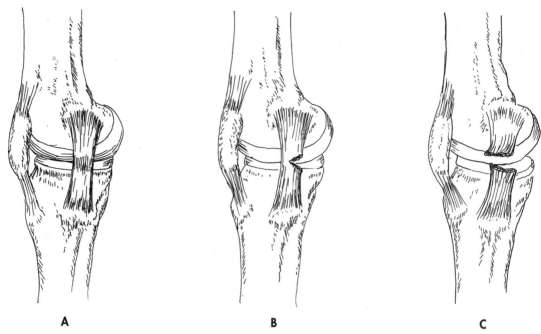

Figure 5-24 Medial collateral tears of the knee. **A**, Grade 1; **B**, Grade 2; **C**, Grade 3.

TABLE 5-8 **Severity of MCL and LCL Tears**

Grade	Opening on Exam	MCL/LCL Test	Instability
1	0 to 5 mm	Minimal	None
2	5 to 10 mm	Partial	Some
3	10 to 15 mm	Significant	Moderate
4	Greater than 15 mm	Complete	Grossly unstable

Modified from Miller M: *Review of orthopaedics,* Philadelphia, 1992, WB Saunders.

ROM. Grade 3 injuries are kept non–weight bearing and the brace is locked for 2 to 3 weeks. Chronic instability may require reconstruction using the semimembranosus tendon (Slocum procedure) or advancing the tibial MCL (Mauck procedure).

For grade 3 MCL tears, many authors advocate locking the brace at 45 degrees of flexion for 2 to 3 weeks, followed by bracing in restricted ROM (0 to 90 degrees). The patient remains non–weight bearing with crutches for 3 weeks. During this immobilization period, isometric exercises (SLRs, quadsets, etc.) are performed. Gentle active ROM exercises may be performed in the brace as tolerated, but restricted weight bearing is continued for 3 months.

LCL injuries usually are caused by a varus stress. Rehabilitation after LCL injury is similar to that after injury of the MCL, but slower healing of LCL usually requires a longer period of brace protection. Complete LCL tears often are managed by operative repair, with or without augmentation with the biceps tendon.

REHABILITATION PROTOCOL

Grades 1 and 2 Injuries of the Medial Collateral Ligament
BROTZMAN AND ROSS

Phase 1	• Apply sturdy rehabilitation brace with settings locked from 15 to 90 degrees.
	• Begin partial weight-bearing ambulation with crutches.
	• Exercise in brace 3 times daily:
	  Isometrics (SLRs, quadriceps sets, VMO exercises)
	  Ankle ROM exercises
	  Active knee flexion to 90 degrees
	  Hip flexion
	  90 to 45 degree knee extension
	  Hip extension
	  Well leg and upper body exercises (aerobic conditioning)
	• Remove brace only to shower.
	• Use icing (cryotherapy) compression dressings early.
	• Prescribe oral NSAIDs.

Phase 2 3 weeks	• Perform exercises out of brace. • Progress knee flexion and extension, TKE, 90 to 0, side step-ups.

	• Begin progressive resistive exercises (PREs) 1 to 10 lbs. • Begin bicycling when ROM is sufficient. • Progress partial weight bearing to full weight bearing, no crutches.
Phase 3 6 weeks	• Initiate negative-resistive work. • Perform PREs with heavy weight. • Use stationary bicycle. • Allow functional activities, including straight-ahead running. • Advance to stadium steps and figure-eight running.
Return to sports	• Confirm painless, stable ROM with no pain on palpation of ligament. • Ensure absence of effusion or instability. • Ensure presence of symmetric muscle strength with uninvolved extremity.

■ *It is important for optimal long-term results that the patient obtain adequate ROM and muscle strength before returning to full activities, including competitive sports. Because individuals heal at different rates, these prerequisites are critical.*

REHABILITATION PROTOCOL

Grades 1 and 2 Injuries of the Medial Collateral Ligament
HOLDEN

GOAL	• Maintenance of cardiovascular reserve and muscle strength and endurance		• Begin ambulation, as tolerated, with crutches. • Apply brace to knee.
TIME OF INJURY	• Use standard first-aid methods. • Use ice and compression dressings. • Employ elevation and knee immobilizer or locked brace.	3 to 7 days	• Continue above activities. • Begin negative-resistive exercises (0 to 35 degrees) with 10 lbs; set determined by symptoms.

1 day	• Ensure early maintenance of muscle tone.
	• Perform quadriceps setting exercises.
	• Perform straight leg raises.
		8 to 14 days	• Individualize negative-resistive exercises:
			  Progressive weight to tolerance
			  Progressive repetitions to fatigue level

2 days	• Perform ROM exercises in whirlpool followed by ice massage.		*Continued*

Grades 1 and 2 Injuries of the Medial Collateral Ligament
HOLDEN

8 to 14 days —cont'd	• Begin cardiovascular/muscle endurance sets (times 10): Jogging, 2 × 120 yards Variable resistance stationary bicycle, 2 minutes • Begin stadium walking: Up bleachers, down steps Progressive to fatigue • Perform whirlpool ROM exercises followed by ice massage.		• Begin acceleration/deceleration speed play. • Begin stadium stair running (to fatigue) up bleachers, down bleachers, down steps. • Perform agility drills (specific to player position).
15 to 21 days	• Initiate terminal extension progressive resistive exercises 10 repetitions × 3 sets • Begin cardiovascular/muscle endurance sets (times 5): 6 × 120 yards Variable resistance stationary bicycle, 5 minutes • Perform figure eight weaving patterns 45 degrees cutting over 20 yards.	4 to 6 weeks	• Ensure full ROM.
		RETURN TO SPORT	• Confirm nontenderness over collateral ligament. • Ensure absence of effusion. • Ensure there is no instability. • Muscle strength should be 95% of opposite side.
		REMAINDER OF SEASON	• Perform PREs on Orthotron (3 times per week). • Use standard MCL taping.

Lateral Retinacular Release SHERMAN

1 day	• Begin ROM exercises and knee strengthening the day of surgery. • Allow weight bearing as tolerated with crutches, typically using crutches 1 to 2 weeks. • Use cryotherapy, compressive wraps, and galvanic stimulation for at least 72 hours for edema control. • Employ capsular mobilization techniques by manipulation of patella to prevent recurrent scarring of the surgical release or suprapatellar adhesions (Fig. 5-34). • Begin quadriceps strengthening: Straight leg raises Quadriceps sets Initiate submaximal exercises at terminal extension, progressing to maximum contraction of the VMO as soon as the patient is able. • Initiate PREs as tolerated.	• Focus on VMO strengthening over next weeks, using VMO biofeedback if required. • Progress PREs. • Continue formal outpatient physical therapy for a minimum of 3 months with active encouragement. Progression of activity: 1. Unassisted walking 2. Swimming 3. Distance walking and cycling 4. Jogging 5. Running 6. Pivoting activities Program parameters: • With program adherence, 90% of patients can perform an isometric straight leg raise without an extensor lag and have at least 90 degrees of flexion with minimal effusion at 1 week. • All patients should have greater than 120 degrees of flexion at 4 weeks.
2 days	• Begin active-assisted and passive ROM exercises for restoration of full flexion. Begin in the sitting position, then use prone techniques to place the lateral capsular attachments on greater stretch.	

Iliotibial Band Friction Syndrome of the Knee in Runners

REHABILITATION RATIONALE

Iliotibial band friction syndrome is the most common cause of lateral knee pain in runners. The iliotibial band is a thickened strip of fascia that extends from the iliac crest to the lateral tibial tubercle, receiving part of the insertion of the tensor fasciae latae and gluteus maximus. A bursa and subsequent inflammatory response develop between the band and bony prominence with repetitive flexion and extension of the knee (such as in downhill running). Usually an inflammatory reaction develops between the iliotibial band and the lateral femoral epicondyle (Fig. 5-25); less often the band is irritated at the lateral tibial prominence.

Factors that contribute to the development of iliotibial friction band syndrome include the following:

• Cavus feet	Increases lateral stresses at iliotibial band
• Varus knee position	Increases lateral stresses at iliotibial band
• Downhill running	Especially aggravates symptoms because the knee is maintained in a flexed position for longer periods than on a flat surface
• "Downhill" leg on a pitched running surface	Runners who run consistently on roads that have a drainage pitch often develop iliotibial band friction syndrome of the downside leg (Noble and Clancy)
• Hard shoes, hard surfaces	Hard running shoes are defined as those having a rearfoot and forefoot impact rating of more than 10 gm and 13 gm, respectively, as tested in 1981 *Runner's World* shoe survey. Hard surfaces include paved roads, but not dirt roads.

Clinical features of iliotibial band friction syndrome include pain and palpable tenderness over the lateral femoral condyle about 2 cm above the joint line during exercise. Pain is exacerbated by downhill running and often is aggravated by repetitive flexion-extension movements (walking down stairs, running, cycling, or skiing). Usually pain becomes so severe that it limits the athlete to a particular distance. Many patients have iliotibial band tightness, which is diagnosed with Ober's test (Fig. 5-26).

Lindenberg classified the pain caused by iliotibial band friction syndrome into four grades according to activity limitation:

1. Pain comes on after run but does not restrict distance or speed.

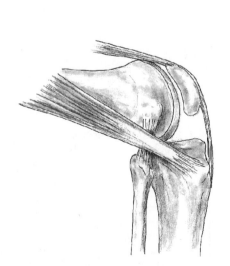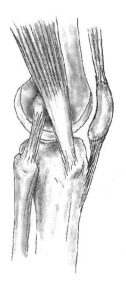

Figure 5-25 As the knee moves from flexion to extension, the iliotibial tract passes from behind to move in front of the lateral femoral epicondyle. The pain experienced by runners with iliotibial tract friction syndrome is caused by the tight band rubbing over the bony prominence of the lateral epicondyle. (Redrawn from Dugas R, D'Ambrosia R: Causes and treatment of common overuse injuries in runners, *J Musculoskel Med* 3(8):113, 1991.)

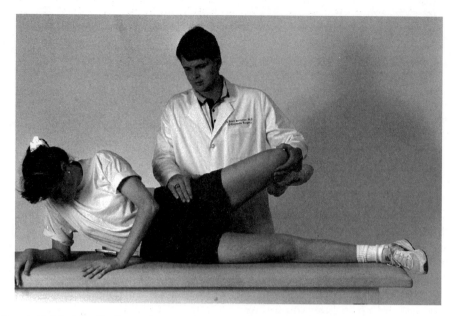

Figure 5-26 **Ober's test** to detect tightness in the iliotibial tract and tensor fasciae latae muscle. Patients are instructed to lie on their sides. The examiner places the upper leg in abduction and some extension so that the iliotibial band crosses the greater trochanter. The knee may be flexed or extended, the latter stretching the iliotibial band more. The pelvis is stabilized and the upper leg is adducted (lowered) toward the floor. With a tight iliotibial band, the leg remains abducted. If normal, the leg adducts (lowers) to the table surface.

2. Pain comes on during run but does not restrict distance or speed.
3. Pain comes on during run and restricts distance or speed.
4. Pain so severe it prevents running.

Natural History

Clancy reports that most runners with iliotibial band friction syndrome must rest from running for 6 weeks.

Our experience indicates that severe inflammation often requires 6 to 8 weeks of rest before symptoms subside and the patient is able to return to running. Patients with acute or mild symptoms usually respond quickly to conservative measures. For recalcitrant symptoms, Noble recommends surgical release of the posterior fibers of the iliotibial band where they overlie the femoral condyle.

REHABILITATION PROTOCOL

Iliotibial Band Friction Syndrome in Runners

- Rest from running until asymptomatic.
- Ice area before and after exercise.
- Prescribe oral NSAIDs.
- Ensure relative rest from running and high flexion-extension activities of the knee (cycling, running, stair descent, skiing).
- Avoid downhill running.
- Avoid running on pitched surfaces with a pitched drainage grade to the road.
- Use soft running shoes rather than hard shoes (see p. 225).
- Use iontophoresis if helpful.
- Give a steroid injection into the bursa if required.

- Perform stretching exercises:
  Iliotibial band stretching
  Two-man Ober stretch (Fig. 5-27)
  Self–Ober stretch (Fig. 5-28)
  Lateral fascial stretch (Fig. 5-29)
  Posterior fascial stretch plus gluteus maximus and piriformis self stretch (Fig. 5-30)
  Standing wall lean for lateral fascial stretch (Fig. 5-31)
  Rectus femoris self stretch (Fig. 5-32)
  Iliopsoas with rectus femoris self-stretch (Fig. 5-33)
- Use lateral heel wedge in the shoe, especially for those with iliotibial band tightness (Clancy and Noble).
- Build in correction in the shoe for a short leg (leg-length discrepancy) if present.

REHABILITATION PROTOCOL—cont'd

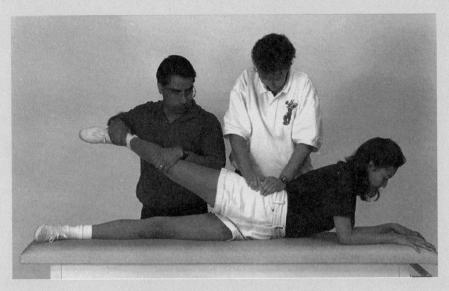

Figure 5-27 Two-man Ober stretch.

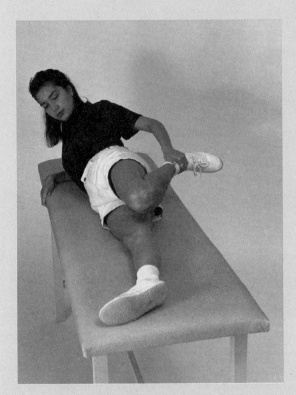

Figure 5-28 Self-Ober stretch.

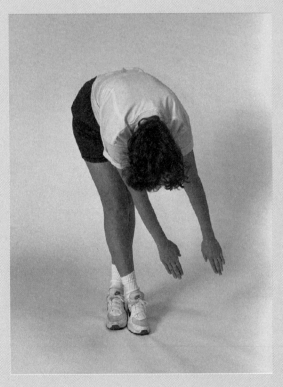

Figure 5-29 Standing lateral fascial stretch. The involved leg is crossed behind the uninvolved leg.

Continued

Iliotibial Band Friction Syndrome in Runners

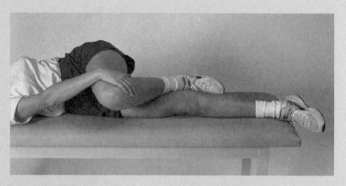

Figure 5-30 Posterior fascial stretch, plus gluteus maximus and piriformis stretch.

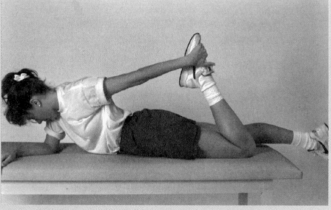

Figure 5-32 Rectus femoris self-stretch.

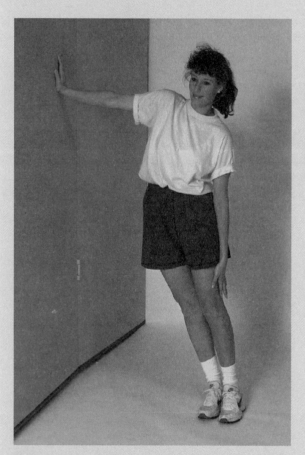

Figure 5-31 Standing wall lean for lateral fascial stretch with the involved leg closest to the wall.

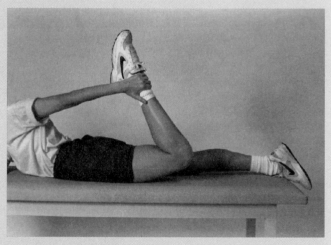

Figure 5-33 Iliopsoas with rectus femoris stretch. Thigh is off the table.

Patellofemoral Disorders

REHABILITATION RATIONALE

Patellofemoral dysfunction, or disorder, may be defined as pain, imbalance, inflammation, and/or instability of any component of the extensor mechanism of the knee. These conditions may result from congenital, traumatic, or mechanical stresses (Shelton and Thigpen).

A careful clinical history and physical examination should be performed to accurately identify the exact syndrome causing the anterior knee pain (see box 5-2).

An individual with patellofemoral pain experiences increased pain when the knee is flexed because the patellofemoral joint reaction force (PFJRF) increases with flexion of the knee from 0.5 times body weight during level walking to 3 to 4 times body weight during stair climbing and 7 to 8 times body weight during squatting (Fig. 5-34).

CHONDROMALACIA PATELLAE

There is some confusion in the literature caused by the (incorrect) interchangeable usage of the terms chondromalacia patellae and anterior knee pain. Chondromalacia patellae is a pathologic description of softening of the articular cartilage on the undersurface of the patella. This does not include the other structures involved in anterior knee pain: the patellar tendon, medial and lateral retinacular structures, and intraarticular structures.

Chondromalacia generally is described in the following four stages:

Stage 1   Articular cartilage shows only softening or blistering.

Stage 2   Fissures appear in the cartilage.

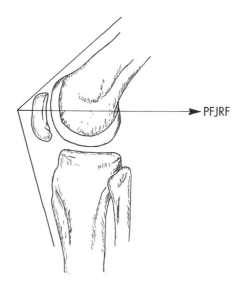

Figure 5-34 Increased patellofemoral joint reaction force (PFJRF) with knee flexion during squatting.

Classification of Patellofemoral Disorders

Trauma (Conditions Caused by Trauma in the Otherwise Normal Knee)

- Acute trauma
  Contusion
  Fracture
     Patella
     Femoral trochlea
     Proximal tibial epiphysis (tubercle)
  Dislocation (rare in normal knee)
  Rupture
     Quadriceps tendon
     Patellar tendon
- Repetitive trauma (overuse syndromes)
  Patellar tendonitis ("jumper's knee")
  Quadriceps tendonitis
  Peripatellar tendonitis (such as anterior knee pain
     in an adolescent due to hamstring contraction)
  Prepatellar bursitis ("housemaid's knee")
  Apophysitis
     Osgood-Schlatter disease
     Sinding-Larsen-Johansson disease
- Late effects of trauma
  Posttraumatic chondromalacia patellae
  Posttraumatic patellofemoral arthritis
  Anterior fat-pad syndrome (posttraumatic fibrosis)
  Reflex sympathetic dystrophy
  Patellar osseous dystrophy
  Acquired patella infera
  Acquired quadriceps fibrosis

Patellofemoral Dysplasia

- Lateral patellar compression syndrome
  With secondary chondromalacia patellae
  With secondary patellofemoral arthritis
- Chronic subluxation of the patella
  With secondary chondromalacia patellae
  With secondary patellofemoral arthritis
- Recurrent dislocation of the patella
  Associated fractures
     Osteochondral (intraarticular)
     Avulsion (extraarticular)
  With secondary chondromalacia patellae
  With secondary patellofemoral arthritis
- Chronic dislocation of the patella
  Congenital
  Acquired

Idiopathic Chondromalacia Patellae Osteochondritis Dissecans

- Patella
- Femoral trochlea

Synovial Plicae (Anatomic Variant Made Symptomatic by Acute or Repetitive Trauma)

- Medial patellar ("shelf")
- Suprapatellar
- Lateral patellar

From Merchant AC: The classification of patellofemoral disorders, *Arthroscopy* 4:235, 1988.

Stage 3 Fibrillation of cartilage occurs, causing a "crab-meat" appearance.
Stage 4 Full cartilage defects are present; subchondral bone is exposed.

PATELLAR TILT VERSUS PATELLAR SUBLUXATION

Patellar tilt and subluxation also are entities separate from patellofemoral pain. Chronic patellar tilt tends to be associated with retinacular tightness and pain because the retinaculum is placed under significant tension with knee flexion.

If a line extending from the lateral articular facet of the patella is parallel to or converges with a line from the lateral condyle of the patellofemoral groove, an abnormal condition exists indicative of increased lateral pressure (Fig. 5-35) (Kramer). In contrast, many patients with a lax extensor retinaculum experience frequent patella subluxation without retinacular pain, but they are more prone to instability problems and dislocation.

PATELLAR FUNCTION AND MECHANICS

The patella links the divergent quadriceps muscle to the common tendon, increasing the quadriceps lever arm and thus its mechanical advantage (McConnell, Ficat). To function efficiently the patella must be properly aligned so that it remains in the trochlear groove of the femur. The ability of the patella to track properly in the trochlear groove depends on the bony structures and the balance of forces of the soft tissues about the joint. Patellar malalignment caused by altered mechanics predisposes an individual to patellofemoral pain.

Lateral forces at the patellofemoral joint are restricted by the medial retinaculum and the VMO; during knee flexion, these are aided by the prominent orientation of the lateral trochlear facet (Fig. 5-36). Any imbalance in these forces may result in patellar maltracking (see box).

Q angle
The Q angle is formed by the intersection of the line of pull of the quadriceps and the patellar tendon measured through the center of the patella. A line is drawn from the anterosuperior iliac spine through the center of the patella and a second line is drawn from the tibial tubercle to the center of the patella (Fig. 5-37). The Q angle is normally less than 10 degrees in men and 15 degrees in women. The upper limit for a normal Q angle is 13 to 15 degrees. An increased Q angle may be associated with increased femoral anteversion, external tibial torsion, and lateral displacement of the tibial tubercle that increases the lateral pull of the patella.

TREATMENT

The literature reports good results in 75% to 85% of cases with nonoperative treatment of patellofemoral disorders (Whittenbecker et al.) Specified periods for conservative trials range from 2 to 6 months. We believe a 6-month trial of conservative treatment is warranted to avoid surgical intervention if at all possible.

REHABILITATION CONSIDERATIONS

The most successful rehabilitation programs customize the specifics of the program to the patient. The

---

Factors Affecting Patellar Alignment (McConnell)

- Increased Q angle
- VMO insufficiency
- Tight lateral structures
- Patella alta: the "superiorly" riding patella rides above the stabilizing structures of the trochlear groove

---

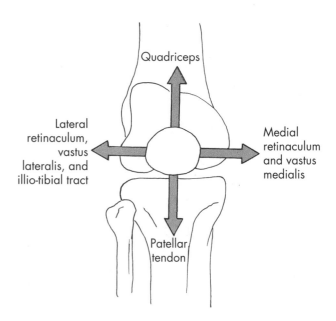

Figure 5-36 Forces around the patella.

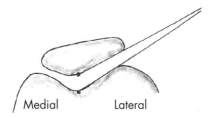

Figure 5-35 Patellar tilt causing an increased pressure on the lateral portion of the patellofemoral surface.

regimen should allow progression without increasing symptoms. Low exercise intensity and high repetitions help achieve this end. Strength, flexibility, endurance, proprioception, and functional training are the key components of the therapeutic exercise program. Medication, relative rest, external support (taping or Palumbo brace), and modalities are helpful adjuncts.

Strengthening

Strengthening programs are directed at increasing the strength of the VMO muscle. This muscle exerts a stabilizing medial force on the patella, predominantly in the last 30 degrees of extension. (Radin, Fulkerson, and Hungerford). The VMO realigns the patella medially and is the only dynamic medial stabilizer.

Isometric exercises such as QS and straight leg raises are most frequently used for strengthening. These exercises produce smaller PFJRF than larger arc exercises and usually are less painful. Soderberg and Cook demonstrated that the rectus femoris was most active during straight leg raises and that the vastus medialis, biceps femoris, and gluteus medius were most active during QS. VMO biofeedback is a useful adjunct in helping the patient properly isolate the VMO (see Fig. 5-3).

The use of hip adductor contractions in conjunction with QS and straight leg raises have been recommended to facilitate VMO strengthening because of the VMO origin near the adductor magnus (Shelton and Thigpen) (Fig. 5-38). Terminal knee extension ex-

ercises (SAQ exercises) also are used to improve quadriceps strengthening in the least efficient portion of the arc of motion (Shelton and Thigpen) (See Fig. 5-21). Closed-chain strengthening techniques are encouraged. Eccentric ankle dorsiflexion exercises have been reported to reduce patellar tendonitis symptoms. (Shelton and Thigpen)

Results of EMG recordings of the VMO are shown in Table 5-9.

Flexibility

Flexibility training has been strongly emphasized as a component in the treatment of patellofemoral disorders. Hamstring tightness may contribute to an increase in patellofemoral joint reaction forces. Tight hamstrings increase knee flexion during running, thus increasing the PFJRF instance (see p. 229); increased peripatellar soft tissue tension from quadriceps tightness may also produce higher PFJRF. Gastrocnemius-soleus inflexibility causes compensatory pronation of the foot, resulting in increased tibial rotation and subsequent additional patellofemoral stress. Iliotibial band tightness can contribute to lateral tracking of the patella.

Some special maneuvers used for determining tightness of these structures are described below.

The *passive patellar tilt* test is performed with the knee extended and the quadriceps relaxed. The examiner lifts the lateral edge of the patella from the lateral femoral condyle (Fig. 5-39). An excessively tight lateral retinaculum is demonstrated by a neutral or negative angle to the horizontal. A preoperative negative passive patellar tilt (therefore excessive lateral tightness) correlates with a successful result after a lateral retinacular release in those who do not respond favorably to conservative measures.

The *patellar glide test* indicates medial or lateral retinacular tightness and/or integrity. With the knee flexed 10 to 30 degrees and the quadriceps relaxed, the patella is divided into longitudinal quadrants. The examiner attempts to displace the patella in a medial direction, then in a lateral direction using the index finger and thumb (Fig. 5-40). This determines lateral and medial parapatellar tightness, respectively. A medial glide of one quadrant is consistent with a tight lateral retinaculum and often correlates with a negative pas-

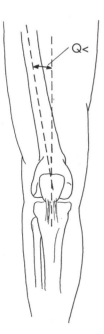

Figure 5-37 Q angle. The Q angle measurement is used to assess the angular alignment of the extensor mechanism. The upper limit of normal is 15 degrees. This angle is formed by the bisection of a line drawn along the femoral shaft and another drawn along the patellar tendon, from the tibial tubercle to the center of the patella.

TABLE 5-9 **EMG Recordings of the VMO**		
	Normal subjects	Patients with patellofemoral pain
VMO:VL ratio	1:1	<1:1
Activity	VMO tonically active	VMO phasically active

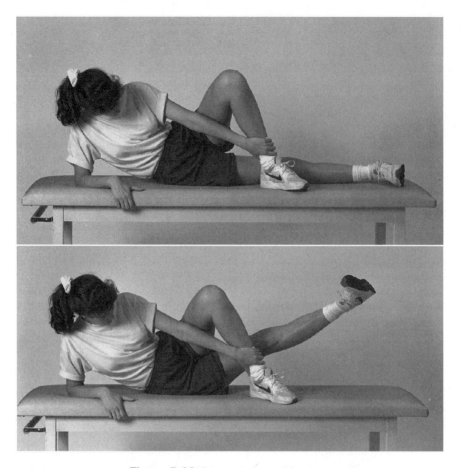

Figure 5-38 Isometric hip adduction.

sive patellar tilt test. A medial glide of three to four quadrants suggests a hypermobile patella. A lateral glide of three quadrants is suggestive of an incompetent medial restraint. A lateral glide of four quadrants (dislocatable patella) is obviously indicative of a deficient medial restraint.

Ober's test for iliotibial band tightness (see Fig. 5-26) is used to evaluate iliotibial band flexibility. It is performed by having the patient side-lying with the lower leg flexed 90 degrees at the knee for support and the pelvis stabilized. With the upper knee flexed at 90 degrees, the hip is brought from flexion/abduction to neutral (in line with the trunk) with neutral rotation and then is allowed to adduct. Both lower extremities are examined for comparison. The involved lower extremity exhibits iliotibial band tightness if the hip cannot adduct beyond neutral as far as the uninvolved side.

Endurance

Most authors encourage endurance training in patients with patellofemoral disorder. Bicycling and swimming are used most often because of their low-impact force on the lower extremities. Ericson and

Nisell advocate a high saddle position during bicycling to minimize PFJRF during cycling. Stair-climber machines can be used to increase endurance, but caution must be taken to avoid increasing symptoms with this method.

Functional Training

The trend of therapeutic exercises for patellofemoral disorder has been toward more functionally oriented activities performed with good VMO control. Several authors advocate a progressive running-agility-drill program that moves from basic to more advanced activities. They emphasize the use of electromyogram (EMG) biofeedback to facilitate VMO control of the patella during functional activities. Again, the absence of patellofemoral symptoms is a key guide to progression.

Rest

Because many forms of patellofemoral disorders are caused by overuse, various levels of rest are recommended as part of the treatment algorithm. Relative rest from activity is obtained by modifying the offending activity or selecting other activities to decrease

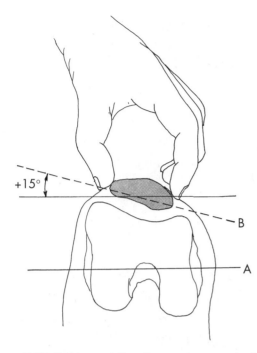

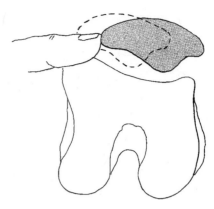

Figure 5-40 Patellar glide test is performed in 30 degrees of flexion. An attempt is made to displace the patella medially and then laterally to determine lateral and medial retinacular tightness, respectively. (Redrawn from Kolowich P: Lateral release of the patella: indications and contraindication, *Am J Sports Med* 14(4):359, 1990.)

Figure 5-39 Passive patellar tilt test. An excessively tight lateral restraint (lateral retinaculum) is demonstrated by a neutral or negative angle to the horizontal. This test is performed with the knee extended and the quadriceps relaxed. (Redrawn from Kolowich P: Lateral release of the patella: indications and contraindication, *Am J Sports Med* 14(4):359, 1990.)

symptoms. Absolute or complete rest is rarely recommended unless conservative treatment fails.

Medication

NSAIDs are often used unless contraindicated. Iontophoresis has had some success. Steroid injection is discouraged because of resultant articular cartilage degradation and possible tendon rupture.

External Support

Several methods have been reported for externally supporting the patella in patients with patellofemoral disorder. Many authors advocate a dynamic patellar stabilizing brace devised by Palumbo. McConnell has designed specific taping procedures to correct faulty patellar posture (see the following section). We have found taping to be helpful, especially when used during the transitional period required for the patient to strengthen the VMO. Taping increases effective quadriceps strength by decreasing pain and VMO inhibition. The actual VMO:vastus lateralis ratio is reported to be improved with patellofemoral taping. McConnell reports that taping applied after evaluation of patellar posture temporarily corrects abnormal tilt, glide, and rotation of the patella, facilitating normal patellar tracking in a pain-free manner. The patient can be taught to do the taping.

McConnell Taping Techniques for Patellofemoral Pain

- Clean, shave, spray with skin prep, and let dry.
- Cover the knee with 4-inch cover roll from midline lateral, over the patella, to under the medial hamstring group. Do not pull the tape tight.
- Outline the patella for better taping orientation. Mark into four quadrants and label.
- Place 6-inch brown Leukotape P over proximal/medial quadrant and apply pressure with the same-side thumb while pulling the tape with opposite-side hand, medial, as tight as possible. This is known as **tilt component** (Fig. 5-41, *A*).
- Place 6" Leukotape P over the proximal/lateral quadrant and, while pulling up on the medial thigh with the same-side hand, pull tape medial with opposite-side hand, again, as tight as possible to the underside of the knee. This is the **glide component** (Fig. 5-41, *B*).
- Place 3-inch tape over distal/medial quadrant, and turn the patella medial to correct external rotation of the inferior pole. Place the tape over the existing tape medial without pulling too tight. There should be no increased inferior pressure on the patella.
- Patient should then perform a **step test** (Fig. 5-41, *D*) to ensure the tape is correcting the patella orientation and that there is no increase in pain with tape. The **tilt component** is performed first, then a step test is applied. The **glide component** (if no improvement) is followed by a step test. If still painful, the **rotation component** is applied (Fig. 5-41, *C*), followed by a step test.
- Patients generally tape every day for 6 weeks, placing the tape on first thing in the morning and removing it last thing before bed. Taping duration

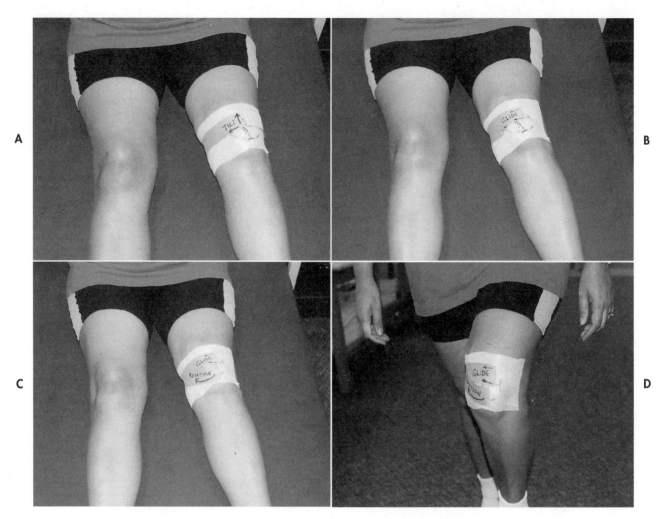

Figure 5-41 McConnell taping is based on an assessment of patellar position and mal-tracking. Three abnormal patellar orientations are examined: **A,** Tilt component, **B,** Glide component, and **C,** Rotation component. **D,** A step-test is performed between each to determine if this lessens the pain.

may be decreased to less time if there is a problem tolerating the tape. The tape should at least be worn during any physical activity.

- The tape must be removed during sleep to allow the skin sufficient time to recover.
- Tape should be removed very slowly. Pulling on the tape will irritate the skin and prevent future taping. Medisolve or Desolvit can be used to aid in tape removal.

Modalities

Because joint distension (effusion) often inhibits quadriceps muscle function (especially VMO), reduction of swelling is important to establish VMO control. Ice has been the most successful modality to reduce pain, inflammation, and swelling. Electrical muscle stimula-

tion (EMS) has shown no significant strength gains over exercise control groups in normal subjects; however, in patients with ACL reconstructions, EMS groups showed improved strength compared with exercise-only groups.

Biomechanics

Excessive pronation of the foot results in compensatory internal tibial rotation, which can increase patellofemoral stress. Abnormal mechanics should be corrected with foot orthotics when appropriate (see Chapter 10). The patient should be evaluated for possible imbalances in strength and flexibility around the hip that may be causing excessive patellofemoral stress due to faulty patterns of movement during functional activities (see box).

Clinical Evaluation of Anterior Knee Pain

Name _____

Age _____ Sex _____

Diagnosis _____

Precautions _____

Treatment protocol _____

Frequency _____ Duration _____

History

Date of injury _____

Date of surgery _____

History of injury _____

_____

Previous injuries/treatments _____

Activity related _____

_____

Intensity/duration _____

_____

Exacerbating factors _____

_____

Complaints: 1. giving way 2. catching 3. popping
4. locking 5. pain 6. pivoting 7. swelling
8. other _____

Difficulties: 1. sitting 2. out of chair 3. night pain
4. ambulation or running 5. stairs 6. job related

Exam

Gait _____

Standing alignment Varus Valgus Recurvatum
Pes planus

Step-up test   Up +/−   Down +/−

Active ROM   R extension _____ Flexion _____
L extension_____ Flexion_____

Girth measurements   Right   Left

MT _____ _____

MVMO _____

MP _____ _____

MC _____ _____

Manual muscle testing   Quadriceps _____

Hamstrings _____

Effusion   0 1+ 2+ 3+ 4+

Patellar tracking   med/lat/normal

Crepitation   med/lat/normal

Patellar orientation _____

Patellar mobility/glide test _____

Patellar tilt _____

Subluxability of patella _____

VMO status   atrophic   feet   normal
pes planus   normal arch   pes cavus

Tendonitis/bursitis _____

REHABILITATION PROTOCOL

Patellofemoral (Anterior) Knee Pain ROSS AND BROTZMAN

- May begin with modalities such as cold pack with interferential electrical stimulation (IF-ES) before exercises to decrease pain and swelling. May also require iontophoresis if tendonitis or reactive plicia is present.
- Perform all exercises with biofeedback over the VMO to ensure proper contraction and increase proprioception of the VMO.
- Patients begin with McConnell taping on the first visit. If the taping is tolerated well, they are instructed in self-taping on the second visit. The patient should be pain-free in the tape before initiating the exercise program.
- The patient is then instructed in open chaintable exercises on the first day. These include QS, straight leg raises, SAQ, hip adduction, flexion, extension and abduction, ankle plantar, and dorsiflexion as well as stretching the quadriceps, hamstrings, tensor, and gastrocnemius. Avoid hamstring stretching if the patient has recurvatum.

- If the patient is pain free with the open-chain exercises, begin closed-chain exercises. These include wall slides, lunges, lateral step-ups, balance board, heel raises, stool laps, hip adduction/SQ in standing, and leg presses.
- If the patient remains pain free with all the above exercises, begin stair-stepper, Fitter, stationary bicycle, and/or Versiclimber for general conditioning and endurance. The patient again receives a cold pack after exercise.
- Exercises are generally performed 3 to 4 times a week with a day's rest for muscle recovery. Repetitions are generally 3 to 4 sets of 10, with increasing resistance as tolerated.
- Allow return to full physical activity while taped if patient is pain free. Perform taping/exercises for approximately 6 weeks. At that time, discontinue the taping and continue the exercises as needed.

REHABILITATION PROTOCOL

Patellofemoral Stress Syndrome   MODIFIED GRIFFIN

Phase 1
1 to 2 days
- Use a knee immobilizer if acutely symptomatic.
- Use ice, IF-ES, and oral antiinflammatories to decrease inflammation and pain.
- Begin QS, straight leg raises, and VMO exercises when pain permits.
- Perform hip adductor/abduction, flexion, and extension exercises.

Phase 2
- Remove immobilizer.
- Fit a patella-stabilizing brace or use McConnell taping.
- Continue ice, IF-ES, especially following exercise.
- Continue oral antiinflammatories if needed.
- Perform straight leg raises, QS, VMO exercises, short arc extensions.
- Begin flexibility exercises for quadriceps, hamstrings, iliotibial band, gastrocnemius, soleus.
- The authors add closed-chain exercises to Griffin's original protocol at this point. This includes lunges, wall slides, lateral step-ups, minisquats, etc. (see previous protocol).
- Start to use bicycle with seat elevated, swim (crawl only), use stair-stepper (small steps done rapidly).

- Begin advanced isotonic exercises for hip flexors, extensors, abductors, adductors, as well as muscle of the lower leg and foot, increasing weight as tolerated, doing 3 sets to 10 and increasing weight by 2 lb.

Phase 3
- Continue using brace or taping.
- Continue quadriceps isotonics from 30 degrees to 0 degrees, increasing weight as tolerated.
- Advance hamstring strengthening exercises.
- Continue bicycling, swimming, stair-stepping, or walking for cardiovascular and muscle endurance; increase duration, then speed.
- Continue flexibility exercises.
- Progress closed-chain activities.

Phase 4
- Add slow return to running if desired; increase distance, then speed.
- Warm up well.
- Use ice following workout.
- Continue aerobic cross training.
- Start to jump, cut, do half squats, kick, and other sport-specific skills if applicable.
- Wear brace or tape for sport participation if desired. Tape up to 6 weeks, then discontinue. Continue brace as needed.

ACUTE PATELLAR DISLOCATION

Rehabilitation Rationale

Mechanism of Injury. Acute patellar dislocation can be caused by a powerful quadriceps contraction imposed on an internally rotated femur, a direct blow to the medial aspect of the patella, or a combination of these mechanisms.

Predisposing Factors. A high incidence of patellofemoral dysplasia has been found in patients with acute dislocations of the patella, and hypoplasia of the lateral femoral condyle has been linked to patellar dislocation (see box).

Classification. Fox and Del Pizzo described five types of patellar dislocation (Fig. 5-42).

Natural History. The average age of patients with patellar dislocation is approximately 20 years. Approximately 20% to 40% of patients with acute dislocations have redislocations. Redislocation is more likely in patients who have patellar dislocation before the age of 15 to 20 years. The results of immobilization versus early ROM after dislocation are the same. Certainly the benefit of immobilization remains unproven. Helbrect and Jackson recommend nonopera-

tive treatment in patients whose postreduction Merchant-view radiograph reveals central tracking of the patella, patients who have no underlying anatomic predisposition to dislocate, and patients who have no evidence of an osteochondral fracture.

Predisposing Factors Contributing to Patellar Dislocation

1. Increased Q angle
2. Genu valgum
3. External rotation of tibia
4. Internal rotation of femur
5. Hypoplastic lateral femoral condyle
6. Patella alta
7. Patellar shape (Wiberg classification)
8. VMO insufficiency
9. Patellar tilt
10. Tight lateral retinaculum
11. Generalized ligamentous laxity

From Fox JM, Del Pizzo W: *The patellofemoral joint*, New York, 1993, McGraw-Hill.

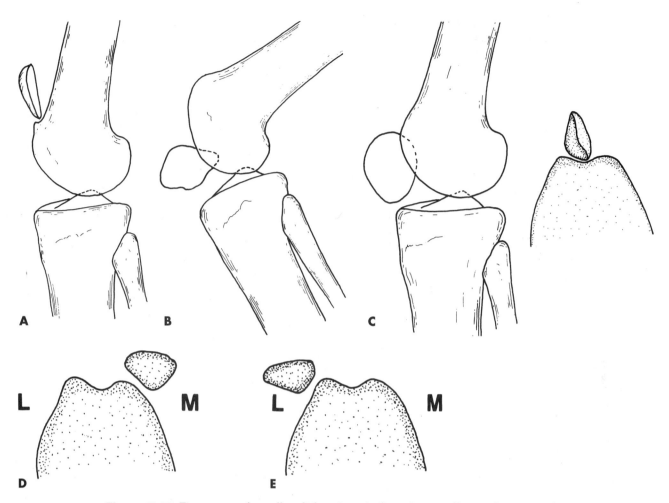

Figure 5-42 Five types of patellar dislocation. **A**, Superior; patella caught on anterior femoral osteophytes. **B**, Horizontal intra-articular. **C**, Vertical intercondylar. **D**, Medial. **E**, Lateral; most common type. (From Fox JM, Del Pizzo WD, editors: *The patellofemoral joint*, New York, 1993, McGraw-Hill.)

REHABILITATION PROTOCOL

Acute Traumatic Patellar Dislocation* FOX AND DEL PIZZO

Phase 1
24 to 48 hours

- Immobilize in knee immobilizer with lateral pad. Use elastic wrap to hold patella against medial retinaculum; use ice, electric stimulation unit, or other modalities to decrease swelling and pain.
- Prescribe antiinflammatory/analgesic medications if needed.
- Use crutches; bear weight as tolerated.
- Attempt isometric QS, hamstring sets, and hip abductors sets; hold each for count of 10; do 3 sets of 10 each.
- May use neuromuscular stimulation unit to help retard atrophy, as well as decrease pain and swelling.

Phase 2
1 to 3 weeks

- May change to patella-stabilizing brace under knee immobilizer.
- Take immobilizer off 3 times a day for ROM 0 to 30 degrees.
- Continue ice and neuromuscular stimulation unit to reduce atrophy.
- Perform QS in full extension.
- Increase to full weight bearing.
- Continue isometric exercises as well as isotonic exercises in 0 to 20 degrees.
- May start short arc extensions 30 to 0 degrees using a rolled towel under the knee.
- Continue isometrics for hamstrings.
- Begin isotonic hip abduction and adduction exercises. *Continued*

*See other protocols for patellar dislocation.

REHABILITATION PROTOCOL—cont'd

Acute Traumatic Patellar Dislocation   FOX AND DEL PIZZO

Phase 2—cont'd

1 to 3 weeks —cont'd
- Progress to 3- to 5-lb weights and do 3 sets of 10 repetitions for each muscle group.
- Perform ROM and strengthening for ankle (dorsi and plantar flexors, as well as invertors and evertors).
- Use cross-leg bicycling for cardiovascular fitness and cross-training effort.
- Perform passive and active assisted knee flexion exercises to 90 degrees.

Phase 3

3 to 6 weeks
- Use patella-stabilizing brace only when swelling and tenderness along medial retinaculum are resolved.
- Perform full ROM exercises.
- Perform stretching exercises for hamstrings, quadriceps, hip abduction, hip adduction, flexion, and extension.
- Advance isotonic quadriceps exercises (from 45 to 0 degrees); progress to 3-lb weight; if patient can do 3 sets of 10 easily, advance to 2 lbs up to 10 to 15 lbs, depending on body weight and prior level of exercise.
- Continue isotonic exercises for all other muscles of lower extremity.
- Use stair-stepper with short steps, walking, or bicycling with elevated seat for cardiovascular fitness when patient has 95 to 100 degrees of knee flexion passively and actively; begin fast stepping side to side and up and down a small step (4 to 6 inches).

Phase 4

6 weeks
- Achieve full ROM.
- Achieve strength equal to noninjured side by advancing isotonic exercises.
- Work for muscular endurance and power by alternating long, slow workouts with short bursts of activity for each muscle group.
- Continue cardiovascular fitness with bicycling, walking, or stair-stepper.
- May attempt to jog and increase running over next 4 to 6 weeks if desired.
- Add skills such as cut, squat.
- Start jumping at 8 to 12 weeks, depending on advancement of other parameters.
- Develop proprioceptive skills in weeks 8 through 10.
- Try step aerobics, functional sports skills, etc.
- Can return to full activity (anticipate 8 to 12 weeks) if ROM is equal to opposite side; no swelling, no pain, strength 95% to 100% of opposite extremity; can hop, skip, squat, and jump without difficulty.

JUMPER'S KNEE

Rehabilitation Rationale

Jumper's knee was first described by Blazina et al. as tendonitis of the patellar tendon or quadriceps tendon at the inferior or superior pole of the patella, respectively. This definition was later broadened to include pathologic conditions at the bone-tendon junction of the patellar tendon on the tibial tuberosity (Fig. 5-43). Repetitive microtrauma results from the frequent use of the extensor mechanism in certain sports, such as volleyball, basketball, track and field (high jumpers, long jumpers, sprinters, runners), and soccer. In adolescents, the same activities and repetitive microtrauma give rise to Osgood-Schlatter or Sinding-Larsen-Johansson diseases (Fig. 5-44).

Jumper's knee represents insertional tendinopathies of the quadriceps and patellar tendons. Patellar tendonitis is the most frequent tendonitis of the knee. It is localized at the lower pole of the patella and most

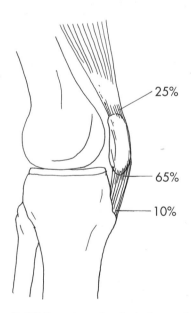

Figure 5-43 Location of pain in jumper's knee.

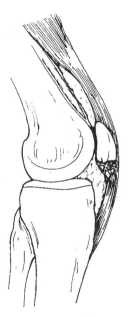

Figure 5-44 Sinding-Larsen-Johansson disease is an osteo-chondritis of the inferior pole of the patella in the skeletally immature. Conservative treatment leads to healing in 3 to 12 months. (From Colosimo A: *Orthop Rev* 19[2]:139, 1990.)

often occurs in patients between the ages of 20 and 40 years. Quadriceps tendonitis is localized at the upper pole of the patella and is more frequent in patients older than 40 years of age. The Stanish classification of jumper's knee is shown in the box.

Stanish Classification of Jumper's Knee

Level 1	No pain
Level 2	Pain with extreme exertion only
Level 3	Pain with exertion and 1 to 2 hours after
Level 4	Pain during any athletic activity and 4 to 6 hours after; performance level decreased
Level 5	Pain immediately after the beginning of sports activity; withdrawal from activity
Level 6	Pain during daily activity

Differential Diagnosis of Jumper's Knee

- Bursitis
  Suprapatellar
  Prepatellar
  Subcutaneous
  Deep infrapatellar
- Patellofemoral arthrosis and chondromalacia
- Fat pad inflammation (Hoffa's disease)
- Meniscal pathology
- Synovial infrapatellar plica
- Osgood-Schlatter and Sinding-Larsen-Johansson diseases (skeletally immature patients)

REHABILITATION PROTOCOL

Prevention of Jumper's Knee DAVID

- Ensure warm-up of the entire body (5 minutes): Bicycle or upper body machine at low intensity or brisk walking
- Perform stretching (15 minutes):
  Quadriceps femoris
  Hamstrings
  Adductors
  Calf
  Iliotibial band
- Exercise:
  Rope jumping (5 minutes)
  Concentric/eccentric quadriceps exercise
  Curwin and Stanish's stop-and-drop program:
    Eccentric exercise program that places maximal stress on the tendon in an effort to increase its strength
    Patient drops to a semisquatting position, controlling the fall with an eccentric contraction

Drop is progressed by increasing the speed of descent until the patient is able to suddenly stop the freely falling body weight using the quadriceps eccentrically
Plyometric exercises
- Apply ice (15 to 20 minutes).
- Repeat stretching.
- Education:
  Frequency of training (reduction in activity when indicated)
  Type of playing surface (avoid hard playing surface)
  Proper shoe type and fit, orthotics if necessary
  Elastic knee supports, McConnell infrapatellar taping, or braces are utilized during training and games; we often use the patellar Aircast
  The reported mechanism of the patellar Aircast brace is compression of the tendon insertions of the patella and stabilization of the patella; during flexion of the knee the compression increases, decreasing the tensile stress and contributing to pain relief

REHABILITATION PROTOCOL

Symptomatic, Acute Jumper's Knee

REST
- As with other problems, a decrease in activity is indicated.
- The amount of inactivity depends on the severity of the injury and individual circumstances (recreational versus professional athlete).
- Cast immobilization is contraindicated. Immobilization results in muscle atrophy and weakened tendon, with recurrence likely when the now-weakened tendon is subjected to high tensile forces.

MEDICATION
- NSAIDs contribute to the conservative treatment of jumper's knee.

- Avoid corticosteroid injections because of potential danger of tendon rupture.
- May use iontophoresis.

BRACING
- Apply patellar Air cast or McConnell infrapatellar taping.

EXERCISE
- Use the same exercise program as outlined for anterior knee pain (Ross and Brotzman Protocol p. 235).

MODALITIES
- May use moist heat massage, ultrasound, phonophoresis, iontophoresis, electrical stimulation, and ice to provide different therapeutic effects that may be of benefit to the patient.

REHABILITATION PROTOCOL

Symptomatic Osgood-Schlatter Disease FOX AND DEL PIZZO

Phase 1
1 to 5 days
- If acutely symptomatic with limp, immobilize until acute symptoms decrease.
- Prescribe oral antiinflammatories if needed to reduce inflammation and pain.
- Apply ice.
- Use crutches if needed.

Phase 2
- Remove from immobilization
- May use an infrapatellar strap or protective brace with inferior horseshoe pad.
- Try interferential electrical stimulation to decrease inflammation if desired (may use in phase 1 also).
- Continue ice or oral antiinflammatories to decrease inflammation.
- Perform straight leg raises.
- Perform resisted plantar flexion of ankle with tubing.
- Begin short arc extension exercises, progressing to 1- to 2-lb weight and advancing in 2-lb increments.
- Begin isotonic exercises for hip flexors, extensors, abductors, adductors, and muscles of the lower leg.
- Achieve full ROM.

- Walk in chest-high water, use water vest, or swim to maintain cardiovascular fitness, or use a bicycle if it does not cause pain.
- Perform stretching exercises for hip and knee muscles.

Phase 3
- Continue to brace and use ice if needed.
- Continue ROM exercises.
- Perform strengthening exercises for hip and knee flexors, extensors, abductors, and adductors; do 3 sets of 10 repetitions, each starting with 3- to 5-lb weights and increasing by 2 lbs when exercise is done easily for the 3 sets.
- Start isometric exercises 0 to 90 degrees and include eccentric exercises for quadriceps; e.g. lift 5 lbs from 90 to 0 degrees knee flexion, then slowly lower weight from 0 to 90 degrees (i.e., eccentric quadriceps activity) as tolerated.

Phase 4
- Add jumping, hopping, stepping.
- Jump off 8-inch step, then jump back up, first slowly and then more rapidly.
- Sport-specific skills where appropriate

Bibliography
ANTERIOR CRUCIATE LIGAMENT

American Academy of Orthopaedic Surgeons: *Knee braces seminar report,* 1985, AAOS.

Amiel D et al: Immobilization effect on collagen turnover in the medial collateral ligament: a comparison between a nine- and twelve-week immobilization period, *Clin Orthop* 172:265, 1983.

Anderson A, Lipscomb A: Analysis of rehabilitation techniques after anterior cruciate reconstruction, *Am J Sports Med* 17:154, 1989.

Andrews JR, Wilke KE: Current concepts in the treatment of anterior cruciate ligament disruption, *J Orthop Sports Phys Ther* 15:279, 1992.

Arnoczky SP, Tallin GB, Marshall JL: Anterior cruciate ligament replacement using patellar tendon: an evaluation of graft revascularization in the dog, *J Bone Joint Surg* 64A:217, 1982.

Barber SD et al: Rehabilitation after ACL reconstruction: function testing, *Sports Med Rehab Series* 15:969, 1992.

Bassett GS, Fleming BW: The Lenox Hill brace and anterolateral rotatory instability, *Am J Sports Med* 11:345, 1983.

Blackburn TA: Rehabilitation of anterior cruciate ligament injuries, *Orthop Clin North Am* 16(2):241, 1985.

Branch TP, Hunter R, Donath M: Dynamic EMG analysis of anterior cruciate-deficient legs with and without bracing during cutting, *Am J Sports Med* 17:35, 1989.

Brewster CE, Moynes DR, Jobe FW: Rehabilitation for anterior cruciate reconstruction, *J Orthop Sports Phys Ther* 5:121, 1983.

Cawley PW, France EP, Paulos LE: Comparison of rehabilitative knee braces: a biomechanical investigation, *Am J Sports Med* 17:141, 1989.

Clancy WG, Nelson DA, Reider B: Anterior cruciate ligament reconstruction using one third of the patellar ligament, augmented by extra-articular tendon transfers, *J Bone Joint Surg* 62A:352, 1982.

Colville MR, Lee CL, Ciullo JV: The Lenox Hill brace: an evaluation of effectiveness in treating knee instability, *Am J Sports Med* 14:257, 1986.

DeCarlo MS et al: Traditional versus accelerated rehabilitation following ACL reconstruction: a one-year follow-up, *J Orthop Sports Phys Ther* 15:309, 1992.

Delitto A et al: Electrically elicited co-contraction of thigh musculature after anterior cruciate ligament surgery: a description and single-case experiment, *Phys Ther* 68:45, 1988.

Delitto A et al: Electrical stimulation versus voluntary exercise in strengthening thigh musculature after anterior cruciate ligament surgery, *Phys Ther* 68:660, 1988.

DePalma BF, Zelko RR: Knee rehabilitation following anterior cruciate ligament injury or surgery, *J Ath Training* 21:200, 1986.

Eriksson G, Haggmark T: Comparison of isometric muscle training and electrical stimulation supplementing isometric muscle training in the recovery after major knee ligament surgery, *Am J Sports Med* 7:169, 1979.

Frndak PA, Berasi CC: Rehabilitation concerns following anterior cruciate ligament reconstruction, *Sports Med* 12:338, 1991.

Fu FH, Woo SL, Irrgang JJ: Current concepts for rehabilitation following anterior cruciate ligament reconstruction, *J Orthop Sports Phys Ther* 15:270, 1992.

Graf B, Uhr F: Complications of intraarticular anterior cruciate reconstruction, *Clin Sports Med* 7:835, 1988.

Hallebrandt FA, Waterland JC: Indirect learning: the influence of uni-manual exercise on related muscle groups of the same and opposite side, *Am J Phys Med Rehabil* 41:45, 1962.

Harner CD et al: Loss of motion following anterior cruciate ligament reconstruction, *Am J Sports Med.*

Henning CE, Lynch MA, Click KR: An in vivo strain gauge study of elongation of the anterior cruciate ligament, *Am J Sports Med* 13:22, 1985.

Hoffmann AA et al: Knee stability in orthotic knee braces, *Am J Sports Med* 12:371, 1984.

Huegel M, Indelicato P: Trends in rehabilitation following anterior cruciate ligament reconstruction, *Clin Sports Med* 7:801, 1988.

Kakkar VV et al: Heparin and dihydroergotamine prophylaxis against thrombo-embolism after hip arthroplasty, *J Bone Joint Surg* 67B:538, 1985.

Karzel RP, Friedman MJ, Ferkel RD: Prosthetic ligament reconstruction of the knee. In DeLee JC, Drez DJ Jr, editors: *Orthopaedic sports medicine: principles and practice,* vol 2, Philadelphia, 1994, WB Saunders.

Kennedy JC, Alexander IJ, Hayes KC: Nerve supply of the human knee and its functional importance, *Am J Sports Med* 10:329, 1982.

Kurosaka M, Yoshiya S, Andrish JT: A biomechanical comparison of different surgical techniques of graft fixation in anterior cruciate ligament reconstruction, *Am J Sports Med* 15:225, 1987.

Lambert KL: Vascularized patellar tendon graft with rigid internal fixation for anterior cruciate ligament insufficiency, *Clin Orthop* 172:85, 1983.

Lephart SM et al: Functional assessment of the anterior cruciate ligament insufficient athlete (abstract), *Med Sci Sports Exerc* (supplement) 20:2, 1988.

Lephart SM et al: Functional performance tests for the anterior cruciate ligament insufficient athlete, *J Ath Training* 26:44, 1991.

McCarthy MR et al: The clinical use of continuous passive motion in physical therapy, *J Orthop Sports Phys Ther* 15:132, 1992.

Millet CW, Drez DJ: Principles of bracing for the anterior cruciate ligament-deficient knee, *Clin Sports Med* 7:827, 1988.

Mohtadi NGH, Webster-Bogaert S, Fowler PJ: Limitation of motion following anterior cruciate ligament reconstruction: a case-control study, *Am J Sports Med* 19:620, 1991.

Nelson KA: The use of knee braces during rehabilitation, *Clin Sports Med* 9:799, 1990.

Newton RA: Joint receptor contributions to reflexive and kinesthetic responses, *Phys Ther* 62:22, 1982.

Nicholas JA, Downing JF: Knee braces that protect against sports injuries, *J Musculoskel Med* 8:15, 1990.

Noyes FR: *Knee braces: seminar report,* Presented at AAOS Annual Meeting, Chicago, Ill, 1985.

Noyes FR, Butler DL, Grood ES: Biomechanical analysis of human ligament grafts used in knee ligament repair and reconstruction, *J Bone Joint Surg* 66A:344, 1984.

Noyes FR et al: Clinical laxity tests and functional stability of the knee: biomechanical concepts, *Clin Orthop* 146:84, 1980.

Noyes FR et al: Advances in the understanding of knee ligament injury, repair, and rehabilitation, *Med Sci Sports Exerc* 16:427, 1984.

Noyes FR, Mangine RE, Barber S: Early knee motion after open and arthroscopic anterior cruciate ligament reconstruction, *Am J Sports Med* 15:149, 1987.

O'Driscoll SW, Keeley FW, Salter RB: The chondrogenic potential of free autogenous periosteal grafts for biological resurfacing of major full surface defects in joint surfaces under the influence of continuous passive motion: an experimental investigation in the rabbit, *J Bone Joint Surg* 68A:1017, 1986.

O'Driscoll SW, Keeley FW, Salter RB: Durability of regenerated articular cartilage produced by free autogenous periosteal grafts in major full-thickness defects in joint surfaces under the influence of continuous passive motion: a follow-up report at one year, *J Bone Joint Surg* 68A:1017, 1988.

O'Driscoll SW, Kumar A, Salter RB: The effect of continuous passive motion on the clearance of a hemarthrosis from a synovial joint, *Clin Orthop* 176:305, 1983.

O'Meara PM, O'Brien WR, Henning CE: Anterior cruciate ligament reconstruction stability with continuous passive motion: the role of isometric graft placement, *Clin Orthop* 277:201, 1992.

Paulos LE et al: Infrapatellar contracture syndrome: an unrecognized cause of knee stiffness with patella entrapment and patella infera, *Am J Sports Med* 15:331, 1987.

Paulos LE, Stern J: *Rehabilitation after anterior cruciate ligament surgery.* In Jackson DW: *The anterior cruciate ligament,* New York, 1993, Raven Press.

Paulos LE, Wnorowski DC, Beck CL: Rehabilitation following knee surgery: recommendations, *Sports Med* 11:257, 1991.

Reynolds L et al: EMG activity of the vastus medialis oblique and vastus lateralis and their role in patellar alignment, *Am J Phys Med* 62:61, 1983.

Risberg MA, Ekeland A: Assessment of functional tests after anterior cruciate ligament surgery, *J Orthop Sports Phys Ther* 19:212, 1994.

Salter RB et al: The biological effect of continuous passive motion on the healing of the full-thickness defects in articular cartilage: an experimental investigation in the rabbit, *J Bone Joint Surg* 62A:1232, 1980.

Salter RB et al: Clinical applications of basic research on continuous passive motion for disorders and injuries of synovial joints: a preliminary report of a feasibility study, *J Orthop Res* 3:325, 1983.

Selkowitz D: Improvement in isometric strength of the quadriceps femoris muscle after training with electrical stimulation, *Phys Ther* 65:186, 1985.

Seto JL, Brewster CE, Lombardo SJ, Tibone JE: Rehabilitation of the knee after anterior cruciate ligament reconstruction, *J Orthop Sports Phys Ther* 11(1):8, July 1989.

Shelbourne KD et al: Arthrofibrosis in acute anterior cruciate ligament reconstruction: the effect of timing of reconstruction and rehabilitation, *Am J Sports Med* 19:332, 1991.

Shelbourne KD, Nitz P: Accelerated rehabilitation after anterior cruciate ligament reconstruction, *Am J Sports Med* 18:292, 1990.

Shelbourne KD, Nitz P: Accelerated rehabilitation after anterior cruciate ligament reconstruction, *J Orthop Sports Phys Ther* 15:256, 1992.

Sisk T et al: Effect of electrical stimulation on quadriceps strength after reconstructive surgery of the anterior cruciate ligament, *Am J Sports Med* 15:215, 1987.

Snyder-Mackler L, Ladin Z, Schepsis AA, Young JC: Electrical stimulation of thigh muscles after reconstruction of anterior cruciate ligament, *J Bone Joint Surg* 73A:1025, 1991.

Spencer J, Hayes K, Alexander I: Knee joint effusion and quadriceps reflex inhibition in man, *Arch Phys Med Rehabil* 65:171, 1984.

Stevenson DV et al: *Rehabilitative knee braces control of terminal knee extension in the ambulatory patient.* Presented at the 34th Annual Meeting of the Orthopaedic Research Society, Atlanta, Feb. 1-4, 1988.

Vargas JH III, Ross DG: Corticosteroids and anterior cruciate ligament repair, *Am J Sports Med* 17:532, 1989.

Warren RF: Primary repair of the anterior cruciate ligament, *Clin Orthop* 172:65, 1983.

Wilcox PG, Jackson DW: Arthroscopic anterior cruciate ligament reconstruction, *Clin Sports Med* 6:513, 1987.

Wilk KE, Andrews JR: Current concepts in the treatment of anterior cruciate ligament disruption, *J Orthop Sports Phys Ther* 15:279, 1992.

Wilk KE, Andrews JR, Clancy WG: Quadriceps muscular strength after removal of the central third patellar tendon for contralateral anterior cruciate ligament reconstruction surgery: a case study, *J Orthop Sports Phys Ther* 18:692, 1993.

MEDIAL COLLATERAL LIGAMENT

Bergfield J: MCL injury, *Am J Sports Med* 7(3):207, 1979.

Clancy W: Functional rehabilitation of the isolated medial collateral ligament sprains, *Am J Sports Med* 7(3):206, 1979.

Holden DL, Eggert AW, Butler JE: Nonoperative treatment of grade I and II medial collateral ligament injuries to the knee, *Am J Sports Med,* 11(5):340, 1983.

Miller MD: *Review of orthopaedics,* Philadelphia, 1992, WB Saunders.

Steadman JR: Rehabilitation of first- and second-degree sprains of the medial collateral ligament, *Am J Sports Med* 7(5):300, 1979.

Torg J: *Rehabilitation of athletic injuries: an atlas of therapeutic exercise,* 1987, New Year Medical Publisher.

ILIOTIBIAL BAND FRICTION SYNDROME

Clancy WG: Symposium on runners' injuries, pt 2: evaluation and treatment of specific injuries, *Am J Sports Med* 8:287, 1980.

Gose J: Iliotibial band tightness *J Orthop Sports Phys Ther* 10:399, 1989.

Graeme Lindenberg et al: Iliotibial band friction syndrome in runners, *Phys Sports Med* 12(5):118, 1984.

Noble CA: The treatment of iliotibial band friction syndrome, *Br J Sports Med* 13:51, 1979.

Renne JW: The iliotibial band friction syndrome, *J Bone Joint Surg* 57A:1110, 1975.

PATELLOFEMORAL DISORDERS

Antich TJ et al: Evaluation of knee extensor mechanism disorders. Clinical presentation of 112 patients, *J Orthop Sports Phys Ther* 8(5):248, 1986.

Colisimo AJ, Bassett FH: Jumper's knee diagnosis and treatment, *Orthop Rev* 19(2):139, 1990.

David JM: Jumper's knee, *J Orthop Sports Phys Ther* 11(4):137, 1989.

Dugas R, D'Ambrosia R: Causes and treatment of common overuse injuries in runners, *J Musculoskel Med* 8:109, 1991.

Eisle MA: A precise approach to anterior knee pain. *Phys Sports Med* 19(6):127, 1991.

Fox JM, Del Pizzo W: *The patellofemoral joint,* New York, 1993, McGraw-Hill.

Grelsamer RP, Cartier P: Comprehensive approach to patellar pathology, *Contemp Orthop* 20(5):493, 1990.

Howkins RJ, Bell RH, Anisette G: Acute patellar dislocations: the natural history, *Am J Sports Med* 14(2):117, 1986.

Hungerford DS, Barry M: Biomechanics of the patellofemoral joint. *Clin Orthop* 144:9, 1979.

Hunter-Griffin, Letha Y: The patellofemoral stress syndrome. Your Patient and Fitness. 3(2):9, 1990.

Kolowich PA et al: Lateral release of the patella: indications and contraindications, *Am J Sports Med* 18(4):359, 1990.

Kramer PG: Patella malignment syndrome: rationale to reduce excessive lateral pressure, *J Orthop Sports Phys Ther* 8(6):301, 1986.

Merchant AC: Classification of patellofemoral disorders, *Arthroscopy* 4(4):235, 1988.

Shelton GL, Thigpen LK: Rehabilitation of patellofemoral dysfunction: a review of literature, *J Orthop Sports Phys Ther* 14(6):243, 1991.

Woodall W, Welsh J: A biomechanical basis for rehabilitation programs involving the patellofemoral joint, *J Orthop Sports Phys Ther* 11:535, 1990.

CHAPTER SIX

Foot and Ankle Rehabilitation

S. BRENT BROTZMAN, MD
JILL BRASEL, PT

Ankle Sprains

REHABILITATION RATIONALE AND BASIC PRINCIPLES

The sprained ankle is the most common injury in sports. Approximately 23,000 people have ankle sprains each day in the United States.

Anatomy

The lateral ankle ligament complex includes the anterior talofibular (ATF), calcaneofibular (CF), and posterior talofibular (PTF) ligaments (Fig. 6-1). The CF and ATF ligaments are synergistic: when one is relaxed, the other is taut. With the ankle plantar flexed, the ATF is more vulnerable to inversion stress; with the ankle dorsiflexed, the CF assumes a more important role.

■ *Because most ankle sprains occur in plantar flexion, the ATF is the most frequently injured ligament in inversion injuries (Fig. 6-2).*

Classification

Rehabilitation of lateral ankle sprains is based on classification of severity (Table 6-1).

Evaluation

The talar tilt test examination is designed to reveal incompetency of the CF ligament (Fig. 6-3). The anterior drawer examination measures the integrity of the ATF ligament (Fig. 6-4).

Stress radiographs, such as the talar tilt test (for CF ligament incompetence), the anterior drawer test (for ATF incompetence), and stress Broden views (for subtalar instability) have been found to have questionable accuracy and reliability in the evaluation of ankle

TABLE 6-1 Classification of Ankle Sprain Severity

Grade	Damage
1	Mild stretching of the fibers within the ligament, but no laxity, little swelling or tenderness
2	Partial tear of the ATF and CF ligaments with mild laxity, mild-to-moderate instability, moderate pain and tenderness, and some loss of motion
3	Complete ruptures of the ATF and CF ligaments that cause an unstable joint, severe swelling, loss of function, and considerably abnormal motion (electromyogram [EMG] studies also document an 80% incidence of peroneal nerve damage in grade 3 sprains, supporting the concept that the lateral peroneal complex provides an inversion restraint)

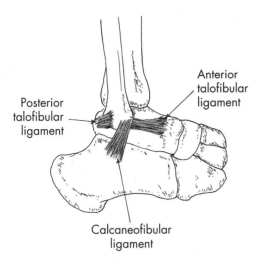

Figure 6-1 Ligaments of the lateral ankle.

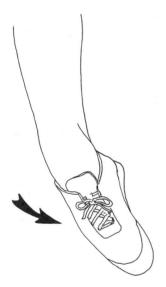

Figure 6-2 The most typical injury mechanism in ankle sprain: plantar flexion, inversion, and adduction.

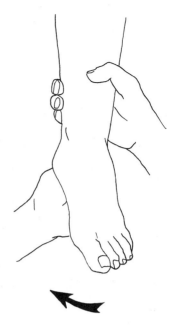

Figure 6-3 The talar tilt (inversion stress) test of the ankle.

sprains because of variable parameters for "normal" (5 to 23 degrees talar tilt), and multiple variations among examiners (limb position, manual pressure, jigs).

Treatment

Most acute ankle sprains can be treated nonoperatively. Seventy-five percent to 100% of patients have good to excellent outcomes whether treated operatively or nonoperatively; those treated nonoperatively generally have fewer complications and more rapid recovery. Initial nonoperative, functional treatment is also supported by the very high success rate of reconstructive procedures for chronic ankle instability, such as those described by Broström and Watson-Jones (Figs. 6-5 and 6-6). Failure of initial nonoperative,

functional treatment still leaves the option of reconstruction with a high success rate.

Competitive athletes should first be treated functionally, with the realization that 10% to 20% may need elective secondary repair (Kannus and Renstrom). Exceptions include ballet dancers and members of the performing arts, whose activities involve "point" and "demipoint" positions (Fig. 6-7). Hamilton recommends open repair of acute grade 3 sprains in these athletes because of a high demand for healing without residual instability and the inadvisability of using a dancer's peroneus brevis for reconstruction of chronic instability.

Functional treatment (which includes only a short period of protection, early range of motion [ROM], and early weight bearing) has been clearly shown to provide the quickest recovery to full ROM and return to physical activity. It does not, however, compromise the late mechanical stability of the ankle more than any other mode of treatment (Kannus and Renstrom).

Van Moppens and Van den Hoogenband observed that at 9 weeks, patients who were immobilized in a cast or who underwent surgery had a higher rate of atrophy of the calf muscles than those who had functional treatment (18% and 22% versus 4%). However, at 6 months the difference was negligible. At 9 weeks, 68% of patients who had functional treatment had been restored to their preinjury levels of activity, compared with 7% of those who underwent operations and 13% of those who had only a cast. At 12 weeks, functional treatment still demonstrated a considerable advantage (81%, 36%, and 7%, respectively). Immobilization in a cast does have the benefits of providing a feeling of security for the patient, immediate pain

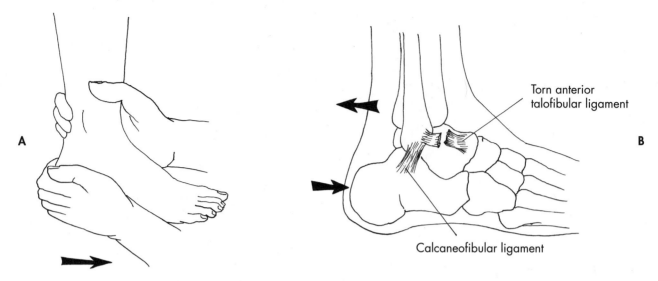

Figure 6-4 **A,** The anterior drawer test of the ankle. **B,** The integrity of the anterior talofibular ligament is assessed by the anterior drawer test. With complete disruption, the talus can be subluxed anteriorly beneath the tibial plafond.

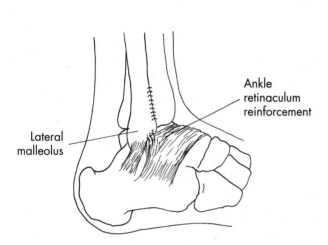

Figure 6-5 Modified Bröstrom ankle reconstruction.

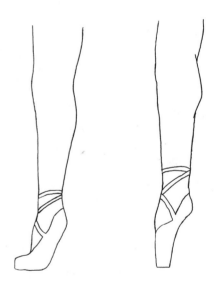

Figure 6-7 Demipointe and pointe in ballet.

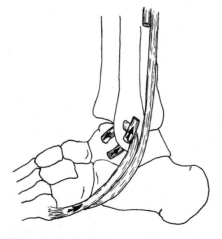

Figure 6-6 The Watson-Jones procedure.

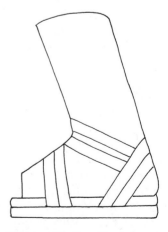

Figure 6-8 Dorsiflexion cast.

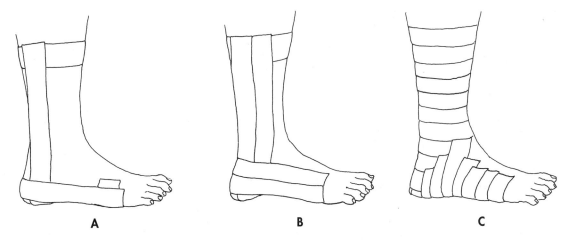

A   B   C

Figure 6-9 **A,** Open basket weave is performed immediately after injury because this technique allows for swelling. This taping provides compression and allows for swelling, but does *not* provide support. The player extends the lower third of the calf past the edge of the table. A heel pad is placed first. Two anchor strips are applied, then horizontal and vertical stirrups are added. **B,** Repeat the vertical stirrup, overlapping half of the previous strip. A second horizontal stirrup is then applied. **C,** Repeat the alternating vertical and horizontal stirrups. A 1-inch opening is left on the dorsum of the foot and leg. Overlap the previous strip by half. The ends are locked with long strips. (Redrawn from *Athletic training and sports medicine,* ed 2, Rosemont, Ill, 1991, AAOS.)

relief, and less need for instruction, but muscle atrophy and stiffness are greater, and recovery is more prolonged. We use casts for noncompliant patients.

Cadaver studies by Smith and Reischle found that 5 to 15 degrees of dorsiflexion were required to reduce an unstable ankle and oppose the ends of the ATF in a cast. To avoid functional lengthening of the ATF ligament and subsequent instability, Smith uses a cast with the ankle slightly dorsiflexed for grade 3 sprains (Fig. 6-8). Others recommend casting with the ankle in slight eversion.

PREVENTATIVE MEASURES

Training Techniques
Two techniques often used by coaches and athletic trainers may help reduce the incidence of inversion ankle sprains:
- Peroneal muscle conditioning program before and during the season
- Teaching players to land with a relatively wide-based gait. This should place the foot a little more lateral to the falling center of gravity and make an inversion stress on the ankle less likely.

Prophylactic Ankle Taping
The efficacy of prophylactic ankle taping has been shown by numerous authors. In a study of 2562 basketball players, Garrick and Requa found a lower incidence of ankle injuries for those who had prophy-

lactic ankle taping. For patients with previous ligament injuries, ankle taping with high-top tennis shoes has been shown to be most effective in preventing reinjury (Lassiter). However, studies have shown that 12% to 50% of the supporting strength is lost in all taping methods after exercise, most occurring in the first few minutes (Rarick).

The open basket weave is one of the most common taping techniques used for acute ankle injuries (Fig. 6-9). The closed basket weave is often used after the risk of swelling has diminished (Fig. 6-10).

The best method of taping remains controversial. Frankeny et al. reported that the Hinton-Boswell method provided the greatest resistance to plantar flexion-inversion movements before and after exercise (Fig. 6-11). However, this method tapes the ankle in relaxed plantar flexion. Placement in dorsiflexion, where the ankle is more stable and extreme plantar flexion is less likely, appears to be a more logical choice. Others have found the basket-weave technique with a combination stirrup and heel lock to be the strongest method.

Braces
Various ankle orthoses have been used in an effort to provide relative external support to the ankle without compromising ankle joint motion. In a study of collegiate football players, Rovere et al. found that lace-on stabilizers were associated with a lower incidence of ankle injury than was taping. However, Bunch found

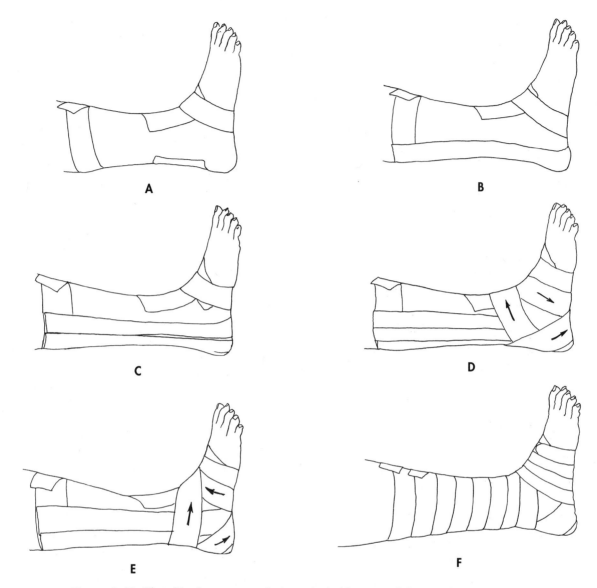

Figure 6-10 Closed basket-weave technique. **A,** Ankle taping following lateral inversion sprains: apply heel and lace pads, then apply two anchor strips. **B,** Apply stirrup strips, beginning on the medial part of the calf and passing under the heel. **C,** Continue applying strips up the lateral aspect of the leg; apply between three and six strips. **D,** Apply two to three heel locks in each direction. **E,** Apply figure-eight strips with force to cause slight foot eversion. **F,** Anchor tape components with fill-in strips, beginning at base stirrups and working up to proximal anchor. (Redrawn from *Athletic training and sports medicine*, ed 2, Rosemont, Ill, 1991, AAOS.)

no significant difference in support between the two after 20 minutes of repeated inversion movements in the lab.

More recent designs include the use of semirigid plastics. Gross et al. demonstrated that these devices limited inversion-eversion motion significantly more than adhesive tape. Examples of these braces include the Aircast Sport Stirrup (Fig. 6-12) and the ALP (Donjoy). Currently there is little agreement in the literature about the effectiveness, support, and subjective comfort of various braces.

REHABILITATION

Ankle Sprains
The initial objective is to minimize swelling and inflammation. Cyriax explains that "the treatment of posttraumatic inflammation is based on the principle that the body's reaction to injury is excessive."

The RICE (rest, ice, compression wrap, elevation) regimen is used for acute injuries (see box, p. 252).

■ *Key recovery factors include protection, early motion and weight bearing, and rehabilitation.*

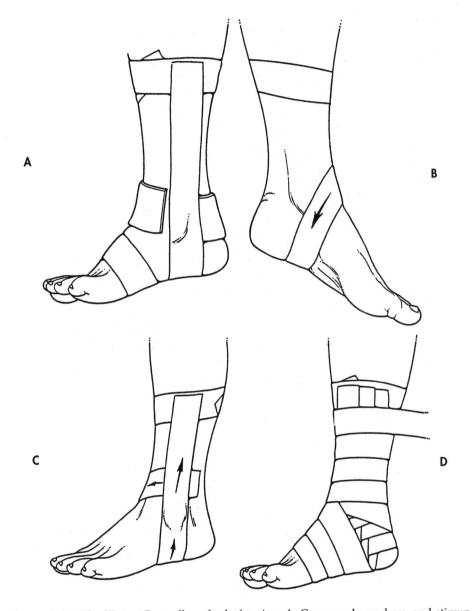

Figure 6-11 The Hinton-Boswell method of taping. **A,** Gauze pads, anchors, and stirrup applied. The anchors are placed at the musculotendinous junction of gastrocnemius and around the arch of the foot. The stirrup is placed medially to laterally, countering inversion forces. **B** and **C,** Two anchors and two stirrups are first applied with the ankle in dorsiflexion. Then, in relaxed plantar flexion, four figures of six are applied overlapping proximally to distally. **D,** Finally, a circular close is used to complete the wrap. (From Frankeny JR: *Clin J Sports Med* 3:1, 1993.)

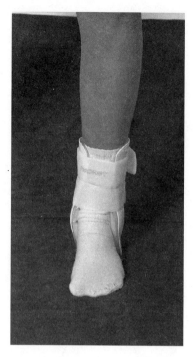

Figure 6-12 Aircast ankle brace.

RICE Regimen

Rest	Avoid activities that cause sharp pain.
	Ensure the availability of crutches if the patient cannot walk without a limp.
	Continue relative rest until the pain and swelling are negligible on weight bearing.
Ice	Ice provides local contraction of blood vessels so that blood flow is reduced to the injured area.
	Reduction of swelling enhances healing.
	Ice provides some pain relief.
	Apply ice for 20 minutes initially every hour, then 3 to 4 times every 24 hours for 72 hours.
Compression	Various compressive dressings combined with ice decrease swelling in the acute inflammatory phase.
Elevation	Sims demonstrated with volumetric testing that elevated limbs have a significant decrease in volumetric displacement because the lymphatics have to work against decreased pressure to return excess fluid.
	Guyton and Ganong demonstrated that as interstitial fluid and pressure increase past certain levels, a critical point is reached that causes collapse of lymphatic vessels.

REHABILITATION PROTOCOL

Acute Ankle Sprain MODIFIED JACKSON PROTOCOL

Jackson outlined a treatment regimen he used successfully for cadets at West Point. His program is divided into three phases. Using this regimen, disability averaged 8 days for mild sprains, 15 days for moderate sprains, and 19 days for severe sprains.

Phase 1
1 day
- Implement RICE regimen.
- Prescribe nonsteroidal antiinflammatory medications (NSAIDs).
- Use crutches if needed; allow weight bearing within limits of pain.

REHABILITATION PROTOCOL—cont'd

Phase 2—Restoration of Motion

Average times for phase 2 are as follows: grade 1 (3 days), grade 2 (4 days), grade 3 (5 to 9 days). (The reader must remember that this population of patients was 18-year-old cadets.)

2 to 12 days

- Begin ankle dorsiflexion and plantar flexion at patient's own pace, preceded by cool whirlpool and an intermittent Jobst pressure stocking (75 mm Hg).
- Use active ROM initially with no resistance to reestablish full ankle flexion and extension at the patient's own pace.
- Later, add rubber tubing resistance as tolerated.
- Begin heel cord stretches.
- Minimize dependent position of leg.
- Allow progressive weight bearing within the limits of pain.
- Initiate the following daily treatments for 1 hour each: 20 minutes cold whirlpool, 20 minutes intermittent pressure stocking, 20 minutes ROM exercises, plus ROM exercises at home.
- Decrease the pressure stocking time as swelling diminishes.
- When patient is walking without a limp, has full painless ankle ROM, and is able to perform toe rise supporting body weight through the injured ankle, progress to phase 3.
- May begin swimming before weight bearing.
- Plantar flexion may be uncomfortable in water for grade 2 or grade 3 sprains with free-style because of resistance created by water.

Phase 3—Agility and Endurance

- Total body conditioning incorporated in each phase, but increased in phase 3.
- Perform strengthening exercises with emphasis on **peroneal tendons** and ankle dorsiflexors, the muscles responsible for actively resisting an inversion-plantar flexion injury.
- Isometric exercises:
   Isometric strengthening against an immobile object or manual resistance (Fig. 6-13):
      Eversion (peroneals)—3 sets of 10
      Dorsiflexion (dorsiflexors)—3 sets of 10
- Perform concentric and eccentric exercises with elastic band:
   Concentric muscle contraction (muscle shortens) against the elastic band (Fig. 6-14, *A*).
   Eccentric contraction (muscle lengthens) during the slow relaxation of the muscle as the elastic band overpowers the deliberately slowly relaxing muscle (Fig. 6-14, *B*).
   This slow muscle relaxation is emphasized to maximize the conditioning benefit of the eccentric contraction.
      Eversion: 3 sets of 10
      Dorsiflexion: 3 sets of 10
- Other exercises:
   Toe raises (Fig. 6-15).
   Step-ups: Patient approaches step from the side, lifts self using the injured extremity, and lands on the uninjured extremity. Patient then attempts to exercise facing the step, moving up and down in a forward/backward position (Fig. 6-16).
   Skipping rope
   Running on level ground
- Use proprioception board (balance board).

Continued

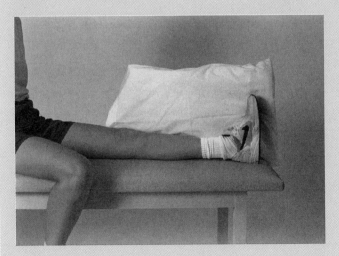

Figure 6-13 Isometric eversion against a fixed object with pillow as a cushion.

REHABILITATION PROTOCOL—cont'd

Acute Ankle Sprain MODIFIED JACKSON PROTOCOL

Phase 3—Agility and Endurance—cont'd
- Initiate BAPS (Biomechanic Ankle Proprioceptive System) (See Fig. 5-13): Trap and DeCarlo demonstrated a reduction in the number of recurrent ankle sprains after the use of proprioceptive/coordination training.

ACTIVITY PROGRESSION
The sequence for progression of activities is as follows:
1. Swimming, aquatic exercises
2. Walking; forward, retro
3. Jogging
4. Running
5. Figure-eights
6. Sport-specific agility drills

While resuming running, the patient should be instructed to run for 5 minutes and walk for several minutes, gradually increasing running time by 5-minute increments. If ankle pain occurs after 20 minutes, instruct the patient to drop back to 15 minutes until comfortable once more.

ORTHOTICS
- Occasionally we use an orthotic with a lateral heel wedge to place the hindfoot in hindfoot valgus in an effort to decrease the incidence of recurrent inversion injury and spraining.
- Patients with a pronated foot (pes planus) have been shown to have a reduced incidence of ankle sprains compared with those with a cavus foot. This fact also supports the use of a lateral heel wedge.

A   B

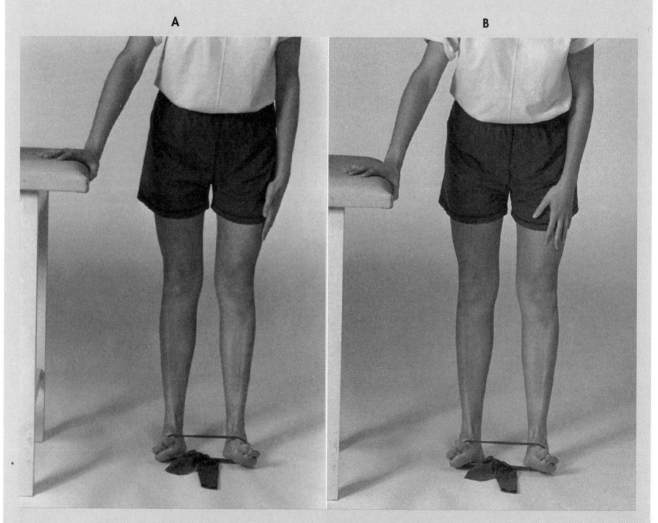

Figure 6-14 A, Concentric contraction (muscle shortens) outward against the band. **B,** Eccentric contraction (muscle lengthens) during slow relaxation of band.

REHABILITATION PROTOCOL—cont'd

RETURN TO COMPETITION

- The athlete may return to competition when there is full muscular control of a painless joint with full ROM and no swelling.
- For 6 months after ankle sprain, athletes are advised to wear high-top shoes with taping or bracing (Aircast).
- Many authors believe taping, bracing, and high-top shoes also help by providing important sensory feedback.

BRACING FOR STABILIZATION OF THE ANKLE

Grade 1 injury
- We generally use an Aircast-type ankle splint in a high-top shoe for 3 to 6 weeks. We replace this with ankle taping and high-top shoes.

Grade 2 injury
- Same.

Grade 3 injury
- For compliant patients, we use a removable walking cast that affords added stability yet allows functional rehabilitation several times a day out of the walking cast. Weight bearing as tolerated (WBAT) with crutches is often required for the first several days. The removable cast may be replaced by an Aircast at 4 to 6 weeks.
- For noncompliant or very young patients, we often use a walking cast despite the increase in atrophy and added time required to return to competition.

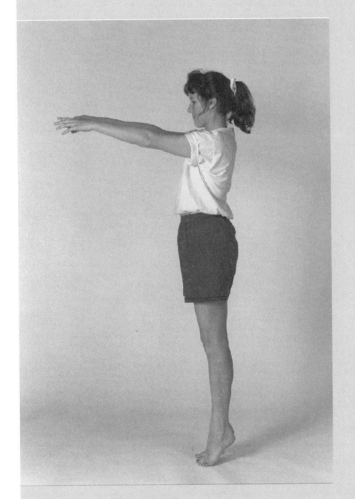

Figure 6-15 Toe raises.

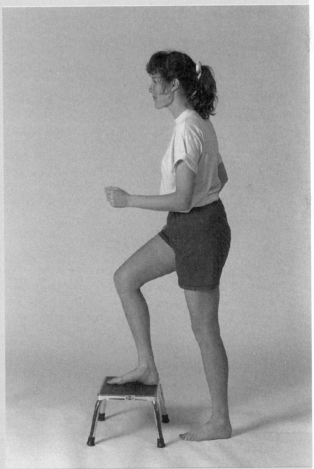

Figure 6-16 Step-ups.

REHABILITATION PROTOCOL

Severe (Grade 3) Ankle Sprains with Removable Walking Boot
MODIFIED LANE PROTOCOL

Requirements
- Adequate immobilization of the ankle
- Accessibility for therapy exercises
- Requires a compliant patient

Advantages
- Fewer complications from disuse and atrophy
- Ease of application
- Early return to sports with a stable ankle mortise

0 to 3 weeks
- Apply ice.
- Elevate.
- Wear walking boot (Fig. 6-17) at all times except during physical therapy.
- Start immediate weight bearing as tolerated in boot (crutches may be required first week).
- Perform daily physical therapy for first week, then 3 times per week for 2 weeks.
- Begin high-voltage galvanic stimulation (HVGS).
- Use Jobst compression combined with elevation.
- May use contrast baths (optional).
- Perform isometric exercises in AFO.
- For first 3 weeks, maintain the ankle joint at 90 degrees at all times in therapy (using tape or other support).
- Avoid eversion or inversion of the ankle.

3 to 5 weeks
- Remove walking boot.
- Change to Aircast-type brace and high-top tennis shoes.
- Initiate gentle ROM and strengthening exercises: Isometric plantar flexion, dorsiflexion, inversion, eversion
  Rubber band exercises, same motions
  Step-ups
  Toe raises
  Calf stretches
  Stationary bicycle
  Swimming if tolerated without pain
- Perform proprioception exercises with balance board at 4 to 5 weeks.
- Avoid adduction and inversion ROM exercises for 6 weeks.

5 to 7 weeks
- Perform agility drills with Aircast or lace-up brace.
- Perform proprioceptive exercises with balance board.
- Continue rubber band eccentric strengthening exercises, concentrating on ankle eversion.
- Perform agility drills:
  Figure-eights
  Backward running
  Cariocas

7 weeks
- Begin sports-related activities with taping or Aircast and high-top shoes.
- Continue taping for 6 to 12 months.
- Continue peroneal eversion rubber band exercises.
- If ankle instability episodes recur despite good compliance, reevaluate exam and clinical situation.

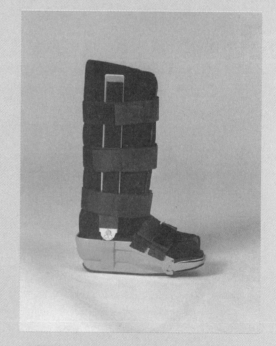

Figure 6-17 Removable walking boot.

REHABILITATION PROTOCOL

After Modified Broström Ankle Ligament Reconstruction
MODIFIED HAMILTON PROTOCOL

0 to 4 days	• Place ankle in anterior/posterior plaster splints in neutral dorsiflexion and discharge patient as non–weight bearing.	6 weeks (Campbell Clinic modification)	• Begin proprioception/balancing activities:

4 to 7 days	• When swelling has subsided, apply a short leg walking cast with the ankle at neutral.
	• Allow weight bearing as tolerated in cast.
			1. Unilateral balancing for timed intervals
			  2. Unilateral balancing with visual cues
			  3. Balancing on one leg and catching of #2 plyoball
			  4. Slide board, increasing distance
			  5. Fitter activity, catching ball

4 weeks	• Remove cast.
	• Apply air splint (Aircast, etc.) for protection, to be worn for 6 to 8 weeks after surgery.
	• Begin gentle ROM exercises of ankle.
	• Begin isometric peroneal strengthening exercises.
	• **Avoid** adduction and inversion until 6 weeks postoperatively.
	• Begin swimming.
			6. Side-to-side bilateral hopping (progress to unilateral)
			  7. Front-to-back bilateral hopping (progress to unilateral)
			  8. Diagonal patterns, hopping
			  9. Minitramp jogging
			 10. Shuttle leg press and rebounding, bilateral and unilateral
			 11. Positive deceleration, ankle everters, Kin-Com.

Continued

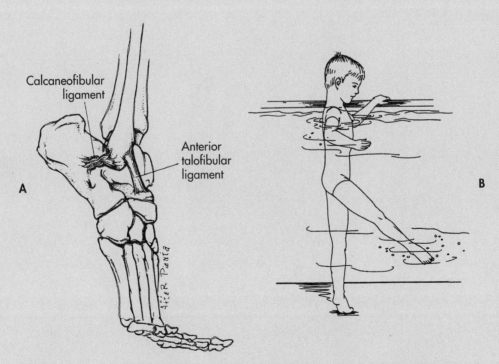

Figure 6-18 A, In plantar flexion, the anterior talofibular ligament is vertically oriented and is particularly vulnerable to inversion forces. Plantar flexion is the position of function for ballet dancers. **B,** During rehabilitation, barré exercises may also be performed in a pool, taking advantage of the buoyancy of water. (From Terry Malone: Rehabilitation of the foot and ankle injuries in ballet dancers, *J Orthop Sports Phys Ther* 11:8, 1990.)

After Modified Broström Ankle Ligament Reconstruction
MODIFIED HAMILTON PROTOCOL

6 weeks (Campbell Clinic modification) —cont'd	• Complete rehabilitation of the peroneals is essential. • Dancers should perform peroneal exercises in full plantar flexion, the position of function in these athletes (Fig. 6-18, *A*). • Early in rehabilitation, pool exercises may be beneficial (Fig. 6-19, *B*).	8 to 12 weeks	• Dancers should perform plantar flexion/eversion exercises with a weighted belt (2 to 20 lbs). • Patient can return to dancing or sports at 8 to 12 weeks after surgery if peroneal strength is normal.

Ankle Fractures

REHABILITATION RATIONALE

Weber classified ankle fractures into three types based on the level of the fibular fracture relative to the tibiotalar joint (plafond) (Fig. 6-19). Type A is distal to the tibiotalar joint; type B is even with the tibiotalar joint; and type C is proximal to the tibiotalar joint. This classification is helpful in making treatment decisions (operative versus nonoperative). The higher the fracture of the fibula, the more extensive the damage to the syndesmosis ligaments, and thus the more likely the ankle mortise will be unstable and require open reduction and internal fixation (Table 6-2).

Treatment Considerations

Anatomic reduction is necessary to restore the normal anatomy of this weight-bearing joint. Ramsey and Hamilton demonstrated that a 1-mm lateral shift of the talus in the mortise reduces the contact area of the ankle by 42%. This has significant implications for development of tibiotalar joint arthritis. Yablon et al. showed the talus follows the lateral malleolus defor-

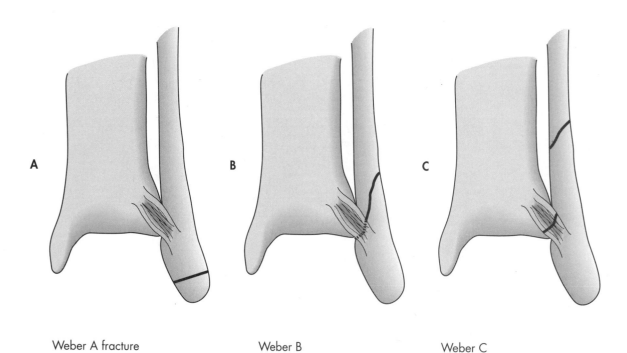

Weber A fracture

Fracture below the syndesmosis

Weber B

Fracture at the syndesmosis

Weber C

Fracture above the syndesmosis (unstable mortise)

Figure 6-19 **A,** Weber type A fracture: fracture below the syndesmosis. **B,** Weber type B fracture: fracture at the syndesmosis. **C,** Weber type C fracture: fracture above the syndesmosis (unstable mortise).

TABLE 6-2 **Types of Ankle Fractures**		
Weber Type	Description	Lauge-Hansen Equivalent (Foot Position at Time of Injury—Direction of Force)
A	Transverse avulsion fracture below level of plafond Syndesmosis intact Ankle mortise stable Typically does not require surgery	Supination—adduction
B	Spiral fracture beginning at the level of the plafond and extending proximally Interosseous ligament usually intact Anterior and posterior inferior tibiofibular ligaments may be torn, depending on the level of the fracture and severity of injury May or may not require surgery, depending on displacement, clinical picture	Supination—eversion
C	Fractured above the syndesmosis Syndesmosis torn, unstable ankle mortise Requires open reduction internal fixation to stabilize ankle mortise	Pronation—eversion Pronation—abduction

Adapted from Mann RA, Coughlin MJ: *Surgery of the foot and ankle*, ed 6, St. Louis, 1993, Mosby.

mity. Ankle stability is related to integrity of the syndesmosis and malleolar ligaments.

Undisplaced fractures with an intact mortise are treated with cast immobilization. Displaced fractures are treated with open reduction and internal fixation, unless an anatomic and stable reduction can be achieved with casting (often the reduction can be obtained, but not maintained).

Early Weight Bearing. Several authors have reported success with early weight bearing as tolerated in a cast after stable operative fixation of ankle fractures. Long-term outcomes with regard to ROM, pain, muscle strength, and function are similar to those after treatment with touchdown weight bearing. Because no long-term advantages have been proved for early weight bearing after operative fixation, we prefer to delay weight bearing and avoid the risk of breakage of hardware or loss of reduction.

Syndesmosis Screw Fixation. Weber type C fractures (and occasionally type B) that disrupt the syndesmosis require syndesmosis screw fixation for stabilization. Although some reports warn against weight bearing before removal of the syndesmosis screw, we often allow patients to bear weight with the screw in place. Many exhibit radiographic evidence of toggling with no symptoms. In these, we remove the screw at the patient's convenience. If the patient is symptomatic, we remove the screw shortly after weight bearing is begun.

REHABILITATION PROTOCOL

After Stable Open Reduction and Internal Fixation of Bimalleolar or Trimalleolar Ankle Fracture

INDICATIONS	• Compliant patient • Stable fixation	2 to 3 weeks	• Evaluate the wound. • If wound is stable and fixation is stable, place highly compliant patients in a removable commercial cast (touchdown weight bearing) and begin gentle, non–weight bearing active ROM exercises:
1 day	• Apply Jones-type dressing (well padded) with posterior splint and stirrup splint for 1 to 2 weeks; avoid equinus (neutral). • Maintain maximal elevation for 48 to 72 hours. • Ensure non–weight bearing with crutches.		Plantar flexion: 4 sets of 15 each day Dorsiflexion: 4 sets of 15 each day Straight leg raises (SLRs) and quadriceps sets for general lower extremity strengthening *Continued*

REHABILITATION PROTOCOL—cont'd

After Stable Open Reduction and Internal Fixation of Bimalleolar or Trimalleolar Ankle Fracture

2 to 3 weeks —cont'd

- Perform gentle towel stretches (especially dorsiflexion) 2 to 3 times a day for ROM (Fig. 6-20).
- Taylor advocates use of a short leg cast with the distal portion of the front of the cast removed (to allow dorsiflexion). He then slips the cast downward so the ankle can be plantar flexed (Fig. 6-21). We have encountered problems with cast fit, rubbing, and abrasions, and we do not use this technique.
- Continue touchdown weight bearing with crutches for 6 weeks. If fixation is very stable, we allow partial weight bearing with crutches at 4 weeks, if this can be done without pain.

6 weeks

- Place patient in a removable commercial walking cast if not already in one and allow weight-bearing ambulation to tolerance for 2 to 4 weeks. Later replace with an Aircast-type ankle splint, to be worn until full ROM and strength are reestablished.
- Remove the brace 4 to 5 times a day for therapy. Begin isometric strengthening exercises (Fig. 6-22):
  Dorsiflexion
  Plantar flexion
  Eversion
  Inversion
- Initiate concomitant Theraband exercises (eccentric strengthening) at this time and progress through bands of incrementally harder resistance (Fig. 6-23).
- Begin stretching exercises for ROM:
  Achilles tendon stretching
  Runners' stretch
  Incline board (Fig. 6-24)
  Peroneal tendon stretching
  Plantar-flexion stretching
- Use joint mobilization if significant capsular tightness and stable fracture are present.
- Do proprioception activities:
  BAPS board or kinesthetic agility training (KAT) device
- Perform toe crawling with towel (Fig. 6-25).
- Perform closed-chain activities:
  Progression as tolerated—
  Wall slides
  Lunges
  Lunges with weight on shoulders
  Stair-climber
- Incorporate stationary bicycling to enhance ROM and aerobic conditioning.
- Use DOT drill.
- After acceptable ROM, proprioception, and strength have been restored, instruct patient on home exercises for progressive closed-chain strengthening and preathletic training drills (if relevant).

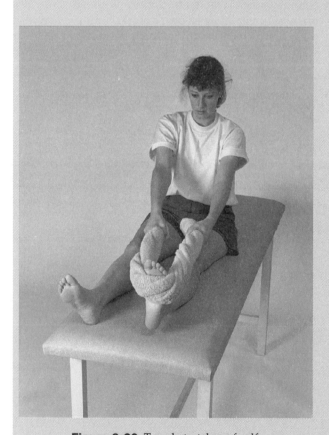

Figure 6-20 Towel stretches of calf.

REHABILITATION PROTOCOL—cont'd

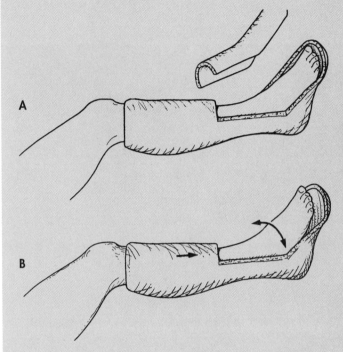

Figure 6-21 A, Distal portion of front of cast removed so that active dorsiflexion at ankle may be carried out. **B,** Cast is later slipped down so that ankle can be plantarflexed in addition. Loose portion of cast is wrapped back in place when exercise period is finished. (Redrawn from Schauwecker F: *The practice of osteosynthesis*, Stuttgart, 1974, Georg Thieme Verlag.)

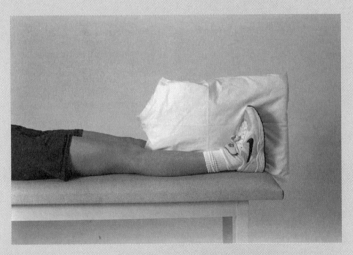

Figure 6-22 Isometric inversion of ankle. With rolled pillow between feet, press medial aspect of feet against pillow. Hold this for 10 seconds, then relax.

After Stable Open Reduction and Internal Fixation of Bimalleolar or Trimalleolar Ankle Fracture

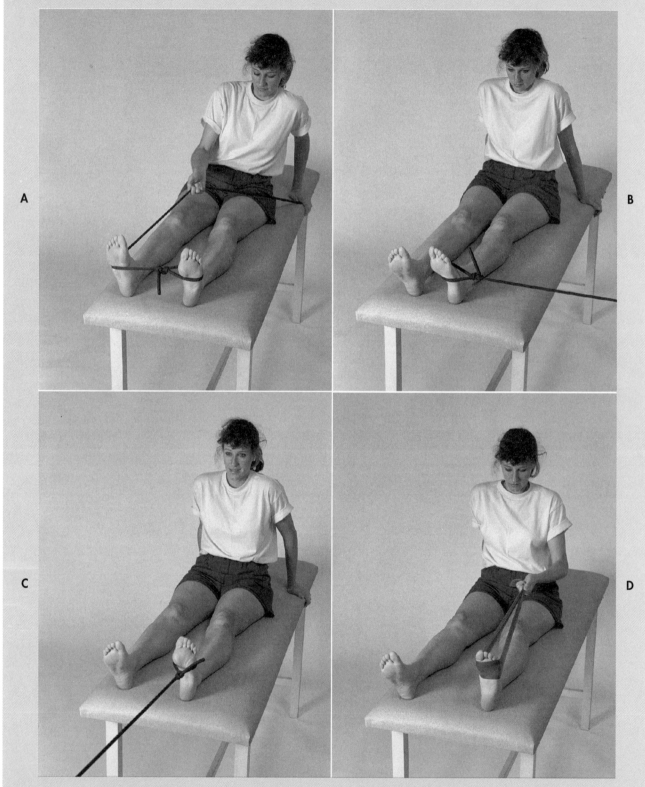

Figure 6-23 **A,** Resisted eversion of ankle. With tubing anchored around uninvolved foot, slowly turn involved foot outward (eversion). This exercise is the most important of this series. **B,** Resisted inversion. Inversion against Theraband. **C,** Resisted dorsiflexion of ankle. Anchor tubing on a stationary object. Pull foot toward body. **D,** Resisted plantar flexion of ankle. Place tubing around foot. Press foot down against tube into dorsiflexion.

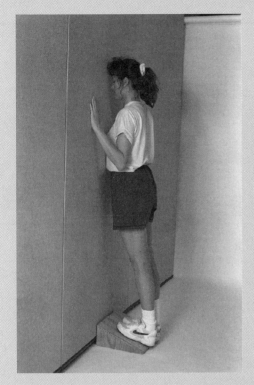

Figure 6-24 Incline board.

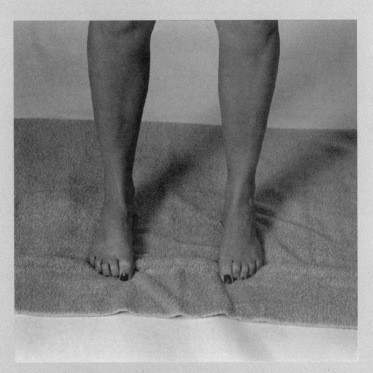

Figure 6-25 Toe crawling with towel. With foot resting on towel, slowly bunch towel by curling toes.

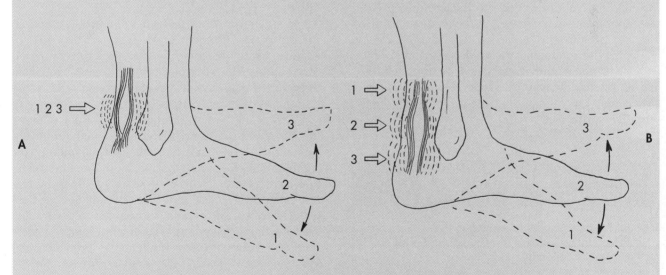

Figure 6-26 Painful arc sign. **A,** In peritendonitis, the tenderness remains in one position despite moving the foot from dorsiflexion to plantar flexion. **B,** In the case of partial tendon rupture or tendonitis, the point of tenderness *moves* as the foot goes from dorsiflexion to plantar flexion. (Redrawn from Williams JGP: *Sports Med* 3:114, 1986.)

DELAYED REHABILITATION PROTOCOL

After Open Reduction and Internal Fixation of Bimalleolar or Trimalleolar Ankle Fracture

INDICATIONS	• Unstable fracture configuration, such as comminuted Weber type C fracture • Noncompliant patient		• Place in well-padded, short leg, non–weight-bearing cast at 1 to 2 weeks. • Maintain in cast for 6 to 7 weeks, non–or touchdown weight bearing. • Instruct in active ROM exercises of knee, straight leg raises.
1 day	• Apply Jones-type dressing (well padded) with posterior splint and stirrup for 2 to 3 days. • Maintain maximal elevation is for 48 to 72 hours. • Ensure non–weight bearing with crutches.	6 weeks	• Initiate exercises of previous protocol (see p. 259) when clinical union is evident.

Achilles Tendonitis and Peritendonitis

REHABILITATION RATIONALE AND BACKGROUND

Puddu et al. classified Achilles tendonitis into three types: pure peritendonitis, peritendonitis with tendonitis, and pure tendonitis. The painful arc sign is helpful in distinguishing peritendonitis from actual tendonitis. The foot is moved from dorsiflexion to plantar flexion (Fig. 6-26, p. 263). In patients with peritendonitis, the tenderness and swelling *remain fixed* in reference to the malleoli (i.e., in the tendon sheath) as the foot goes from dorsiflexion to plantar flexion. In patients with tendonitis, the tenderness and swelling *move* with the tendon as the foot goes from dorsiflexion to plantar flexion. Magnetic resonance imaging (MRI) also may help to distinguish peritendonitis from tendonitis (see box).

Differential Diagnosis of Achilles Tendonitis

• Partial rupture of Achilles tendon
• Retrocalcaneal bursitis (of retrocalcaneal bursa)
• Haglund's deformity (pump bump)
• Calcaneal apophysitis (skeletally immature—Sever's apophysitis)
• Calcaneal exostosis
• Calcaneal stress fracture
• Calcaneal fracture
• Posterior tibial tendon tendonitis (medial pain)
• Plantar fasciitis (inferior heel pain)

Anatomy

The blood supply to the tendon is via its investing mesotenon, with the richest supply emerging anteriorly (Schatzker). Lagergren and Lindholm found decreased vascularity in the Achilles tendon 2 to 6 cm above the insertion of the tendon.

The location of Achilles tendonitis is either at the insertion, in an area 2 to 6 cm proximal to the insertion (relative avascular zone), or at the musculotendinous junction ("tennis leg").

Etiology

Approximately 80% of patients with Achilles tendonitis are males. Clement et al. reported that 75% of Achilles tendonitis could be attributed to training errors (Table 6-3). Multiple authors report functional overpronation as a common etiologic factor in Achilles tendon disorders (Fig. 6-27, *A*).

Clement and Smart, through observations of slow-motion cinematography, determined that prolonged pronation causes tibial internal rotation, pulling the Achilles tendon medially. At push off, there is a resultant bowstring or "whipping" effect, pulling the tendon laterally (Fig. 6-27, *B*). This whipping action contributes to microtears and subsequent degeneration. These authors also describe conflicting rotatory forces imparted to the tibia by simultaneous pronation and knee extension, causing vascular impairment by blanching or "wringing out" of the vessels in the zone of relative tendon avascularity. This leads to subsequent degenerative changes (Fig. 6-28). Kvist also found markedly limited total passive subtalar joint mobility or ankle dorsiflexion limitation in 70% of athletes with insertional pain and in 58% of athletes with peritendonitis, compared with 44% of control athletes.

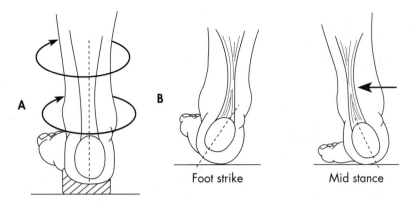

Figure 6-27 A, Correction of functional overpronation by medial rearfoot post minimizes potential for postulated vascular wringing. **B,** Whipping action of the Achilles tendon produced by overpronation. (From Clement D et al: *Am J Sports Med* 12(3):181, 1981.)

TABLE 6-3 **Most Prevalent Etiologic Factors (N = 109)**	
Factor	Patients
Training Errors	82
1. Sudden increase in mileage	13
2. Single severe session	11
3. Increase in intensity	6
4. Hill training	4
5. Return from layoff	4
6. Combination	44
Alignment Factors	
1. Varus, with functional pronation	61
2. Valgus, pes cavus foot	6
Gastrocnemius/Soleus	
Insufficiency in strength and flexibility	41
Ineffective footwear	11

From Clement et al: *Am J Sports Med* 12:179, 1984.

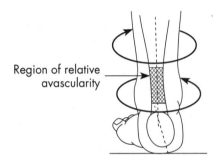

Figure 6-28 External tibial rotation produced by knee extension conflicting with internal tibial rotation produced by prolonged pronation. This results in "wringing out" of vessels in the zone of relative avascularity. (From Clement et al: *Am J Sports Med* 12(3).

Achilles tendon overuse injuries can be best characterized as a spectrum of disease ranging from inflammation of the paratendinous tissue (paratendonitis), to structural degeneration of the tendon (tendonosis), and finally tendon rupture.

REHABILITATION PROTOCOL

Achilles Tendonitis in Running Athletes

CORRECTION OF TRAINING ERRORS	• Achilles tendonitis usually is related to a too rapid increase in frequency, duration, and intensity of training.	• Stop interval training. • Change from hard to soft running surface. • Begin stretching program before and after exercise (Fig. 6-29); stress compliance. • Soften or cut out portion of a hard heel counter if causing posterior heel pain. *Continued*
MODIFICATION OF RUNNING PROGRAM	• Stop hill running. • Decrease mileage significantly or initiate relative rest. • Increase cross-training in low-impact sports, such as swimming.	

REHABILITATION PROTOCOL—cont'd
Achilles Tendonitis in Running Athletes

TREATMENT OF TENDONITIS

- Prescribe oral nonsteroidal antiinflammatories unless contraindicated.
- Begin ice/cryotherapy:
    Ice after exercise
    Ice before exercise if soreness persists with exercise
- Use iontophoresis.
- Avoid cortisone injections (weakening and possible rupture of tendon).
- Perform biomechanical foot and footwear correction if necessary (see Chapter 10).
- Restore normal limb alignment if necessary.
- Correct overpronation with biomechanical orthoses (see Chapter 10).

- Some patients benefit from elevation of heel with small heel lift (¼ to ⅜ inch) to decrease excursion of tendon.
- Shoewear:
    Firm, close-fitting heel counters
    Wide heel base for rearfoot stability
    12 to 15 mm for heel wedge
    Flexible sole to allow extension of metatarsophalangeal (MTP) joints at pushoff. (This will keep the lever arm from ankle to forefoot from being lengthened, which would otherwise increase the strain on the Achilles tendon.)
    Avoid stiff-soled shoes; these increase the work of the muscle-tendon complex.

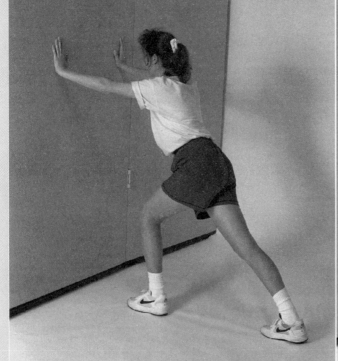
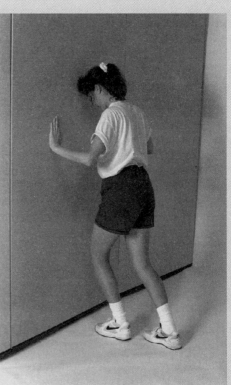

Figure 6-29 A, Gastrocnemius stretch. Patient keeps the back leg straight, with heel on floor and turned slightly outward. Lean into wall until a stretch is felt in the affected calf. Hold 15 seconds and repeat five times. Perform three to five sessions per day. **B,** Soleus stretch. Patient keeps the back leg slightly bent, with heel on floor and turned slightly outward. Lean into wall until a stretch is felt in calf. Hold 15 seconds and repeat five times. Perform three to five sessions per day.

REHABILITATION PROTOCOL

Mild Acute Achilles Tendonitis MODIFIED DELEE PROTOCOL

INDICATIONS
- Onset of symptoms less than 1 to 2 weeks prior
- Still able to perform activities (sports) despite pain

TREATMENT
- Prescribe oral nonsteroidal antiinflammatory medicine.
- Ensure 2 weeks of rest from the aggravating activity.

- Counsel on training and correct errors (p. 265).
- Begin stretching regimen for gastrocnemius and soleus complex.
- Begin eccentric exercise program 7 to 10 days after pain has subsided (see Table 6-4).

TABLE 6-4 **Example of Toe-Raise Eccentric Exercise Program for Achilles Tendonitis (REYNOLDS)**

Phase	Sets/Reps	Speed	Weight	Frequency	Function*
1	3/10	Slow	Body	2×/day	ADLs sx-free
2	4/10	Mod	Body	2×/day	Mod walk up to 15 min sx-free
3	5/10	Fast	Body	2×/day	Fast walk up to 20 min sx-free
4	6/10	Slow	Body + 10 lbs	2×/day	Walk/jog 5 min/1 min sx-free up to 20 min
5	7/10	Mod	Body + 10 lbs	2×/day	Walk/jog 5 min/3 min sx-free up to 20 min
6	8/10	Fast	Body + 10 lbs	2×/day	Walk/jog 5 min/5 min sx-free up to 25 min

*Sx, symptom; min, minutes; mod, moderate.
From Reynolds *J Orthop Sports Phys Ther* 13(4):175, 1991.

■ *The highest stress on the Achilles tendon during sports occurs during eccentric contraction of gastrocnemius and soleus complex; for example, pushing off the weight-bearing foot and simultaneously extending the knee, such as in uphill running. Thus, eccentric exercises should be used for rehabilitation of athletes who will undergo these stresses in their sports.*

REHABILITATION PROTOCOL

Eccentric Strengthening of Achilles Tendon REYNOLDS

- Pain is the rate-limiting factor.
- Ensure that each level of progression is performed symptom free before progressing to the next level.
- The progression should be slow to allow healing, rather than attempting to force a more rapid recovery and prolonging rehabilitation.
- Perform a toe raise on a 4-inch box or step. Both legs perform a toe raise. Once maximum plantar flexion is achieved, lift the uninvolved leg and lower the involved leg into dorsiflexion.
- Increase speed, sets, and weight to tolerance.
- Table 6-4 shows an example of an eccentric exercise program.
- Warm up–cool down before exercises:
   5- to 10-minute warmup
   Stretching: three 30-second stretches of the gastrocnemius and soleus.

   Stretch after the exercises and apply ice for 15 minutes with the ankle in a slightly dorsiflexed position
- Aquatic therapy is useful if the athlete is unable to bear full weight. Use a submersed brick to provide elevation. Submersion can begin at shoulder height and progress to waist height.
- A cycle ergometer (using lower extremities and moving upper extremities on the handle) is a useful cardiovascular adjunct.
- When the patient has reached phase 6, begin a walk/jog program. Perform frequent stops to stretch.
- Increase total walk/jog time to 1 hour. At this point, decrease jog duration and increase intensity.

Severe Achilles Tendonitis

Typically these patients have attempted to "run through" their pain and have had no success. The ankle is tender on palpation and the patient is unable to perform usual activity.

REHABILITATION PROTOCOL

Severe Achilles Tendonitis   BROTZMAN, RICHARDSON

- Stop running completely.
- Immobilize in a cast, commercial removable walking cast, or prefabricated AFO (depending on patient's compliance), to treat severe inflammation.
- Immobilization may range from 2 to 6 weeks, depending on severity of inflammation (usually around 3 weeks).
- May perform one-legged bicycling with uninvolved leg for cardiovascular fitness.
- Remove from cast when nontender to palpation.
- Initiate the following measures:
    Gentle stretching exercises 2 to 3 times daily
    Oral nonsteroidal antiinflammatory medications if not contraindicated

Cryotherapy
Slow, painless progression of activities:
1. Swimming
2. Bicycling
3. Walking
4. Light jogging
5. Eccentric exercises:
    Aquatic exercises utilizing toe raises in pool
    Toe raises with heel hanging over edge of stair
    Progressively increase speed of heel drop
    Rest if becomes symptomatic
6. Return to activity in graduated manner.

NOTE: The protocol above takes into account the notoriously poor compliance of runners who are asked to quit running. We typically use a fiberglass cast that cannot be removed easily by the patient.

REHABILITATION PROTOCOL

Severe Achilles Tendonitis   DELEE

- Stop the precipitating cause (running, etc.)
- Program of "modified rest":
  Stop precipating event (e.g., interval training, sprints)
  Allow patient to maintain aerobic fitness with alternative activities (e.g., swimming)
  Continue modified rest for 7 to 10 days after Achilles tendon pain has subsided
- Daily program of gastrocnemius and soleus stretching and strengthening exercises:
  Gastrocnemius and soleus stretches before and after exercises
- Initiate strengthening when pain has subsided:

  Toe raises with heel hanging over edge of a chair
  Move ankle through full ROM
  Begin eccentric exercise by progressively increasing the speed of the heel drop
- Correct functional components of foot malalignment with orthotic if needed.
- At 2 weeks after symptoms subside, begin a gradual return to the preinjury level of activity with a progressive, staged running program that increases intensity and duration.
- Return to sport is based on severity and duration of symptoms.

Achilles Tendonitis in Ballet Dancers

Virtually all ballet dancers experience Achilles tendonitis several times during their career. A major factor contributing to Achilles tendonitis in ballet dancers appears to be dancing surfaces with poor shock absorption (especially primary training floor). Palazzi,

Rivas, and Mujaca found that 45% of Achilles problems occurred in dancers using cement floors, 23% in those using linoleum, and 4% in those using wood. Many dancers develop symptoms when performing on harder surfaces during a tour.

Other contributing factors include tight heel cords

and pronation of the feet. Improper form also increases the likelihood of Achilles tendonitis. Common errors include rolling in ("sickling") or rolling out during pliés or relevés, not keeping knees out over toes during pliés, and too much turn-out coming from ankles rather than hips, leading to heel valgus and excessive pronation. Repetitive en pointe, demipoint, or plié positions typically produce symptoms of overuse of the Achilles tendon.

Symptoms usually include pain on plié and landing from jumps, inflammation, swelling along the tendon, tenderness, and occasionally induration, crepitance, and nodularity (see box).

Treatment Considerations
Progression is likely if proper treatment is not begun. Elite ballet dancers cannot refrain from dancing for extended periods because of loss of flexibility and level of skill. Thus, any treatment program should involve relative rest and activity modification.

Classification of Symptoms (Palazzi)

1 Pain only after dance
2 Pain initially with dance that decreases after warmup and reappears after dancing
3 Pain during and after dance
4 Rupture

REHABILITATION PROTOCOL

Achilles Tendonitis in Ballet Dancers

Grades 1 and 2 Injuries
- Reduce intensity and duration of practice.
- Use soft training surface (not cement or linoleum).
- Place ¼- to ⅜-inch heel lifts in a soft, well-padded running shoe.
- Perform gastrocnemius and soleus stretching regimen several times a day, plus before and after activity.
- Prescribe oral nonsteroidal antiinflammatory medication.
- Use cryotherapy before and after exercises.
- Use modalities as tolerated (iontophoresis)
- During recovery phase begin Reynolds' eccentric strengthening exercises (Table 6-4, p. 267), plus concentric exercises.

- Use Achilles taping techniques to decrease tension forces on the tendon (Fig. 6-30).
- As pain and tenderness to palpation decrease, begin gradual return to original dance regimen.

Grade 3 Injuries
- Discontinue dancing.
- Deep-water aquatic Reynolds' program beginning with shoulder-high water (see Table 6-4, p. 267).
- Perform stretching exercises for flexibility of the gastrocnemius and soleus muscles.
- Well-leg bicycling, if unilateral involvement, for cardiovascular conditioning.
- Monitor and progress in response to clinical examination.
Continued

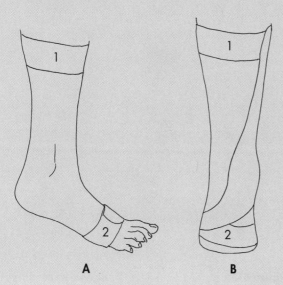

A   **B**

Figure 6-30 Achilles tendon taping. **A,** Begin procedure with two anchor strips, below the metatarsal head and at midcalf. **B,** Apply a longitudinal strip from the first metatarsal head to the gastrocnemius muscle.

Continued

REHABILITATION PROTOCOL—cont'd
Achilles Tendonitis in Ballet Dancers

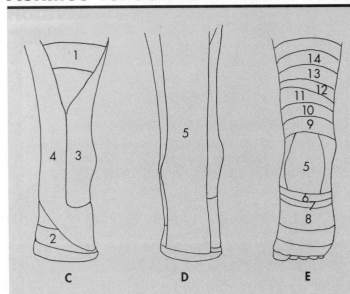

Figure 6-30—cont'd   C, Apply a second longitudinal strip, from the fifth metatarsal head to the gastrocnemius muscle. **D,** Center a third longitudinal strip between the first two, from the metatarsal arch to the posterior aspect of the calf. **E,** Using circular strips, close off the forefoot and the lower part of the calf. (From *Athletic training and sports med*, AAOS, 684, 1991.)

Turf Toe

REHABILITATION RATIONALE AND BASIC PRINCIPLES

The term turf toe includes a range of injuries to the capsuloligamentous complex of the first MTP joint. The mechanism of injury is hyperextension of the MTP joint (Fig. 6-31).

Predisposing factors include hard artificial playing surfaces (AstroTurf), soft-soled athletic shoes that allow hyperextension of the forefoot (Fig. 6-32), and occasionally a preexisting limited ROM of the first MTP joint.

Important diagnostic information includes the mechanism of injury, type of playing surface, type of shoe, exact location of pain, and the sensation of sub-

Figure 6-31 Hyperextension of first metatarsophalangeal joint.

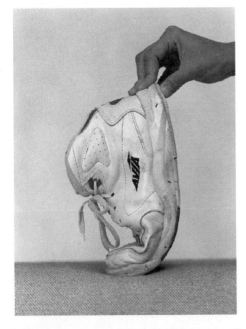

Figure 6-32 A shoe with a highly flexible insole offers little protection for a hyperextension injury.

luxation of the joint at the time of injury. Physical examination should note the presence or absence of ecchymosis and swelling around the MTP joint, ROM of the MTP, and localized tenderness of the sesamoids as well as of the dorsal or medial capsule.

In addition to the standard three views of the foot, medial and axial sesamoid views should be obtained (Fig. 6-33).

PREVENTION OF INJURY

Stiffening of the forefoot of the shoe or use of a rigid orthosis may prevent turf toe. Several commercial orthoses are available that have a semirigid forefoot plate (steel spring plate) (Fig. 6-34). Normal active ROM of the first MTP is approximately 80 degrees, with 25 degrees of passive motion available (Fig. 6-35). At least 60 degrees of dorsiflexion is considered normal in barefoot walking. Stiff-soled shoe wear can restrict MTP joint dorsiflexion to 25 to 30 degrees without noticeably affecting gait (Clanton; Butler).

A stiff-soled shoe with a steel-plate insert is recommended to avoid reinjury by resisting hyperextension of the first MTP joint. After injury, a change to a wider or longer shoe may be necessary. Artificial turf shoes with more cleats of shorter length provide greater stability when bearing weight directly, as well as allowing sideward release with high shear forces (Sammarco).

Some authors advocate taping the first MTP joint in patients with turf toe to restrict dorsiflexion (Fig. 6-36). We have had limited success with this method, except when used with a stiff soled shoe for mild grade I injuries. This method loses significant support after the first 10 to 15 minutes of activity.

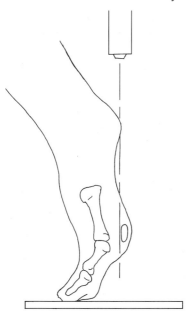

Figure 6-33 Sesamoid radiographic view.

DIFFERENTIAL DIAGNOSIS

Differential diagnosis and long-term sequelae of turf toe are shown in the box.

Treatment

Both treatment and rehabilitation of turf toe are based on the severity of injury (types I through III), as indicated by the Clanton classification system (Table 6-5).

Patients may return to sports when the swelling of the MTP joint has resolved and may return to competition when full, painless ROM from 0 to 90 degrees has been obtained.

Typical time lost from sports for each type of injury is shown in Table 6-6.

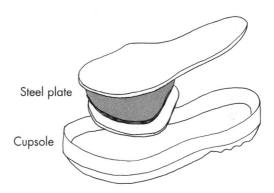

Figure 6-34 An exploded rendering of a shoe showing a plate of spring steel in the forefoot to prevent turf toe injuries.

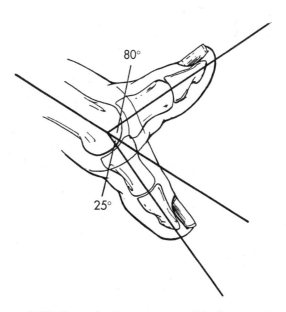

Figure 6-35 Normal active extension of the first metatarsophalangeal joint averages 80 degrees. Active plantar flexion averages 20 to 25 degrees. This excursion may decrease with advancing age. Also, 25 degrees of passive motion is available. (From Delee JC, Drez D Jr: *Orthopedic sports medicine: principles and practice*, Philadelphia, 1994, WB Saunders.)

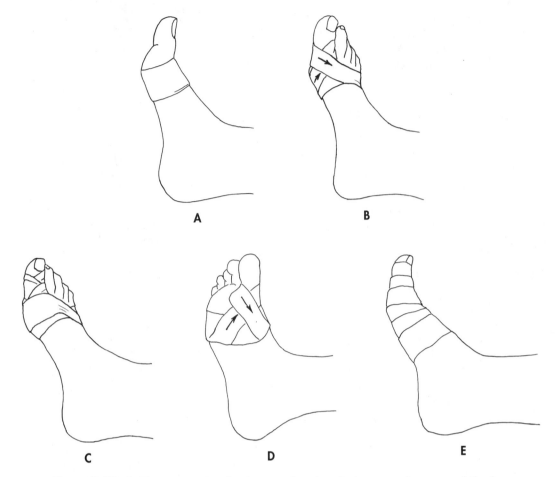

Figure 6-36 A, Great toe taping: begin procedure by placing an anchor around the fore-foot, encircling the metatarsals. **B,** Apply half figure-eight taping at the first MTP joint and encircle the great toe. **C,** To prevent extension, repeat the figure-eight procedure two to three times. **D,** Begin figure-eight taping of the first MTP joint and encircle the great toe. **E,** Close in the toe and forefoot with overlapping strips applied distal to proximal. (Redrawn from Athletic training and sports medicine. AAOS 687, Fig. 43-33, *A-E*.)

TABLE 6-5 Clanton Classification of Turf Toe Injury and Treatment

Type	Objective Findings	Pathologic Condition	Treatment
I	No ecchymosis Minimal or no swelling Localized plantar or medial tenderness	Stretching of capsuloligamentous complex	Ice/elevation NSAIDs Rigid insole Continued participation in athletics
II	Diffuse tenderness Ecchymosis Pain, restriction of motion	Partial tear of capsuloligamentous complex	Same as type I Restriction of athletic activity for 7 to 145 days, depending on clinical course (see guidelines below under return to sports)
III	Severe tenderness to palpation Considerable ecchymosis and swelling Marked restriction of motion	Tear of capsuloligamentous complex Compression injury of articular surface	Same as type II Crutches and limited weight bearing If MTP dislocated, reduction and immobilization initially with cast Restriction of athletic activity (see guidelines)

Modified from Clanton TO. In Brotzman SB, Graves SG: *Orthopaedic knowledge update: sports medicine*, Griffin LY, editor, Rosemont, Ill, 1993, AAOS.

TABLE 6-6 Time Lost From Sports for Turf Toe Injury—Average

Type	Time Loss
I	Continued participation with rigid insole
II	1 day to 2 weeks
III	3 to 10 weeks

GENERAL REHABILITATION PRINCIPLES

- Rehabilitation includes using early icing and elevation, NSAIDs, restriction from sports, and in some instances limited weight bearing.
- Begin active and passive ROM exercises of the MTP joint (both non–weight bearing and weight bearing) as soon as a decrease in symptoms allows (see protocol below).

Turf Toe: Diagnosis and Long-term Sequelae

Differential Diagnosis
- Sesamoid fracture
- Flexor hallucis brevis tendonitis
- Bursitis over the tibial sesamoid
- Sesamoiditis
- Osteochondritis
- Sesamoid-metatarsal degenerative arthritis
- Partite sesamoids with stress fracture
- Chondromalacia MTP joint

Long-Term Sequelae
- Metatarsalgia
- Bunion
- Hallux rigidus
- Ligament calcification

REHABILITATION PROTOCOL

Turf Toe (Non–Weight-Bearing Exercise Program)   SAMMARCO

Start by doing each exercise 10 times. Increase repetitions by 5 each day, up to a total of 30 repetitions. Do program 3 times daily. Exercise slowly and to the maximum stretch.

PULLING EXERCISES
- Sit on floor with legs straight out in front. Place a towel around ball of foot. Grasp both ends of towel with hands, pulling foot toward knee. Stretch to the count of 5. Release.
- Same as above, except pull more with right hand to bring foot to right, then pull with left hand to bring foot to left.
- Repeat both with knee bent about 30 degrees.

FLEXING EXERCISES
- Sit on floor with legs straight out in front. Flex foot upward, toward face, curling toes under at the same time, then point the foot downward, bringing toes up at the same time. The sequence is foot up, toes down, foot down, toes up.
- Sit on floor with legs straight out in front, placing both heel and ball of foot flat against a wall. Flex toes toward face. Hold to count of 5. Relax.
- Repeat both with knee bent about 30 degrees.

SLIDING EXERCISES
- Sit in chair with knee bent and foot flat on floor under knee. Keeping heel and ball of foot on floor, raise toes. Keeping toes up, slide foot back a few inches, relax toes. Then raise toes again and slide foot back a few more inches. Keep raising the toes and sliding foot back until it is no longer possible to keep heel on floor while raising the toes.
- From starting position, slide foot forward as far as possible, keeping both toes and heel in contact with floor. Keeping heel on floor and knee straight, flex foot up toward knee. Then point foot, pressing toes onto floor. Repeat, except keep toes curled while stretching and pointing foot.
- From starting position, "claw" the toes, inching foot forward as toes claw; then release. Separate toes between clawing. Inch out as far as possible, then slide back and start again.

PRESSING EXERCISE
- Sit in chair with knee bent and foot flat on floor under knee. Raise heel, keeping toes flat on floor; then press down again. Lean upper body forward for increased stretch.

Continued

REHABILITATION PROTOCOL—cont'd

Turf Toe (Non–Weight-Bearing Exercise Program)   SAMMARCO

ROLLING EXERCISES

- Sit in chair with knee bent and foot flat on the floor under knee. Turn inside edge of foot toward face (supinate), keeping outside edge on floor. Hold to the count of 5. Then flatten foot and bring outside edge toward face (pronate), keeping inside edge on floor, including big toe. Hold to count of 5. Do not let knee move during this exercise.
- From starting position, raise big toe, then next toe, progressing to little toe. Reverse, going from little toe to big toe.

- From starting position, slightly lift heel, putting weight on lateral borders of foot. Roll from little toe to big toe, then back through heel without letting heel touch the floor, making a complete circle around ball of foot. Repeat and reverse.

If edema and stiffness persist, contrast, whirlpool, and ultrasound with cold compression may be used as adjuncts. These modalities are aimed at decreasing edema, increasing motion, and mobilizing scar until symptoms subside.

Heel Pain

REHABILITATION RATIONALE

Heel pain is best classified by anatomic location (see box).

This section discusses plantar fasciitis (inferior heel pain). Posterior heel pain is discussed in the section on Achilles tendonitis (p. 264).

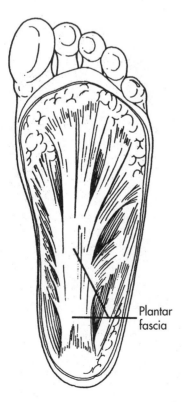

Figure 6-37 Plantar fascia of the foot.

Differential Diagnosis of Heel Pain

Plantar (Inferior)
Plantar fasciitis/plantar fascia rupture
Calcaneal spur
Fat pad syndrome
Calcaneal periostitis
Compression of the nerve to the abductor digiti quinti

Medial
Tarsal tunnel syndrome
Medial calcaneal neuritis
Posterior tibial tendon disorders

Lateral
Lateral calcaneal neuritis
Peroneal tendon disorders

Posterior
Retrocalcaneal bursitis
Calcaneal apophysitis (skeletally immature)
Haglund's deformity
Calcaneal exostosis

Diffuse
Calcaneal stress fracture
Calcaneal fracture

Other
Systemic disorder (often bilateral)
Reiter's syndrome
Ankylosing spondylitis
Lupus
Gouty arthropathy
Pseudogout
Rheumatoid arthritis
Systemic lupus erythematosus

Modified from Doxey: *J Orthop Sports Phys Ther* 9(1):26, 1987.

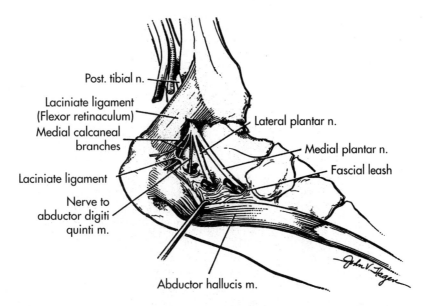

Figure 6-38 Site of entrapment of the posterior tibial nerve and its branches, demonstrating possible entrapment beneath the laciniate ligament and at the point where the nerve passes through the fascia of the abductor hallucis muscle. (From Baxter DE, Thigpen CM: *Foot Ankle Int* 5(1):16, Copyright American Orthopaedic Foot and Ankle Society, 1984. From Delee JC, Drez D Jr: *Orthopedic sports medicine: principles and practice*, Philadelphia, 1994, WB Saunders.)

Anatomy and Pathomechanics

The plantar fascia is a dense, fibrous connective tissue structure originating from the medial tuberosity of the calcaneus. Of its three portions—medial, lateral, and central bands—the largest is the central portion (Fig. 6-37). The central portion of the fascia originates from the medial process of the calcaneal tuberosity superficial to the origin of the flexor digitorum brevis, quadratus plantae, and abductor hallicus muscle. The fascia extends through the medial longitudinal arch into individual bundles and inserts into each proximal phalanx (Doxey).

The medial calcaneal nerve supplies sensation to the medial heel. The nerve to the abductor digiti minimi may be compressed by the intrinsic muscles of the foot. Some studies, such as those by Baxter and Thigpen, suggest that nerve entrapment (abductor digiti quinti) plays a role in inferior heel pain (Fig. 6-38).

The plantar fascia is an important static support for the longitudinal arch of the foot (Schepsis et al.). Strain on the longitudinal arch exerts its maximal pull on the plantar fascia, especially its origin on the medial process of the calcaneal tuberosity. The plantar fascia elongates with increased loads to act as a shock absorber, but its ability to elongate is limited (especially with decreasing elasticity common with age) (Noyes). Passive extension of the MTP joints pulls the plantar fascia distally and also increases the height of the arch of the foot (Fig. 6-39).

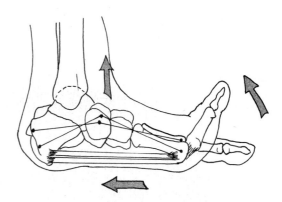

Figure 6-39 The windlass effect: dorsiflexion of the metatarsal phalangeal joints results in increased arch height. (Redrawn from Sport research review article.)

Etiology

Inferior, subcalcaneal pain may well represent a spectrum of pathologic entities including plantar fasciitis, nerve entrapment of the abductor digiti quinti nerve, periostitis, and subcalcaneal bursitis.

Plantar fasciitis is more common in sports that involve running and also is frequent in dancers, tennis players, basketball players, and nonathletes whose occupations require prolonged weight bearing. Direct repetitive microtrauma with heel strike to the ligamentous and nerve structures has been implicated, especially in middle-aged, overweight, nonathletic individuals who stand on hard, unyielding surfaces, as well as in long-distance runners.

Some anatomic features seem to make plantar fasciitis more likely. Mann and Inman noted that in patients with pes planus, heel pronation increased the tension on the plantar fascia, predisposing the patient to heel pain. Pronation of the subtalar joint everts the calcaneus and lengthens the plantar fascia. A tight gastrocnemius (with increased compensatory pronation) also predisposes patients to plantar fasciitis. Cavus feet with relative rigidity have been noted to place more stress on the loaded plantar fascia. Several studies have shown an association with plantar fasciitis and obesity. However, other researchers have not obtained similar findings.

Bone spurs may be associated with plantar fasciitis, but are not believed to be the cause of it. Many studies show no clear association between spurs and plantar fasciitis. Studies of patients with plantar fasciitis report that 10% to 70% have an associated ipsilateral calcaneal spur; however, most also have a spur on the contralateral asymptomatic foot. Anatomic studies have shown the spur is located at the short flexor origin rather than at the plantar fascia origin, casting further doubt on its role in contributing to heel pain.

Diagnosis

Bilateral plantar fasciitis symptoms require ruling out systemic disorders such as Reiter's syndrome, ankylosing spondylitis, gouty arthropathy, and systemic lupus erythematosus. A high index of suspicion for a systemic disorder should accompany bilateral heel pain in a young male aged 15 to 35 years (Table 6-7).

Signs and Symptoms

The classic presentation of plantar fasciitis includes a gradual, insidious onset of inferomedial heel pain at

TABLE 6-7 Causes of Inflammation of the Plantar Fascia

Primary Inflammation	Secondary Inflammation
Idiopathic	Local inflammatory conditions
Local factors	Sprain of the foot
Abnormal foot alignment	Chronic disorders
Cavus foot	Posterior tibialis tendonitis
Planovalgus foot	
Pronated foot	Nerve entrapment
Increased loading of the plantar fascia	Posterior tibial nerve (tarsal tunnel syndrome)
Tight Achilles tendon	Medial calcaneal branch of the posterior tibial nerve
Fat pad atrophy	
Osteopenia of the calcaneus	Nerve to the abductor digiti quinti
Systemic factors	Bony disorders
Overweight	Accessory navicular
Systemic disease	Tarsal coalition
Inflammatory arthritis	Subtalar instability
Gout	Calcaneal periostitis
Sarcoidosis	Calcaneal apophysitis
Hyperlipoproteinemia	Fracture
Training errors	Haglund's deformity
Overuse	Subcalcaneal bursitis
Incorrect training	Retrocalcaneal bursitis
Incorrect footware	Systemic inflammatory conditions
Hard surface	Inflammatory arthritis
	Gout
	Infection
	Gonorrhea
	Tuberculosis

From Noyes FE, Demaio M, Mangine RE: *Orthopedics* 16(10):1154, 1993.

TABLE 6-8 Anatomic Palpatory Signs of Heel Pain Syndromes

Diagnosis	Anatomic Location of Pain
Plantar fasciitis	Origin of plantar aponeurosis at medial calcaneal tubercle
Fat pad syndrome	Plantar fat pad (bottom and sides)
Calcaneal periostitis	Diffuse plantar and medial/lateral calcaneal borders
Posterior tibial tendon disorders	Over the medial midtarsal area at the navicular, which may radiate proximally behind the medial malleolus
Peroneal tendon disorders	Lateral calcaneus and peroneal tubercle
Tarsal tunnel syndrome	Diffuse plantar foot that may radiate distally with tingling, burning, and numbness
Medial calcaneal neuritis	Well localized to the anterior half of the medial plantar heel pad and medial side of heel; does not radiate into distal foot
Lateral calcaneal neuritis	Heel pain that radiates laterally, more poorly localized
Calcaneal stress fracture	Diffuse pain over entire calcaneus
Calcaneal apophysitis	Generalized over posterior heel, especially the sides
Generalized arthritis	Poorly localized but generally over the entire heel pad

From Doxey GE: *J Orthop Sports Phys Ther* 9(1):30, 1987.

the insertion of the plantar fascia. Pain is worse with rising in the morning or ambulation and may be exacerbated by climbing stairs or doing toe raises. Morning stiffness is also common.

Evaluation of patients with inferior heel pain includes the following:

- History and examination (Table 6-8)
- Biomechanical assessment of foot:
  Pronated or pes planus foot
  Cavus-type foot
  Assessment of fat pad (signs of atrophy)
  Presence of tight Achilles tendon
- Evaluation for possible training errors in runners

(rapid mileage increase, running on steep hills, poor running shoes, improper techniques, etc.)
- Radiographic assessment with 45-degree oblique view and standard three views of foot
- Bone scan if recalcitrant pain (more than 6 weeks after treatment initiated) or suspected stress fracture from history
- Rheumatologic workup for patients with suspected underlying systemic process (patients with bilateral heel pain, recalcitrant symptoms, associated sacroiliac joint or multiple joint pain) (Table 6-9)
- EMG studies if clinical suspicion of nerve entrapment

TABLE 6-9 Subcalcaneal Pain Syndromes

	Rheumatoid Arthritis	Reiter's Syndrome	Ankylosing Spondylitis	Hyperlipoproteinemia Type II	Gout
	Retrocalcaneal bursitis is the most common lesion	Plantar fasciitis	Plantar fasciitis	Plantar nodules and fasciitis	Plantar fasciitis
Signs	Cocking up of toes Subluxation of metatarsal heads Fibular deviation of toes 2 to 4 Swelling of tibiotalar joint Loss of subtalar motion	Acute diffuse swelling of digits Pain at medial calcaneal tuberosity or swelling over Achilles insertion Low back pain	May follow Reiter's syndrome Limited chest expansion Low back pain Painful sacroiliac joints	Xanthomatous nodules in plantar fascia	Tophi Swelling of ankle Pain Metatarsal pain and swelling
Radiograph of foot	Changes at metatarsal joint and interphalangeal joints of the great toe	Enthesopathy, periostitis	Enthesopathy, periostitis	Asymmetric arthritis of small and large joints	Bony erosion calcific tophi

From Noyes FE, Demaio M, Mangine RE: *Orthopedics* 16(10):115, 1993.

REHABILITATION PROTOCOL
Plantar Fasciitis

Plantar Fascia Stretching
- To stretch the plantar fascia the patient sits with the knees bent and feet flat on floor. The tops of the toes are gently bent up with the hand.
- With the ankle dorsiflexed, pull the toes back toward the ankle. Hold the stretch in a sustained fashion for 10 seconds, repeating 10 times a day. The stretch should be felt in the plantar fascia (Fig. 6-40).

Achilles Stretching
- Runner's stretch
- Incline board

Steroid Injections
- Patients often receive good response from injection of steroid and long-acting anesthetic into area of plantar fascia insertion.

Continued

REHABILITATION PROTOCOL—cont'd

Plantar Fasciitis

Steroid Injections—cont'd
- We do not use more than 2 to 3 injections over the initial 2 to 4 weeks.
- The possible risks of injection must be discussed with the patient and possible harmful long-term sequelae weighed against short-term benefits:
    Possible plantar fascia rupture with subsequent loss of medial longitudinal arch
    Fat pad atrophy
    Allergic reaction to medication
    Low risk of infection
    Fairly painful injection

Heel Inserts
- Soft, spongy bilateral heel cups (e.g., Viscoheels) or soft, semirigid orthotic if biomechanical correction needed.

Special Treatment Considerations for Runners With Plantar Fasciitis
- Maintain relative rest until asymptomatic.
- James et al. recommend a 6-week timetable, starting with jogging a 7.5- to 8-minute-pace per mile 15 minutes a day for the first week back. Five minutes are added to the daily schedule until 40 minutes of painless nonstop running is achieved (DeMaio and James).
- Other running modifications include decreasing velocity, shortening stride length, and decreasing heel contact.
- Train on soft surfaces (such as grass) to diminish impact.
- Training shoes should have the following:
    A firm heel counter to control the hindfoot
    A well-molded Achilles pad
    A beveled and flared heel to help control heel stability
    A soft cushion with the heel 12 to 15 mm higher than the sole
    Sole of the shoe under the forefoot with significant midsole cushion, but flexible over the metatarsal heads.

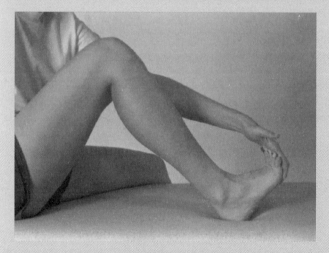

Figure 6-40 To stretch the plantar fascia, the patient sits with the knees bent and feet flat on floor. The tops of the toes are gently bent upward with the hand. Plantar fascia stretch. With the ankle dorsiflexed, pull the toes back toward the ankle. Hold the stretch in a sustained fashion for 10 seconds, repeating 10 times a day. The stretch should be felt in the plantar fascia.

REHABILITATION PROTOCOL

Evaluation-Based Rehabilitation Protocol for Plantar Fasciitis
MODIFIED PROTOCOL DE MAIO AND DREZ

	Weeks 1 to 4	Weeks 4 to 8 of Treatment	Weeks 8 to 12 of Treatment
Evaluation	• Confirm fascial origin of pain. • Evaluate for contributing factors: Overuse/training errors Biomechanics of foot (planus) Status of Achilles tendon (tight) Shoes (cushioning, appropriate fit) Body habitus X-ray Rule out inflammatory arthritis, nerve entrapment, stress fracture (see previous page).	• Persistent pain • Confirm proper fit of orthotics. • Confirm diagnosis with review of history and physical exam • Review treatment regimen and assess patient's compliance	• Persistent pain • Medical workup • Bone scan Possible EMG if nerve entrapment is suspected. Rheumatoid profile lab and workup to rule out inflammatory arthritis Repeat x-rays
Treatment	• Use ice massage of insertion (antiinflammatory effect). • Prescribe NSAIDs unless contraindicated. • Modify shoe. • Fit soft, viscoelastic heel inserts. • Apply soft or semirigid orthotic if biomechanical correction needed. • Perform Achilles tendon and plantar fascia stretching (p. 278). • Reduce weight. • Modify activity (stop running for 6 weeks). • Maintain cardiovascular fitness (swimming, upper body exercise).	• Assess need for steroid injection (note risks). • Perform ice massage. • Taper NSAIDs. • Establish maintenance program. • Maintain fitness program. • With improvement, gradually return to previous activity. • Review training errors again with corrections.	• Use night splinting to decrease plantar flexion at night (Figure 6-41) • May use short leg walking cast for 4 to 6 weeks (or removable walking boot for highly compliant patient; removed only for bathing). • Use steroid injection (see risks). • In patients whose symptoms diminish, return to 4- to 8-week protocol. • Persistent symptoms for 6 months may require operative intervention
Goals	• Decrease inflammation • Relative rest • Correct underlying contributing factors • Increase flexibility	• Return to previous level of function • Prevent recurrence	• Confirm diagnosis

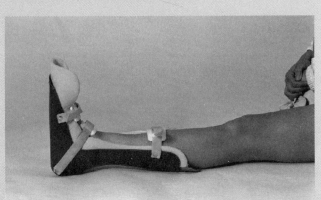

Figure 6-41 Position of night splint during patient use.

RUPTURE OF THE PLANTAR FASCIA

Rupture of the plantar fascia typically results in long-term loss of the medial arch of the foot. Treatment is nonoperative. Because unprotected weight bearing is painful in the acute phase, the patient is placed touch-down to weight bearing as tolerated with a removable walking cast and crutches. The acute phase often lasts 3 to 6 weeks. Protected weight bearing with a firm shoe and/or orthotic is begun after the acute phase subsides. Passive stretching exercises, local massage, and modalities are often begun after subsidence of acute pain. A custom-made semirigid or soft orthotic in subtalar neutral (see Chapter 10) is worn for support of the longitudinal arch of the foot.

Bibliography
ANKLE SPRAINS

Boruta PM et al: Foot fellow review: acute lateral ligament injuries: a literature review, *Foot Ankle Int* 11:2, Oct. 1990, pp. 107-113.

Frankeny JR: *Clin J Sports Med* 3:1, 1993.

Garrick JG, Requa RK: Epidemiology of women's gymnastic injuries, *Am J Sports Med* 14:67, 1986.

Hamilton WG: Sprained ankles in ballet dancers. *Foot Ankle Int* 3(2):99, 1982.

Jackson DW, Ashley RL, Powell JW: Ankle sprains in young athletes. *Clin Orthop* 101:201, 1974.

Kannus P, Renstrom P: Current concepts review: treatment of acute tears of the lateral ligaments of the ankle *J Bone Joint Surg* 73A(2):305, 1991.

Lane SE: Severe ankle sprains: treatment with an ankle-foot orthosis, *Phys Sports Med* 18(11):43, 1990.

Malone TR, Hardaker WT: Rehabilitation of foot and ankle injuries in ballet dancers, *J Orthop Sports Phys Ther* 11(8):355, 1990.

Mann RA, Coughlin MJ: *Surgery of the foot and ankle*, ed 6, St. Louis, 1993, Mosby–Year Book.

Requa R, Garrick JG: Injuries in interscholastic wrestling, *Phys Sports Med* 9:44, 1981.

Rovere GD, Clarke TJ, Yates CS: Retrospective comparison of taping and ankle stabilizers in preventing ankle injuries, *Am J Sports Med* 16:228, 1988.

Sims D: Effects of positioning on ankle edema, *J Orthop Sports Phys Ther* 8(1):30, 1986.

Smith R, Reischle SF: Treatment of ankle sprains in young athletes, *Am J Sports Med* 14(6):465, 1986.

VanMoppens FI, Van Den Hoogenband CR: Diagnostic and therapeutic aspects of inversion trauma of the ankle joint, thesis, University of Maastricht, The Netherlands, 1982.

ANKLE FRACTURES

Ahl T, Dalen N, Selvik G: Mobilization after operation of ankle fractures: good results of early motion and weight bearing, *Acta Orthop Scand* 59(3):302, 1988.

Bauer M et al: Supination-eversion fractures of the ankle joint: changes in incidence over 30 years, *Foot Ankle Int* 8(1):26, 1987.

Burwell HN, Charnley AD: The treatment of displaced fractures at the ankle by rigid internal fixation and early joint movement, *J Bone Joint Surg* 47B(4):634, 1965.

Finsen V et al: Early postoperative weight-bearing and muscle activity in patients who have a fracture of the ankle, *J Bone Joint Surg* 71A:23, 1989.

Kristiansen T, George D: Operative treatment of ankle fractures, *Surgical rounds of orthopaedics* 15, 1990.

Morris M, Chandler RW: Fractures of the ankle, *Techniques orthop* 2(3):10, 1987.

Ramsey PL, Hamilton W: Changes in tibiotalar area contact caused by lateral talarshift, *J Bone Joint Surg* 58(A):356, 1976.

ACHILLES TENDONITIS

Clement D, Taunton J, Smart G: Achilles tendinitis and peritendinitis: etiology and treatment, *Am J Sports Med* 12:179, 1984.

Delee JC, Drez D Jr: *Orthopedic sports medicine: principles and practice*, Philadelphia, 1994, WB Saunders.

Jozsa L, Kvist M, Bálint BJ: The role of recreational sport activity in Achilles tendon rupture: a study of 292 cases, *Am J Sports Med* 17:338, 1989.

Kvist H, Kvist M: The operative treatment of chronic calcaneal paratenonitis, *J Bone Joint Surg* 62(B): 353, 1980.

Lagergren C, Lindholm A: Vascular distribution in the Achilles tendon—an angiographic and microangiographic study, *Acta Chir Scand* 116:491, 1988.

Leach R, James S, Wasilewski S: Achilles tendinitis, *Am J Sports Med* 9:93, 1981.

Leach RE, Schepsis AA, Takai H: Achilles tendinitis, *Phys Sports Med* 19(8):87, 1991.

Puddy G, Ippolitoe Postacchini F: A classification of Achilles tendon disease, *Am J Sports Med* 4:145, 1976.

Reynolds NL, Worrell TW: Chronic Achilles peritendinitis: etiology, pathophysiology, and treatment, *J Orthop Sports Phys Ther* 13(4):171, 1991.

Stanish WD, Rubinovich RM, Curwin S: Eccentric exercise in chronic tendinitis. *Clin Orthop* 208:65, 1986.

Williams JGP: Achilles tendinitis, *Sports Med* 3:114, 1986.

TURF TOE

Clanton TO, Butler JE, Eggert A: Injuries to the metatarsophalangeal joint in athletes, *Foot Ankle Int* 7:162, 1986.

Cooper DL, Fair J: Turf toe, *Phys Sports Med* 6:139, 1978.

Mann RA, Coughlin MJ: *Surgery of the foot and ankle*, ed 6, St Louis, 1993, Mosby–Year Book.

Mullis DL, Miller WE: A disabling sports injury of the great toe, *Foot Ankle Int* 22, 1980.

Rodeo SA et al: Turf toe: an analysis of metatarsophalangeal joint sprains in professional football players, *Am J Sports Med* 18:280, 1990.

Sammarco GJ: How I manage turf toe, *Phys Sports Med* 16:113, 1988.

PLANTAR FASCIITIS/HEEL PAIN

Baxter DE, Thigpen CM: Heel pain: operative results, *Foot Ankle Int* 5:16, 1984.

Berman DL: Diagnosing and treating heel injuries in runners, *Phys Asst* 331.

Demaio M et al: Plantar fasciitis, Sports medicine rehabilitation series, *Orthopedics* 16(10):1153, 1992.

Doxey GE: Calcaneal pain: a review of various disorders, *J Orthop Sports Phys Ther* 9:925, 1987.

Dreeban SM, Mann RA: Heel pain: sorting through the differential diagnosis, *J Musculoskel Med* 9:21, 1992.

Graham CE: Painful heel syndrome, *J Musculoskel Med* 3:42, 1986.

Jahss MH et al: Investigations into the fat pads of the sole of the foot: anatomy and histology, *Foot Ankle Int* 13:233, 1992.

James SL, Bates BT, Osternig LR: Injuries to runners, *Am J Sports Med* 6:40, 1978.

Kosmahl EM, Kosmahl HE: Painful plantar heel, plantar fasciitis, and calcaneal spur: etiology and treatment, *J Orthop Sports Phys Ther* 9:17, 1987.

Leach RE, Schepsis A: When hindfoot pain slows the athlete, *J Musculoskel Med* 9, 1992.

Leach RE, Seavey MS, Salter DK: Results of surgery in athletes with plantar fasciitis, *Foot Ankle Int* 7:156, 1986.

Noyes FE, DeMaio M, Mangine RE: Heel pain, *Orthopedics* 16(10):1154, 1993.

Schepsis AA, Leach RE, Goryzca J: Plantar fasciitis, *Clin Orthop* 266:185, 1991.

Tanner SM, Harvey JS: How we manage plantar fasciitis, *Phys Sports Med* 16(8):39, 1988.

Wapner KL, Sharkey PF: The use of night splints for treatment of recalcitrant plantar fasciitis, *Foot Ankle Int* 12(3):135, 1991.

CHAPTER SEVEN

Rehabilitation After Total Joint Arthroplasty

HUGH U. CAMERON, MD

S. BRENT BROTZMAN, MD

MARYLYLE BOOLOS, PT

Total Hip Arthroplasty

REHABILITATION RATIONALE

The original primary indication for total hip arthroplasty of incapacitating pain in the patient older than 65 years of age, refractory to all medical and surgical therapy, has been expanded after the documented, remarkable success of total hip arthroplasty (Fig. 7-1) in a variety of disorders (see boxes).

DEEP VEIN THROMBOSIS (DVT) PROPHYLAXIS

Thromboembolic disease is the most common cause of serious complications after total hip arthroplasty. The mortality caused by emboli in total hip arthroplasty patients who do not receive prophylactic medication is reported to be 5 times greater than that after abdominal and thoracic surgery. It is the most common cause of death occurring within 3 months of surgery. Kakkar found 29% of thrombi developed before postoperative day 12, and 23% developed between 12 and 24 days after surgery. Thus, the risk of DVT appears to be highest during the first 3 weeks after surgery.

Disorders of the Hip Joint for Which Total Hip Arthroplasty May Be Indicated

Arthritis
  Rheumatoid
  Juvenile rheumatoid (Still's disease)
  Pyogenic
Ankylosing spondylitis
Avascular necrosis
  Postfracture or dislocation
  Idiopathic
Bone tumor
Cassion disease
Degenerative joint disease
  Osteoarthritis
Developmental dysplasia of the hip
Failed hip reconstruction
  Cup arthroplasty
  Femoral head prosthesis
  Girdlestone procedure
  Resurfacing arthroplasty
  Total hip replacement

Fracture or dislocation
  Acetabulum
  Proximal femur
Fusion or pseudarthrosis of hip
Gaucher's disease
Hemoglobinopathies (sickle cell disease)
Hemophilia
Hereditary disorders
Legg-Calvé-Perthes disease (LCPD)
Osteomyelitis (remote, not active)
  Hematogenous
  Postoperative
Osteotomy
Renal disease
  Cortisone induced
  Alcoholism
Slipped capital femoral epiphysis
Tuberculosis

Contraindications to Total Hip Arthroplasty

Absolute Contraindications

1. Active infection in the joint, unless carrying out a revision either as an immediate exchange or an interval procedure
2. Systemic infection or sepsis
3. Neuropathic joint
4. Malignant tumors that do not allow adequate fixation of the components

Relative Contraindications

1. Localized infection, especially bladder, skin, chest, or other local regions
2. Absent or relative insufficiency of the abductor musculature
3. Progressive neurologic deficit
4. Any process rapidly destroying bone
5. Patients requiring extensive dental or urologic procedures, such as transurethral resection of the prostate, should have this performed before total joint replacement

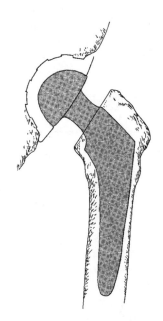

Figure 7-1 Total hip replacement.

Numerous studies have shown clotting in the calf or thigh veins in up to 50% of patients after elective surgery; 80% to 90% of the thromboses occur in the limb that has undergone surgery. Calf thrombi alone are unlikely to produce clinically apparent pulmonary emboli; these typically arise from larger, more proximal veins. From 5% to 23% of calf vein DVTs propagate proximally.

Several factors increase the risk of thromboembolism:

- Prior episode of thromboembolism
- Prior venous surgery and varicose veins
- Previous orthopaedic surgery
- Advanced age
- Malignancy
- Congestive heart failure and chronic lower extremity swelling
- Immobilization
- Obesity
- Oral contraceptives and hormones
- Excessive blood loss and transfusion

Spinal and epidural anesthesia carry a lower risk of DVT than does general anesthesia (13% versus 27%).

The best method of prophylaxis remains controversial. Much of the literature is difficult to interpret because of variability in reporting calf or thigh thrombi, clinical methods used to detect pulmonary embolism and DVT, and a large variation in pharmacologic protocol. Multiple pharmacologic agents are available for prophylaxis. The data from comparison studies vary widely. The most commonly used agents are low-dose warfarin, low-dose heparin, adjusted-dose heparin, dextran, and aspirin. Duration of therapy is also a source of disagreement in the literature.

Most authors recommend early ambulation, leg elevation, and the use of graded pressure stockings, but the effectiveness of these stockings is not well documented. External sequential pneumatic compression devices may decrease the overall incidence of DVT, but are less effective in reducing the formation of the more proximal thrombi. We routinely use low-dose Coumadin, which is carefully monitored; sequential compression stockings; and early mobilization. Listed in the box are several common regimens of pharmacologic DVT prophylaxis.

GOALS OF REHABILITATION PROGRAM AFTER TOTAL HIP ARTHROPLASTY

- Guard against dislocation of the implant.
- Gain functional strength.
- Strengthen hip and knee musculature.
- Prevent bed-rest hazards (e.g., thrombophlebitis, pulmonary embolism, decubiti, pneumonia).
- Teach independent transfers and ambulation with assistive devices.
- Obtain pain-free range of motion (ROM) within precaution limits.
- ■ *Rehabilitation considerations in cemented and cementless techniques*
  - *Cemented total hip*
    Weight bearing to tolerance (WBTT) with walker immediately after surgery

Pharmacologic DVT Prophylaxis

Warfarin (Coumadin)

Most commonly used pharmacologic method of prophylaxis (55%)

Vitamin K antagonist

Delay in onset of action of 2 to 3 days

Multiple studies have proven the efficacy of warfarin for prophylaxis. The rate of DVT is reduced to 17% to 21%, proximal DVT reduced to 2% to 6.9%, and fatal pulmonary emboli 0% to 0.2%.

Regimen #1

5 to 10 mg PO the night before surgery

5 mg PO the next evening

Dosage adjusted to maintain prothrombin time of 1.3 to 1.5 times controls or international normalized ratio (INR) of 2 to 3

Regimen #2

Warfarin begun 10 to 14 days prior to surgery

Prothrombin time is regulated 1.5 to 3 seconds longer than controls

Postoperatively prothrombin time is increased to 1.5 times control

Duration of therapy remains a source of disagreement in the literature. Suggested durations range from 2 weeks to 6 months. The most common regimen is 3 weeks of therapy.

Disadvantages of Warfarin (Coumadin)

Severe side effects such as bleeding (Morrey reports the incidence of bleeding ranges from 3.4% to 25%). Mild bleeding is treated with warfarin withdrawal and parenteral vitamin K. Severe bleeding is treated with fresh frozen plasma.

Delay of onset

Requires close laboratory monitoring

Other side effects include skin necrosis, fever, nausea, dermatitis, urticaria, diarrhea, and abdominal cramping.

Low-Dose Heparin

Binds antithrombin III

Protocols range from 5000 IU subcutaneously two to three times daily to 7500 IU subcutaneously two times daily

Advantage is that coagulation parameters do not have to be monitored

Effective in general surgery, but these findings are *not* supported by the orthopaedic literature for surgery of the lower extremities.

Aspirin

Inhibits cycloxygenase system, inhibiting platelet aggregation

Review of the literature shows no statistically significant difference of DVT between controls (46%) and aspirin prophylaxis (40%).

Complications of aspirin prophylaxis include gastric irritation and increased bleeding time.

We do *not* advocate use of aspirin for DVT prophylaxis.

Lovinox

Undergoing current clinical trials in the U.S.

A good review of DVT prophylaxis may be found in Frymoyer JW, editor: *Orthopedic knowledge update, No 4*, 1993, AAOS.

- *Noncemented total hip*

  Touchdown weight bearing (TDWB) for 6 to 8 weeks with walker. Some authors prefer partial weight bearing (PWB) of 60 to 80 lbs.

Most surgeons treat cemented and cementless hip devices quite differently. The cement is as strong as it is ever going to be within 15 minutes of insertion. Some surgeons believe that some weight-bearing protection should be provided until the bone at the interface with the cement, which has been damaged by mechanical or thermal trauma, has reconstituted with the development of a periimplant bone plate. This phenomenon takes about 6 weeks. Most surgeons, however, believe that the initial stability obtained with cement is adequate to allow immediate, full, unprotected weight bearing.

With noncemented hip prostheses the initial fixation is press fit. Maximum implant fixation is unlikely to be achieved until some tissue on-growth or in-growth into the implant has been established.

Whereas fixation by 6 weeks is usually adequate, maximum stability is probably not achieved until approximately 6 months. For these reasons many surgeons advocate non–weight bearing or toe-touch weight bearing for the first 6 weeks. Some believe that the initial stability achieved is adequate to allow weight bearing as tolerated.

It must be remembered that straight leg raising can produce very large loads in the hip, and many surgeons prefer to avoid this, as well as side leg lifting in the lying position for the same time frame. Even vigorous isometric contractions of the hip abductors should be practiced with caution.

Initial rotational resistance of a noncemented hip may be low, and it may be preferable to protect the hip from large rotational forces for 6 weeks or so. The most common rotational load comes when arising from a seated position so that pushing off with the hands is strongly recommended.

Even after full weight bearing is established, it is

essential that the patient continue to use a cane in the contralateral hand until limp stops. This helps to prevent or avoid the development of a Trendelenburg gait, which may be difficult to eradicate at a later date. In some very difficult revisions where implant or bone stability has been difficult to establish, the patient may be advised to continue to use a cane indefinitely. In general, when the patient gets up and walks away forgetting about the cane, it can safely be discarded.

The routines outlined here are general routines and may need to be tailored to specific patients. For example, weight bearing should be limited to touch if any osteotomy of the femur has been carried out. Osteotomies can be classified as alignment correction osteotomies, either angular or rotational; shortening osteotomies, such as calcar episiotomy or subtrochanteric shortening; and exposure osteotomies, such as a trochanteric osteotomy or slide, an extended trochanteric osteotomy or slide, or a window.

Expansion osteotomies allow the insertion of a larger prosthesis. Reduction osteotomies allow narrowing of the proximal femur. In these groups weight bearing should be delayed until some union is present. These patients should also avoid straight leg raising and side leg lifting until, in the opinion of the surgeon, it is safe to do so.

Treatment may also have to be adjusted because of inadequate initial fixation. In revision surgery a very stable press fit of the acetabular component may be difficult to achieve, and multiple screw fixation may be required. Under those circumstances caution should be exercised in rehabilitation.

Treatment might also have to be adjusted because of stability. Revision recurrent dislocations may require the use of an abduction brace to prevent adduction and flexion to more than 80 degrees for varying periods of up to 6 months. Similarly, significant leg shortening through the hip at the time of revision, with or without a constrained socket, should be protected for 3 to 6 months with an abduction brace until the soft tissues tighten up.

These considerations should be reviewed and integrated into a specific rehabilitation protocol tailored to the individual patient.

REHABILITATION PROTOCOL

Total Hip Arthroplasty

Preoperative
- Instruct on precautions for hip dislocation
- Transfer instructions:
  In and out of bed
  Chair:
    Depth-of-chair restrictions: avoid deep chairs. We also instruct patients to look at the ceiling as they sit down to minimize trunk flexion.
    Sitting: avoid crossing legs.
    Rising from chair: scoot to edge of the chair, then rise.
    Use of elevated commode seat: elevated seat is placed on commode at a slant, with higher part at the back, to aid in rising.
- Ambulation: instruct on use of anticipated assistive device (walker).
- Exercises: demonstrate day-1 exercises (see below).

Postoperative
- Out of bed in stroke chair twice a day with assistance 1 or 2 days postoperative. Do **NOT** use a low chair.
- Begin ambulation with assistive device twice a day (walker) 1 or 2 days postoperatively with assistance from therapist.
  Cemented prosthesis: WBAT with walker for at least 6 weeks, then use a cane in the contralateral hand for 4 to 6 months.

  Cementless technique: TDWB with walker for 6 to 8 weeks (some authors recommend 12 weeks), then use a cane in the contralateral hand for 4 to 6 months. A wheelchair may be used for long distances with careful avoidance of excessive hip flexion of more than 80 degrees while in the wheelchair. Therapist must check to ensure that the foot rests are long enough. Place a triangular cushion in the chair, with the highest point posterior, to avoid excessive hip flexion.

Isometric exercises (review parameters, p. 286)
- Straight leg raises: tighten knee and lift leg off bed, keeping the knee straight. Flex the opposite knee to aid this exercise. Straight leg raises are more important after total knee arthroplasty than after total hip arthroplasty.
- Quadriceps sets: tighten quadriceps by pushing knee down and hold for a count of 4.
- Gluteal sets: squeeze buttocks together and hold for a count of 4.
- Ankle pumps: pump ankle up and down repeatedly.
- Isometric abduction with self-resistance while lying. Later, wrap a Theraband around the knees and perform abduction against the Theraband.

Continued

Total Hip Arthroplasty

Isometric exercises—cont'd

- 4-point exercise:
  Bend knee up while standing
  Straighten knee
  Bend knee back
  Return foot to starting position
- Hip abduction/adduction:
  Supine position: abduct (slide leg out to side) and back keeping toes pointed up. Make sure leg is not externally rotated or gluteus medius will not be strengthened.
  Standing position: move leg out to side and back. Do not lean over the side.
  Side-lying position: Lying on side, patient abducts the leg against gravity (Fig. 7-2). The patient should be turned 30 degrees toward prone to utilize the gluteus maximus and medius muscles. Most patients would otherwise tend to rotate toward the supine position, thus abducting with the tensor fascia femoris.

■ *Cameron emphasizes that hip abductor strengthening is the most important single exercise that will allow the patient to return to ambulation without a limp. The type of surgical approach (e.g., trochanteric osteotomy) and implant fixation (cement) dictates the timing of initiating hip abduction exercises (see pp. 286 and 287).*

Stretching exercises

- 1 or 2 days postoperatively, begin daily Thomas stretch tests to avoid flexion contracture of the hip. Pull the uninvolved knee up to the chest while lying supine in bed. At the same time, push the involved leg into extension against the bed. The hip extension stretches the anterior capsule and hip flexors of the involved hip and aids with previous flexion contracture and avoidance of postoperative contracture. Perform this stretch 5 to 6 times per session, 6 times a day (Fig. 7-3).

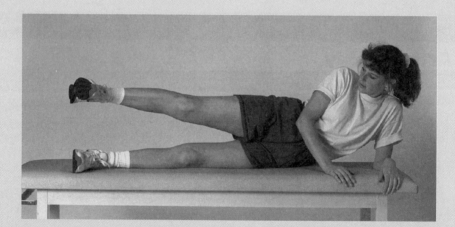

Figure 7-2 Side-lying hip abduction. Postoperatively, lying on side, lift involved extremity 8 to 10 inches away from floor. The patient should turn the body 30 degrees toward prone.

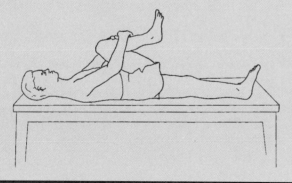

Figure 7-3 Thomas stretch tests: patient lying supine in bed, holding one knee flexed to chest, the other leg perfectly straight, pressing down on bed.

REHABILITATION PROTOCOL—cont'd

Stretching exercises—cont'd

- May begin stationary exercise bicycling with a high seat 4 to 7 days postoperatively. To mount the bicycle, the patient stands facing the side of the bicycle and places one hand on the center of the handle bars and the other on the seat. Place the uninvolved leg over the bar and onto the floor so that the seat is straddled. Protect the involved leg from full weight bearing by pressure on the hands. With both hands on the handle bars and partial weight on the involved leg, place the uninvolved leg on the pedal. Stand on the uninvolved leg to sit on the seat. Then turn the pedals so that the involved leg can be placed on the pedal at the bottom of the arc.

  Until successful completion of a full arc on the bicycle, the seat should be set as high as possible. Initially most patients find it easier to pedal backward until they can complete a revolution. The seat may be progressively lowered to increase hip flexion within safe parameters.

  Initially the patient should ride the bicycle with minimal tension at 15 miles per hour, 2 to 4 times a day. We leave a stationary bicycle on the floor for use in the room. By 6 to 8 weeks, may increase the tension until fatigue occurs after approximately 10 to 15 minutes of riding.

- May also perform extension stretching of the anterior capsule (to avoid hip flexion contracture) by extending the involved leg while the uninvolved leg is mildly flexed at the hip and knee, supported by a walker (the therapist stabilizes the walker). Thrust the pelvis forward and the shoulders backward for a sustained stretch of the anterior capsule (Fig. 7-4).

- Observe and correct gait faults because many of these faults involve the patient's avoidance of stretching the anterior structures of the hip secondary to pain (p. 300).

Abduction pillow

- Keep an abduction pillow between legs while in bed.
- ■ NOTE: *Many surgeons use a knee immobilizer on the ipsilateral knee during the first week to avoid possible prosthesis dislocation. Use the abduction pillow while asleep or resting in bed for 5 to 6 weeks; it may then be safely discontinued.*

Bathroom rehabilitation

- Permit bathroom privileges with assistance and elevated commode seat.
- Teach bathroom transfers when patient is ambulating 10 to 20 feet outside of room.
- Use elevated commode seat at all times.

Assistive devices

Occupational therapist brings these and instructs patient on assistive activities of daily living (ADLs):

"Reacher" or "grabber" to help retrieve objects on the floor or assist with socks or stockings

Shoe horn and loosely fitting shoes or loafers

Transfers

Bed to chair:

  Avoid leaning forward to get out of chair or off bed.

  Slide hips forward first then come to standing.

  Do not cross legs when pivoting from supine to bedside position.

  Nurse or therapist assists until safe, secure transfers.

Bathroom:

  Use elevated toilet seat with assistance.

  Continue assistance until able to perform safe, secure transfers.

Transfer to home

- Instruct patient to travel in the back seat of a 4-door sedan, sitting or reclining lengthwise across the seat, leaning on 1 to 2 pillows under head and shoulders.
- Avoid sitting in conventional fashion (hip flexed more than 90 degrees) to avoid posterior dislocation in the event of a sudden stop.
- Urge those without a 4-door sedan to sit on 2 pillows with the seat reclined (minimize flexion of hip).
- Adhere to these principles for 6 weeks until soft tissue stabilization is achieved (Steinberg, et al.).
- May begin driving 6 weeks postoperatively.
- Review hip precautions and instructions with patient (see boxes).

Continued

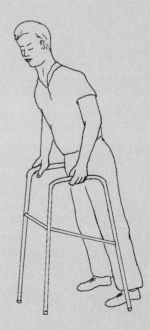

Figure 7-4 Extension stretch while standing.

REHABILITATION PROTOCOL—cont'd

Total Hip Arthroplasty

TABLE 7-1 Campbell Clinic Protocol Total Hip Replacement

Date	Preop	OR	POD 1	POD 2	POD 3	POD 4
Unit	Outpatient	Ortho Unit/ OR	Ortho Unit			
Consults	Medicine Anesthesia Physical therapy		Respiratory therapy Start PT bid.	Social Service Dietary Service		OT consult for ADL evaluation
Tests	T & Cross 2 units (autologous) Routine lab CXR/ECG Hip films	HCT (6-8 hours postop) AP/Lat Hip in RR	HCT or CBC Big 7 PT, PTT	Same	Same	PT; PTT if ordered
Treatments	Betadine scrub, shower or bath bid; if allergic, use Hibiclens	Perform preop total hip shave. Install egg crate to bed. Perform incentive spirometry q2 hours.	pRBCs if HCT low	Discontinue hemovac, if anemic FeSO4 or equivalent with meals.	Discontinue hemovac if not already done, PCA, and IV fluid.	Discontinue PCA if not already done.
Meds	Continue home meds	Home meds, IV antibiotics Antiauseants LOC/AOC Sedative PCA or IM pain meds plus PO	Continue from day 1, plus Coumadin or Love-nox.	Continue all, but stop IV antibiotics.	Continue, but encourage PO pain meds.	Continue, but stop PCA and go to PO pain meds.
Diet	NPO post midnight	Postop advance diet as tolerated to regular, ADA, etc.		Dietary consult (only if needed)		
Activity	Place elevated commode seat on toilet. Place reacher at bedside.	Abduction pillow Logroll q2 hr Ankle pumps	Sit up in stroke chair bid. Perform isometric exercises. Stand with assistance. Ambulate with assistance.	Sit up in stroke chair bid Progress to ambulation with assistance bid. Perform exercises with assistance.		Start bathroom privileges. Assess home needs, limitations, and equipment needs.
Teaching	Provide preop THA instruction. Discuss THA precautions with patient and family. Review hip and lower extremity exercises.	Begin leg exercises, ankle pumps, quadriceps sets, SLRs, and isometric exercises.	Reinforce THA precautions and exercises. Assess for hazards of dislocation and prevent them. Assess availability of elevated toilet seat, reacher, abduction pillow, and knee immobilizer. Warn against use of low chairs. Reinforce use of stroke chair.	Continue to reinforce THA precautions and exercises.		

REHABILITATION PROTOCOL—cont'd

TABLE 7-1 Campbell Clinic Protocol Total Hip Replacement—cont'd

POD 5	POD 6	POD 7	POD 8	POD 9	POD 10	POD 11
	Evaluate for possible transfer to rehab unit.					
	Lower extremity renous flow studies if on DVT protocol.		Continue to monitor PT and PTT.			
Continue as POD 4.	Continue as POD 4.	Continue as POD 4.	Continue as POD 4.	Continue as POD 4.	Continue as POD 4.	Continue home meds and PO pain meds. Discontinue antinauseants, LOC/AOC, Coumadin or Lovi-nox, and Sedative.
Increase ambulation and bathroom privileges.			Begin step rehab.		Evaluate needs and equipment requirements again.	Discharge criteria—Patient must perform independent ambulation with assistive device; independent transfers, including bathroom, and patient must understand THA precautions.
		Review home restrictions and THA precautions.			Reinforce do's and dont's at home with patient and family, e.g., don't cross legs, no driving for 6 weeks, etc.	

Total Hip Arthroplasty

Exercise progression

- Hip abduction: progress exercises from isometric abduction against self-resistance to Theraband wrapped around the knees. At 5 to 6 weeks, begin standing hip abduction exercises with pulleys, sports cord, or weights. Also may perform side-stepping with a sports cord around the hips, as well as lateral step-ups with a low step, if clinically safe (see Fig. 5-14).

Progress hip abduction exercises until the patient exhibits a normal gait with good abductor strength. Our progression for a postoperative cemented prosthesis with no trochanteric osteotomy generally follows the outline below.

1. Supine isometric abduction against hand or bedrail (2 or 3 days)
2. Supine abduction sliding the involved leg out and back
3. Side-lying abduction with the involved leg on top and abduction against gravity (see Fig. 7-2)
4. Standing abduction moving the leg out to side and back (Fig. 7-12)

5. Theraband (C) exercises, sports cord, and step-ups (5 to 6 weeks)

Perform prone-lying extension exercises of the hip to strengthen the gluteus maximus (Fig. 7-13). These may be performed with the knee flexed (to isolate the gluteus maximus) and with the knee extended to strengthen the hamstrings and gluteus maximus.

■ *Note: This exercise progression is slower in certain patients (see pp. 286 and 287)*

General strengthening exercises: develop endurance, cardiovascular exercise, and general strengthening of all extremities.

■ *We use the Campbell Clinic algorithm and the Primary Total Hip Replacement Care Pathway by Cameron shown in Tables 7-1 and 7-2. These regimens should be modified as required to fit the patient's individual clinical needs.*

Discharge Instructions

- Continue previous exercises (pp. 287 and 288) and ambulation activities.
- Continue to observe hip precautions.
- Install elevated toilet seat in home.
- Supply walker for home.
- Review rehabilitation specific to home situation (steps, stairwells, narrow doorways, etc.).
- Ensure home physical therapy and/or home nursing care has been arranged.
- Orient family to patient's needs, abilities, and limitations, and review hip precautions with family members.
- Reiterate avoidance of driving for 6 weeks (most cars have very low seats).
- Give patient a prescription for prophylactic antibiotics that may be needed eventually for dental or urologic procedure.

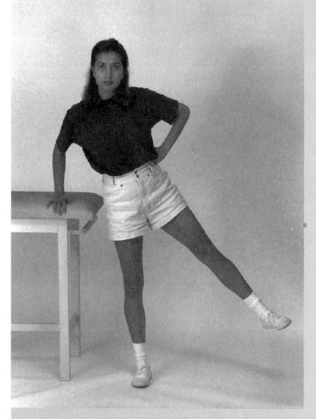

Figure 7-12 Standing abduction moving the leg out to side and back.

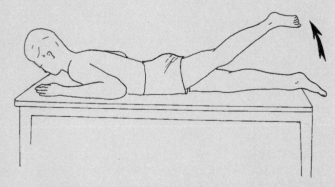

Figure 7-13 Prone-lying extension exercises of the hip are performed to strengthen the gluteus maximus. Lying prone, the patient lifts the leg 8 to 10 inches from the floor, keeping knee locked.

Precautions (Posterior Surgical Approach)

Do not lie on side that has undergone surgery until receiving clearance to do so from your surgeon.

Avoid crossing legs or internally rotating involved limb.

Keep abduction pillow between legs when in bed.

Keep legs separated when sitting.

Avoid low chairs that cause significant flexion of hip; knees should always be lower than hips.

Avoid low toilet (use elevated commode seat).

Avoid bending over to pick up objects (use a reacher); do not let hand pass knee.

Avoid sitting forward to pull up blankets (use a reacher).

Avoid leaning over to get out of chair; slide hips forward first, then come to standing.

Avoid standing with toes turned in.

Patient Instructions (Posterior Surgical Approach)

Do Not Bend Over too Far
Do not let your hand pass your knee.
Use your reacher.

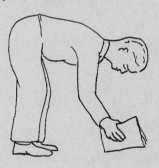

Do Not Lean Over to Get Up
Instead, slide hips forward first, then come to standing.

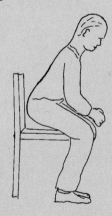

Do Not Pull Blankets up Like This
Use your reacher.

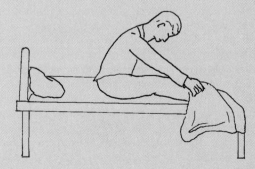

Do Not Sit Low on Toilet or Chair
You must use a toilet seat.
Build up a low chair with pillows.

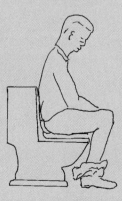

Total Hip Arthroplasty

Patient Instructions (Posterior Surgical Approach)—cont'd

Do Not Stand With Toes Turned in
Do not let knees roll inward while sitting.

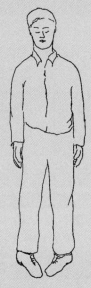

Do Not Cross Your Legs
While sitting, standing, or lying down.

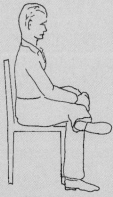

Do Not Lie Down Without a Pillow Between Legs
You do not want to cross or turn your legs inward.

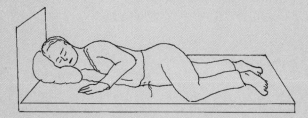

You have been instructed to **avoid:**
1. Crossing your legs or bringing them together—adduction.
2. Bringing knees too close to your chest—extreme hip flexion (you can bend until your hand gets to your knee).
3. Turning foot in toward other leg (internal rotation).

Listed below are several positions that could be part of your everyday activities. Remember to apply the above precautions.
1. When sitting, sit with knees comfortably apart.
2. Avoid sitting in low chairs and, especially, over-stuffed sofas or chairs.
3. Do not lie on the involved side until cleared by your doctor.
4. When lying on the uninvolved side always have a large pillow or two small pillows between your knees. Have the knees in a slightly bent position.
5. Continue to use your elevated commode seat after you have been discharged from the hospital, until cleared by the doctor (usually around 6 to 10 weeks).
6. Do not cross legs while walking, especially when turning.
7. Avoid bending past 80 degrees (touching feet, pulling up pants, picking up something off of floor, pulling up blankets while in bed, etc.).
8. Sit in a slightly reclined position—avoid leaning forward when sitting or on commode. Do not let shoulders get ahead of hips when sitting or coming to stand.
9. Avoid raising knee higher than hip when sitting in a chair.
10. Do not try to get into a bathtub for a bath, unless using a tub chair.
11. *Going up and down stairs:*
    Up—step up with uninvolved leg, keeping crutches on the step below until both feet are on the step above, then bring both crutches up on the step.
    Down—place crutches on the step below, step down with the involved leg, and then with the uninvolved leg.
12. Continue to use your crutches/walker until you return to see your doctor.
13. Avoid sitting for longer than 1 hour before standing and stretching.
14. You can return to driving 6 weeks after surgery only if you have good control over the involved leg and can move your extremity from accelerator to brake with little effort.
15. Place nightstand on the same side of the bed as the uninvolved leg. Avoid twisting the trunk toward the involved side, which would be the same as turning the leg inward.
16. Try to lie flat in bed at least 15 to 30 minutes per day to prevent tightness in front part of hip.
17. If you find you have increased swelling in the involved leg after going home, try propping foot up (remembering to lean back)—if swelling persists, contact your doctor. Also contact your doctor if you develop calf tenderness. Remember that as long as there is touch weight bearing only, the muscles are not acting to pump blood up the leg, so the leg is likely to swell somewhat until full weight bearing is established. This swelling usually disappears during the night.

TABLE 7-2 Orthopaedic and Arthritic Hospital: Primary Total Hip Replacement Care Pathway (CAMERON)

Components of care Year 19 ___	PRE-ADMISSION		Day prior ☐ PRE-OP - DAY 0 Same day ☐		OPERATING ROOM - DAY 0	
	INTERVENTIONS (M/D)	OUTCOMES	INTERVENTIONS (M/D)	OUTCOMES	INTERVENTIONS (M/D)	OUTCOMES

Treatments Assessment Intervention Evaluation Teaching occurs c̄ each pt contact during hospital stay	Forward pre-adm package
	
	Screen pre-adm documentation
	Pop ◯ Non pop ◯
	Consult -internist ◯
	   -anaes ⬡
	   ___ ◯
	Complete Ed/consents/tests
	Confirm date of surgery
	
	Screen/explain/solicit clinical trials. Research consult ◯
	Review Pt
	   Care Pathway
		Pre-adm package returned ☐
		
		Consults completed ☐
		Consent completed ☐
		
		Medically prepared ☐
		Surgery booked
		
		(If applicable clinical trial sticker)
		
		Outcomes verb by pt/family ☐
			Pre-op anaes visit
			Pre-op Hx & physical
			Assess/confirm baseline status of:
			- NVS
			
			- Surgical site
			
			- VS
				Pre-op routine completed (Pre-op Information Record/Checklist)	Perform surgery
					
					Monitor physiological parameters
						Operative extremity warm c̄ pedal pulse
						Surgical intervention uneventful
						
						Haemodynamic stablity

Medications	Screens meds A&S Consult Pharmacy ⬡ Ed: meds pre-op Ed: antibiotic coverage Ed: pain management Ed: prophylactic Tx for DVT/PE	Accurate meds profile obtained Meds to be D/C verb Purpose verb Strategies verb Purpose verb	Update meds, A&S Verify pt own meds Draw blood -INR	Pt own meds used	Admin anaes & meds Admin prophylactic antibiotic ✽	Anaesthetic interventions s̄ complications **Antibiotic rec'd pre-op** ☐
Fluid/Nutrition/ Elimination	Screen A&S, therapeutic diets, restrictions & needs Consult RD ⬡ Ed: NPO Ed/consent autologous ✽ transfusion Ed: bowel routine	Nutritional needs identified Bowel habits identified	Provide fluids as ordered	No solid foods consumed Haemodynamic stability	Start IV Replace fluids Admin blood ◯ Estimate BL Monitor output	BL ≤600 mL ☐
Activity	Ed: correct positioning Ed: DB&C/F&A exercises Ed: possible equip needs for D/C home	Importance of correct positioning verb Demo Knowledge of possible equip. needed verb	Answer questions re: positioning		Position abduction wedge/pillow(s) **Approach** Anterior ◯ Anterolateral ◯ Posterolateral ◯ **Category** Cemented ◯ Uncemented ◯ Hybrid ⬡	Joint integrity maintained
Psychosocial	Assess anxiety level & address fears Consult SW ◯	Fear of hospitalization minimized for pt/family	Orient unit routines Reinforce Ed Monitor anxiety level Provide emotional support	Feelings/fears vented		
Discharge	Confirm Rehab Hosp pre-registration or D/C plans (transportation) Confirm pre-booking of appts	Requirements, expectations known by pt/family ☐ Rehab Hosp ◯ Home ◯ c̄ HC ◯ Appts booked ☐				
Signatures	RN		RN	RN		RN
	SW		RN	RN		ANAES
✽ REFER TO POLICY/ PROCEDURE/ GUIDELINE			RN	RN		MD

Continued

TABLE 7-2 Orthopaedic and Arthritic Hospital: Primary Total Hip Replacement Care Pathway—cont'd

RECOVERY ROOM - DAY 0		POST OP - DAY 0	SCU ☐ In-pt ☐
INTERVENTIONS	OUTCOMES	INTERVENTIONS	OUTCOMES
(M/D)		(M/D)	
Evaluate level of conciousness, VS & haemodynamic status Consult X-ray ◯ Lab ◯ Other _____	RR score of 7 met ☐		N D E
Assess NVS ✱	NVS changes identified ☐ →		Satisfactory NVS ☐☐☐ Purpose of reporting NVS verb
Monitor dsg/haemovac ✱	Minimal bleeding ☐ →		Minimal bleeding ☐☐☐
Assess VS ✱	VS stable ☐ →		
Monitor HR	No evidence of new dysrhythmias ☐ →		☐☐☐ →
Admin O₂ as ordered ✱ Monitor SaO₂ ECG prn	O₂ maintained ≥ 95% ☐ →	S →	
Assess airway (D/C mechanical airway) Detect laryngeal spasms Assess heat loss	Airway patent ☐ → Comfort demo/verb	C U →	☐☐☐
Admin meds ✱ Check level of anaes	No adverse drug reactions Awake, responds to stimuli	→	→
Admin analgesic IV	Comfort level maintained ☐	→ PCA ✱ ◯ Ed: Admin analgesic IV IM SC	Use of/demo PCA Comfort level maintained ☐☐☐
		Anticoagulant ✱ protocol ◯ daily order ◯	Anticoagulation rec'd
Assess N&V Admin antiemetic	No aspiration	→	N&V minimized ☐☐☐☐
Monitor intake	NPO maintained	Monitor/balance fluid intake ✱	CF diet tolerated
Maintain IV	Haemodynamic stability	→	
Admin blood ◯		Admin blood ◯	
Monitor output		Monitor/balance fluid output ✱ Insert catheter as ordered	Adequate amount clear amber ☐☐☐ odourless urine voided
Assess bowel sounds		Assess/Ed: bowel sounds	
Apply Slings & Springs ✱	Joint integrity maintained	→ → Bedrest positioning p r n Skin care p r n	→ → Absence of skin pressure areas
Re-Ed: DB&C/F&A exercises	Satisfactory breath sounds & circulation ☐ →	→	→
Determine orientation to person place & time Ed: transfer location SCU ◯ In-pt ◯	Pt orientated ☐		Pt orientated ☐☐☐
		Monitor anxiety level Provide emotional support	Feelings/fears vented
		Night	
Nurse	PT	RN	PT
		Day	
		RN	
		Evening	
		RN	
	ANAES	RPN	MD

TABLE 7-2 Orthopaedic and Arthritic Hospital: Primary Total Hip Replacement Care Pathway—cont'd

DAY 1	SCU ☐	In-pt ☐	DAY 2		DAY 3	
INTERVENTIONS	OUTCOMES		INTERVENTIONS	OUTCOMES	INTERVENTIONS	OUTCOMES
(M/D)			(M/D)		(M/D)	
Assess NVS	Satisfactory NVS	N D E ☐☐☐			Check dsg & Ed:	
Monitor dsg/haemovac	Minimal bleeding		Reduce dsg & remove haemovac		→	
			Ice pack prn	Swelling minimized N D E ☐☐☐	→	Swelling minimized N D E ☐☐☐
Assess VS	VS stable ☐☐☐		→	→	→	→
Review Pt Care Pathway	Outcomes verb by pt/family		→	→	→	→
Admin meds	No adverse drug reactions		→	→	→	→
Verify pt own meds	Pt own meds used					
PCA ⬡			D/C PCA	Adequate pain control verb ☐☐☐	Admin PO analgesic	Adequate pain control verb ☐☐☐
Admin analgesic IV IM SC	Comfort level maintained ☐☐☐		Admin analgesic			
Anticoagulant	Anticoagulation rec'd		→	Anticoagulation rec'd	→	Anticoagulation rec'd
Draw blood - INR			→		→	
			Ed: report unresolved unusual pain &/or swelling	Awareness verb		
Assess N&V Admin antiemetic	N&V minimized		→	No N&V		
Monitor diet & fluid intake	CF to light diet tolerated		High fiber diet Consult RD ⬡	50% of meal consumed ☐☐☐	→	75% of meal consumed ☐☐☐
Maintain IV if required Draw blood - Hgb Admin blood ⬡	Asymptomatic if Hgb ↓ ☐☐☐		D/C IV Admin blood ⬡	Asymptomatic if Hgb ↓ ☐☐☐	Draw blood - Hgb	→
Monitor/balance output	Adequate amount clear amber odourless urine voided ☐☐☐			→		→
Assess/Ed: B. Sounds Admin/Ed: stool softener prn	B. Sounds present ☐☐☐		Monitor bowel function →	No S/S ileus Impact of ↓ activity & analgesic on bowel function verb	→ →	Pt's Normal bowel function present ☐☐☐
Ed: safe positoning & use of S&S D/C S&S when desired	Joint integrity maintained		Reinforce positioning D/C wedge if applicable Maintain pillows	Correct positioning verb/demo	→	→
Ed: ROM & strengthening exercises ✲	Exercises recalled &/or demo		Add exercises ✲	→	→	→
Ed: transfer techniques			Reinforce transfer techniques re bed chair	Transferred c̄ assistance ☐☐☐		Correct transfer techniques recalled/demo ☐☐☐
May amb c̄ _____			Ed: amb c̄ _____ WB _____	Amb c̄ assistance/ supervision ☐☐☐	Progress amb	Amb c̄ supervision ☐☐☐
WB _____ Assist sitting edge of bed	Sat c̄ assistance			Sat chair ≤ 45 minutes per sitting	Increase sitting tolerance	→
					Recognize satisfaction/ dissatisfaction &/or knowledge deficiency Implement appropriate action	Satisfaction c̄ care verb ☐☐☐
Monitor anxiety level Provide emotional support	Feelings/fears vented		→ →	→		
					Team reassess pt's progress & confirm D/C arrangement	D/C plan unchanged ☐☐☐
Night			Night		Night	
RN		PT	RN	PT	RN	PT
Day			Day		Day	
RN			RN		RN	SW
Evening			Evening		Evening	
RN			RN		RN	
RPN		MD	RPN	MD	RPN	MD

Continued

Total Hip Arthroplasty

TABLE 7-2 Orthopaedic and Arthritic Hospital: Primary Total Hip Replacement Care Pathway—cont'd

DAY 4		DAY 5		DAY 6	
INTERVENTIONS (M/D)	OUTCOMES	INTERVENTIONS (M/D)	OUTCOMES	INTERVENTIONS (M/D)	OUTCOMES
Check incision line	Swelling minimized	→	→	→	Well approximated c̄ no oozing N D E ▢▢▢
Ice pack prn	Swelling minimized				
Assess VS	VS stable				
Review Pt Care Pathway	Outcomes verb by pt/family	→	→	→	→
Admin meds	No adverse drug reactions	→	→	→	→
					No S/S infection ▢▢▢
Admin PO analgesic	Adequate pain control verb N D E ▢▢▢	→	→	→	→
Anticoagulant	Anticoagulation rec'd	→	Anticoagulation rec'd	→	Anticoagulation rec'd
Draw blood - INR		→		→	No S/S DVT/PE ▢▢▢
High fiber diet	75% of meal consumed	→	High fiber diet tolerated	Offer DAT	Diet tolerated
	Asymptomatic if Hgb↓		→		→
	Adequate amount clear amber odourless urine voided		→		No S/S of UTI ▢▢▢
Monitor BM	Pt's normal bowel function present	Monitor BM Supp/fleet if no BM	→		→
Admin/Ed: stool softener prn					
Laxative if no BM					
Reinforce positioning	Correct positioning verb/demo	→	→		→
Add exercises	Exercises recalled &/or demo	→	→	→	→
Reinforce transfer techniques	Independent in transfers ▢▢▢	→	Continued independent transfers ▢▢▢		→
Progress amb	Safe independent amb ▢▢▢	Progress amb aid if able ↑ amb distance	Continued safe independent amb ▢▢▢	Focus on amb pattern	Amb independent c̄ D/C aid ▢▢▢
				IF HOME, Ed: stair technique	→
	Sitting independently				
		IF HOME, Ed/demo safe ADL equip & techniques	IF HOME, knowledge of ADL, equip & safe use verb		
Recognize satisfaction/ dissatisfaction &/or knowledge deficiency	Satisfaction c̄ care verb ▢▢▢	→	→	→	→
Implement appropriate action					
		Inform SW if plan changes	D/C plan unchanged ▢▢▢	→	→
IF HOME c̄HC, initiate HC referral			HC assessment completed		
Night		Night		Night	
RN	PT	RN	PT	RN	PT
Day		Day		Day	
RN		RN		RN	
Evening		Evening		Evening	
RN		RN		RN	
RPN	MD	RPN	MD	RPN	MD

TABLE 7-2 Orthopaedic and Arthritic Hospital: Primary Total Hip Replacement Care Pathway—cont'd

Components of care Year 19___	DAY 7 INTERVENTIONS (M/D)	DAY 7 OUTCOMES	DAY 8 INTERVENTIONS (M/D)	DAY 8 OUTCOMES	Post D/C checklist
Treatments Assessment Intervention Evaluation Teaching occurs c̄ contact during hospital stay	Order/facilitate suture removal Ed: D/C incision care	Well approximated c̄ no oozing Suture removal plan verb [N D E] →	→	→	
	Review Pt Care Pathway	Outcomes verb by pt/family [□□□] →		Outcomes verb by pt/family [□□□]	
Medications	Admin meds	No adverse drug reactions →	→	→	Infection ⬡
	Admin PO analgesic	Adequate pain control verb →	→	→	
	Anticoagulant Draw blood - INR	Anticoagulation rec'd →	Ed: prescription		DVT/PE ⬡
Fluid/ Nutrition/ Elimination	Offer DAT	Diet tolerated →	→	→	
	Draw blood - Hgb	Asymptomatic if Hgb↓			
		No S/S of UTI	→	→	UTI ⬡
		Pt's normol bowel function present	→	→	
Activity	Discuss post D/C positioning concerns	Correct positioning verb			
	Review D/C independent exercise program	Exercises to be continued verb			
		Continued independent transfers			
	Focus on amb pattern	Proper gait pattern described	IF HOME, discuss walking speed & D/C activities	IF HOME, D/C guidelines verb [□□□]	
	IF HOME, reinforce stair technique	IF HOME, independent stairs [□□□]			
	IF HOME, reinforce importance of ADL equip	IF HOME, organization of equip verb [□□□]			
Psychosocial	Recognize satifaction/ dissatisfaction &/or knowledge deficiency Implement appropriate action	Satsifaction c̄ care verb →	→	→	
Discharge	Ed: Clinical D/C instructions	Clinical D/C instructions verb	Ed: Appts	D/C according to pre-adm plan [□□□]	Appts 6 wk _____
	Bill payment	Bill paid			3 mo _____
	IF HOME c̄ HC, confirm home services	Transportation confirmed [□□□]			6 mo _____
	IF REHAB HOSP, confirm plans	D/C plans confirmed [□□□]	IF REHAB HOSP forward info & Care Pathway		Rehab Hosp report on chart ⬡
Signatures	Night _____ RN _____	_____ PT	Night _____ RN _____	_____ PT	Care Pathway D/C on DAY ____
	Day _____ RN		Day _____ RN		Care Pathway completed on DAY ____
	Evening _____ RN		Evening _____ RN		LOS _____
*REFER TO POLICY/ PROCEDURE/ GUIDELINE	_____ RPN	_____ MD	_____ RPN	_____ MD	Reason _____ _____

Managing problems

Trendelenburg gait (weak hip abductors):

Concentrate on hip abduction exercises to strengthen abductors.

Evaluate leg-length discrepancy.

Have patient stand on involved leg while flexing opposite (uninvolved) knee 30 degrees. If opposite hip drops, have patient try to lift and hold in an effort to reeducate and work the gluteus medius muscle (hip abductor).

Flexion contracture of the hip:

AVOID placing pillows under the knee after surgery.

Walking backward helps stretch flexion contracture. Perform the Thomas stretch test for a total of 30 stretches a day (5 stretches 6 times per day). Pull the uninvolved knee to the chest while supine. Push the involved leg into extension against the bed. This stretches the anterior capsule and hip flexors of the involved leg.

Gait Faults

Gait faults should be watched for and corrected. Chandler points out that most gait faults are either caused by or contribute to flexion deformities at the hip.

The first and most common gait fault occurs when the patient takes a large step with the involved leg and a short step with the uninvolved leg. The patient does this to avoid extension of the involved leg, which causes a stretching discomfort in the groin. The patient should be taught to concentrate on taking longer strides with the uninvolved extremity.

A second common gait fault occurs when the patient breaks the knee in late stance phase. Again, this is done to avoid extension of the hip. It is associated with flexion of the knee and early and excessive heel rise at late stance phase. The patient should be instructed to keep the heel on the ground in late stance phase.

A third common gait fault occurs when the patient flexes forward at the waist in mid and late stance. Once again the patient is attempting to avoid hip extension. To correct this, teach the patient to thrust the pelvis forward and the shoulders backward during mid and late stance phase of gait.

One additional fault, a limp, occasionally arises simply as a habit that can be difficult to break. A full-length mirror is a useful adjunct in gait training because it allows patients to observe themselves while walking toward it.

All of these gait faults are corrected with observation and teaching, as well as with increased stretching exercises to aid hip extension (e.g., Thomas test stretching).

Therapist may stretch in the Thomas test position or with the patient hanging the involved leg laterally off the table as the therapist stabilizes the pelvis and gently stretches the anterior hip structures (Fig. 7-14).

Other Important Rehabilitation Parameters:

Stair training:

Going up stairs: step up first with the uninvolved leg, keeping crutches on the step below until both feet are on the step above, then bring both crutches up on the step.

Position of Instability (Cameron)

- Posterior dislocation: flexion, adduction, and internal rotation
- Anterior dislocation: extension, adduction, and external rotation

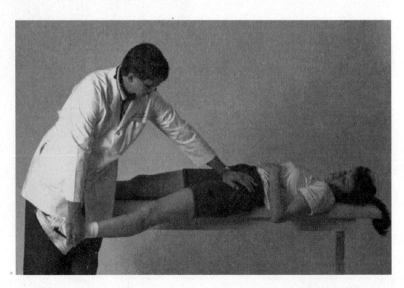

Figure 7-14 Therapist stretching the anterior hip structures in the Thomas test position.

Going down stairs: place crutches on the step below, then step down with the involved leg, then with the uninvolved leg.

Restraints of home environment and activities of daily living (ADLs):

Assess home environment and activities of daily living for unique rehabilitation problems:

Assess home equipment needs

Assess unique barriers to mobility

Institute a home exercise program that may be realistically performed

Stair Training

The good go up to heaven: "Good" extremity goes first upstairs.

The bad go down to hell: "Bad" or involved extremity goes first downstairs.

Cane:

We also advocate the long-term use of a cane in the contralateral hand to minimize daily forces across the hip arthroplasty and, it is hoped, to prolong implant longevity (Fig. 7-15). (See Table 7-1.)

Prophylactic antibiotics for future dental and genitourinary procedures:

To avoid possible hematogenous seeding of joint prostheses after transient bacteremias caused by invasive dental procedures or urologic procedures, most orthopaedists recommend antibiotic prophylaxis. No conclusive research data has established the true risk of infection of joint replacements after dental bacteremias. Significant disagreement exists in the dental literature. Because of the catastrophic nature of a total joint infection, we advocate prophylactic antibiotic use for dental procedures, genitourinary procedures, or purulent skin infections (see box). Potentially high-risk patients (see

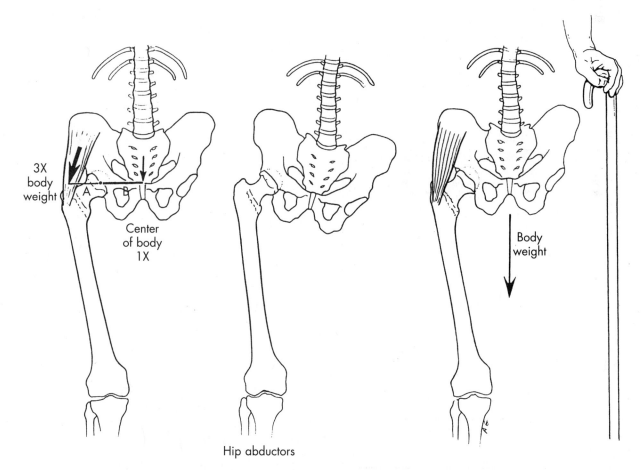

Hip abductors

Figure 7-15 The use of a cane redirects the force across the hip. Without the cane, the resultant force across the hip is about 3 times body weight, because the force of the abductors acts on the greater trochanter to offset body weight and levels the pelvis in single stance. (From Kyle RF: Fractures of the hip. In Gustilo RB, Kyle RF, Templeman D: *Fractures and dislocations,* St Louis, 1993, Mosby.)

Antibiotic Regimens Suggested for Prophylaxis of High-Risk Dental Patients With Total Joint Replacements

Standard Regimens
- Cephradine (Anspor or Velosef)
  1 gm orally 1 hour prior to dental procedure
- Cephalexin (Keflex)
  1 gm orally 1 hour prior, 500 mg 6 hours later
- Cephalexin (Keflex)
  2 gm orally 1 hour prior, 1 gm 6 hours later
- Cephalexin (Keflex)
  1 gm orally 1 hour prior, 500 mg 4 hours later

Allergic to Penicillin or Cephalosporins
- Clindamycin
  600 mg orally 1 hour prior to dental procedure
- Clindamycin
  300 mg orally 1 hour prior to dental procedure
- Clindamycin
  600 mg orally 1 hour before dental procedure, 600 mg 6 hours later
- Erythromycin
  500 mg orally 1 hour prior, 500 mg 4 hours later

From Little JW: *J Am Dent Assoc* 125:1376, 1994.

Patients with Increased Risk of Infection Following Total Joint Replacements

Predisposing Conditions
- Rheumatoid arthritis
- Steroid use
- Use of other agents causing immunosuppression
- Insulin-dependent diabetes
- Hemophilia
- Hemoglobinopathies such as sickle cell disease

Local Factors
- Complications associated with joint prosthesis
  Replacement of prosthesis
  Loose prosthesis
- History of previous infection

Acute Infection Located at Distant Sites
- Skin
- Other

Modified from Little JW: *J Am Dent Assoc* 125:1376, 1994.

box) should have concomitant gingival sulcus irrigation and mouth rinsing with chlorhexidine solution before periodontal procedures or extractions.

Total Knee Arthroplasty

REHABILITATION RATIONALE

Indications for total knee arthroplasty include disabling knee pain with functional impairment and radiographic evidence of significant arthritic involvement, and failed conservative measures, including ambulatory aids (cane), nonsteroidal antiinflammatory medications (NSAIDs), and life-style modification (Fig. 7-16).

Contraindications for total knee arthroplasty:
Absolute
- Recent or current joint infection—unless carrying out an infected revision
- Sepsis or systemic infection
- Neuropathic arthropathy
- Painful solid knee fusion (Painful healed knee fusions are usually due to reflex sympathetic dystrophy. Reflex sympathetic dystrophy is not helped by additional surgery.)

Relative contraindications
- Severe osteoporosis
- Debilitated poor health
- Nonfunctioning extensor mechanism
- Painless, well-functioning arthrodesis
- Significant peripheral vascular disease

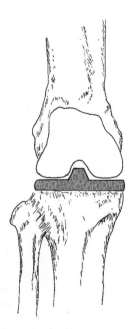

Figure 7-16 Total knee arthroplasty.

GOALS OF REHABILITATION AFTER TOTAL KNEE ARTHROPLASTY

- Prevent hazards of bedrest (DVT, pulmonary embolism [PE], pressure ulcers, etc.).
- Assist with adequate and functional ROM:
  Strengthen knee musculature
  Assist patient in achieving functional independent ADLs
- Independent ambulation with an assistive device

REHABILITATION RATIONALE

Many surgeons use an identical routine, whether implants are cemented or noncemented, the rationale being that the initial fixation of noncemented femoral components is in general so good that loosening is a very uncommon occurrence. The tibial component is largely loaded in compression. The stability achieved with pegs and screws may not be adequate to prevent micromotion (which may prevent bone ingrowth of up to 100 microns). Stem fixation may reduce the micromotion to a level such that full, immediate weight bearing can be allowed. To date the literature is silent on this issue. The progression of weight bearing at present, therefore, is based solely on the surgeon's discretion.

The guidelines given here are general guidelines and may have to be tailored to individual patients. Concomitant osteotomies or significant structural bone grafting should be an indication for limited

weight bearing until union has been achieved. Similarly, if the bone is extremely osteoporotic, a delay in full weight bearing until the periimplant bone plate develops may be indicated.

Exposure problems requiring tibial tubercle osteotomy or a quadriceps tendon division may indicate that straight leg raising be avoided until adequate healing has been achieved, which may take 4 to 8 weeks.

PERIOPERATIVE REHABILITATION CONSIDERATIONS

Component design, fixation method, bone quality, and operative technique (osteotomy, extensor mechanism technique) will all affect perioperative rehabilitation. Implants can be posterior cruciate sacrificing, posterior cruciate sacrificing with substitution, or posterior cruciate retaining. See the box for advantages and disadvantages of these component designs.

Ninety degrees of flexion is generally considered the minimum requirement for ADLs. Those from cultures such as Japan and Korea may prefer a much greater range of movement as may the followers of Islam. Flexion of 90 degrees is generally required to descend stairs (Fox). Flexion of at least 105 degrees is required to arise easily from a low chair (Fox). Patients with less than 100 to 115 degrees of flexion preoperatively tend to increase their motion postoperatively.

Orthopaedic Knowledge Update (OKU) #4 asserts that a flexion contracture of 20 degrees or less immediately after surgery often corrects with physical therapy. Therefore, they recommend that the inability to obtain full extension intraoperatively is not an absolute indication for further bone resection, as long as attention

---

Classification of Tricompartmental Total Knee Implants

Constraint
Unconstrained
Relies heavily on soft tissue integrity to provide joint stability
Rarely used in total knee arthroplasty

Semiconstrained
Most knee prostheses fall into this group
With judicious soft tissue releases and proper implant selection, flexion contractures up to 45 degrees and angular deformities up to 25 degrees can be corrected

Fully Constrained
Fully constrained in one or more planes of motion
Because of restriction of motion in one or more planes of motion, implant stresses are very high with potentially higher incidence of loosening, excessive wear, and breakage
Reserved for severe instability and severe deformity too large for semiconstrained implants.

Fixation Method for Total Knee Implants

Cemented
Used for older, more sedentary patients

Porous Ingrowth
Theoretically, porous ingrowth fixation should not deteriorate with time (unlike cemented fixation) and is thus the ideal choice for younger or more active candidates

Hybrid Technique
Noncemented "ingrowth" femoral and patellar component with a cemented tibial component
Frequently used because of failure to achieve fixation with some of the original porous-coated tibial components as reported in the literature

TABLE 7-3 Campbell Clinic Protocol Total Knee Arthroplasty Patient

Date	Preoperative	Operative day	POD1	POD2	POD3	POD4
Unit	Outpatient/ preoperative	OrthoUnit/OR/ PACU				
Consults	-Med evaluation and clear -Anesthesia -Resp. therapy ————	————	-Social service -PT consult to start activity bid ————	Dietary consult if needed ————	————→DC	
Tests	-EKTA or Big 7 -CBC, PT & APTT, UA, T&C 2-4 PRBCs (autologous) -CXR, EKG, AP & Lat surg knee (standing film)	-Hct (6-8hrs p-op) -AP & Lat total knee x-ray	-Hct or CBC -Big 7 or EKTA if ordered PT & APTT	Hct or CBC PT & APTT	Hct or CBC PT & APTT	PT & APTT if ordered
Treatments	Betadine scrub-shower or bath bid	-Total knee prep -Egg crate-bed to OR -Postop O$_2$ if need -Autotransfusion or Hemovac -Incentive spirometry q 2 hours	PRBCs as needed Continue O$_2$ and IV	DC Hemovac or Constavac per MD	-DC drain -DC IV fluids if no PCA	
Meds	Continue home meds	Home meds ——— IV antibiotics— Antinausea IM prn ——— AOC/LOC——— Sedative HS prn——— Pain med, IM or PCA——— PO pain med— if needed	———— Cont. 24-48hr— ———— ———— Anticoagulant per MD ———— ———— ————	———— ———→DC ———— ———— Anticoagulant per MD ———— ———— ———→	———— ———— ———— ———— ———— ———→DC Encourage PO pain med	———— ———— ———— ———— -DC IM, PCA & IV fluids -PO pain med
Diet	NPO p Md	Preop NPO Postop advance to diet as tolerated	Progress diet as tolerated			
Activity		-Postop: bed rest turn q 2 hr -Start ankle pumps -When asleep at night use knee immobilizer and pillow under ankle for extension of knee	-Up in chair bid, w/leg elevated -Stand, ambulate per MD w/assistive device and knee immobilizer Continue exercises (see p. 309)	Up in chair bid Progress amb. w/assist, WBTT for cemented -TDWB for uncemented	Start CPM inc. CPM (5-10° daily) (if MD uses CPM) -Avoid more than 40 degrees flexion in first 3 days	-Start active ROM w/MD order -PROM exercises knee
Teaching	Preop booklet review Postop routines	Postop reinforce preop teaching & leg exercises		Reinforce activity prog & position		Encourage knee flexion while sitting
Discharge Planning	-Assess home environment -Formulate DC plan		-Notify social services of home needs		Assess need for skilled nursing unit or *rehabilitation unit*	

POD5	POD6	POD7	POD8	POD9	POD10	POD11

PT to tid

OT consult for ADL
    eval. & equipment

Venous flow studies,
    if ordered for
    protocol

						→DC	
						→DC	Discharge meds
						→DC	

| | | | | | |→DC | |

| | | | | | |→DC | Pain med PO |

POD7	POD9	POD10	POD11
-Inc. knee flexion	Step & stair	Review home	Discharge Criteria
-Goal is 0 to 90	rehabilitation	exercise prog.	-Independent
degrees prior to		Assess home needs &	ambulation
D/C from		equipment	w/assistive device
rehabilitation			-Dev. independent
			transfers including
			bathroom
			-Understands TKA
			precautions
			-0 to 90 degrees ROM

Review home instruct

Reinforce home do's
  & don'ts

Finalize placement
  referrals

Assess equipment &
  home needs

is paid to posterior capsular release and posterior femoral osteophyte excision.

Continuous Passive Motion (CPM)

There is conflicting data on the long-term effects of continuous passive motion (CPM) on ROM, DVT, pulmonary emboli, and pain relief. Several studies have shown a shorter period of hospitalization with the use of CPM by shortening the length of time required to achieve 90 degrees of flexion. However, an increased incidence of wound complications also has been reported. Reports vary on whether there is any long-term (1 year) improvement of postoperative flexion in patients receiving CPM versus those not receiving CPM.

■ *Transcutaneous oxygen tension of the skin near the incision for total knee replacement has been shown to decrease significantly after the knee is flexed more than 40 degrees. Therefore, a CPM rate of 1 cycle per minute and a maximum flexion limited to 40 degrees for the first 3 days is recommended.*

If a CPM unit is used, the leg seldom comes out into full extension. Such a device must be removed several times a day so that the patient can work to prevent the development of a fixed flexion deformity.

Manipulation

The usual site of adhesions is the suprapatellar pouch. If a manipulation is to be carried out, it is better done early. An early (e.g., around 2 weeks) manipulation can be carried out with minimal force. Adhesions begin to gain in strength after this time, and a late (e.g., around 4 weeks) manipulation may require considerable force, potentially leading to complications.

Deep Vein Thrombosis (DVT) Prophylaxis

The incidence of DVT after total knee arthroplasty is much higher than originally suspected. Based on clinical detection, the DVT rate after total knee arthroplasty ranges from 1% to 10%; however, more sensitive techniques (radioactive fibrinogen scans) have revealed a much higher incidence (50% to 70%). Prophylactic treatment is indicated (p. 286).

Rehabilitation of Patients With "Hybrid" Ingrowth Implants Versus Those With Cemented Total Knee Implants

Cemented Total Knee Arthroplasty

- Ability for weight bearing as tolerated with walker from 1 day postoperatively

"Hybrid" or Ingrowth Total Knee Arthroplasty

- TDWB only with walker for first 6 weeks
- Next 6 weeks begin crutch walking with weight bearing as tolerated

Note: Surgeon's preference may be different.

PCL—Sacrifice or Retain

Advantages of Preserving the PCL

- Potentially restores more normal knee kinematics, resulting in a more normal stair climbing ability compared to those with PCL sacrificing knees.

Disadvantages of Preserving the PCL

- Excessive rollback of the femur on the tibia if too tight
- The preoperative joint line must be reproduced.
- More difficult collateral ligament balancing.
- More difficulty in correcting large flexion contractures.

Total Knee Arthroplasty—Outline

Preoperative (physical therapy)

- Review transfers with patient:
  Bed-to-chair transfers
  Bathroom transfers
  Tub transfers with tub chair at home
- Teach postoperative knee exercises and give patient handout.
- Teach ambulation with assistive device (walker): TDWB or WBAT for total knee arthroplasty at the discretion of the surgeon.
- Review precautions:
  To prevent possible dislocation, Insall recommends avoiding hamstring exercises in a sitting position when using a posterior stabilized prosthesis (cruciate sacrificing).

Inpatient Rehabilitation Goals

- 0 to 90 degrees ROM in the first 2 weeks before discharge from an inpatient (hospital or rehabilitation unit) setting
- Rapid return of quadriceps control and strength to enable patient to ambulate without knee immobilizer
- Safety during ambulation with walker and transfers
- Rapid mobilization to minimize risks of bed rest

Because of tradeoffs between early restoration of knee ROM (especially flexion) and wound stability in the early postoperative period, two separate protocols are used at the Campbell Clinic, according to surgeon preference. Both of these protocols are presented.

REHABILITATION PROTOCOL

Total Knee Arthroplasty—"Accelerated"

Day 1
- Initiate isometric exercises (p. 309).
  Straight leg raises
  Quad sets
- Ambulate twice a day with knee immobilizer, assistance, and walker.

■ NOTE: *Use immobilizer during ambulation until patient is able to perform 3 straight leg raises in succession out of the immobilizer.*

- Cemented prosthesis:
  WBAT with walker
- Noncemented prosthesis:
  TDWB with walker
- Transfer out of bed and into chair twice a day with leg in full extension on stool or another chair (see Fig. 5-4).
- **CPM machine:**
  Do not allow more than 40 degrees of flexion on settings until after 3 days
  Usually 1 cycle per minute
  Progress 5 to 10 degrees a day as tolerated
  Do not record passive ROM measurements from CPM machine, but rather from patient because these may differ 5 to 10 degrees.
- Initiate active ROM and active-assisted ROM exercises (p. 309).
- During sleep, replace the knee immobilizer and place a pillow under the ankle to help knee extension.

2 days to
2 weeks
- Proceed with Campbell Clinic total knee arthroplasty protocol (see Table 7-3).
- Continue isometric exercises throughout rehabilitation.
- Use vastus medialis oblique (VMO) biofeedback if patient is having difficulty

with quadriceps strengthening or control (see Fig. 5-3).
- Begin gentle passive ROM exercises for knee ROM:
  Knee extension (Fig. 7-17)
  Knee flexion
  Heel slides
  Wall slides
- Begin patellar mobilization techniques when incision stable (postoperative day 3 to 5) to avoid contracture (see Fig. 5-11).
- Perform active hip abduction and adduction exercises.
- Continue active and active-assisted knee ROM exercises.
- Continue and progress these exercises until 6 weeks after surgery. Give home exercises with outpatient physical therapist following patient 2 to 3 times per week.
- Provide discharge instructions. Plan discharge when ROM of involved knee is from 0 to 90 degrees and patient can independently execute transfers and ambulation.

10 days to
3 weeks
- Continue previous exercises.
- Continue use of walker until otherwise instructed by physician.
- Ensure that home physical therapy and/or home nursing care has been arranged.
- Prescribe prophylactic antibiotics for possible eventual dental or urologic procedures (p. 302).
- Do not permit driving for 4 to 6 weeks.
- Provide walker for home and equipment/supplies as needed.

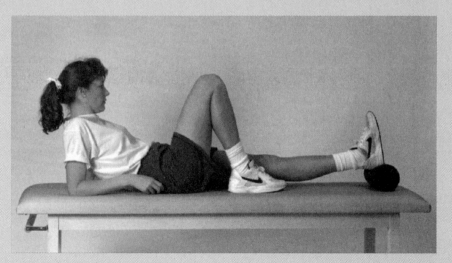

Figure 7-17 Passive ROM exercises for knee extension. Place towel under foot. Slow, sustained push with hands downward on quadriceps.

Continued

REHABILITATION PROTOCOL—cont'd

Total Knee Arthroplasty—"Accelerated"

10 days to
3 weeks
—cont'd

- Orient family to patient's needs, abilities, and limitations.
- Review tub transfers:

  Many patients lack sufficient strength, ROM, or agility to step over tub for showering

  Place tub chair as far back in tub as possible, facing the faucets. Patient backs up to the tub, sits on the chair, and then lifts the leg over.

  Tub mats and nonslip stickers for tub-floor traction also are recommended.

6 weeks

- Begin weight bearing as tolerated with ambulatory aid, if this has not already begun.
- Perform wall slides; progress to lunges (see Figs. 5-2 and 5-17).
- Perform quadriceps dips or step-ups (Fig. 7-18).

- Begin closed-chain knee exercises on total gym and progress over 4 to 5 weeks:
  Bilateral lower extremities
  Single leg exercises (see Fig. 5-12)
  Incline
- Progress stationary bicycling.
- Perform lap-stool exercises (hamstring strengthening) (Fig. 7-19).
- Cone walking: progress from 4- to 6- to 8-inch cones.
- Use McConnell taping of patella to unload patellofemoral stress if patellofemoral symptoms occur with exercise.
- Continue home physical therapy exercises.

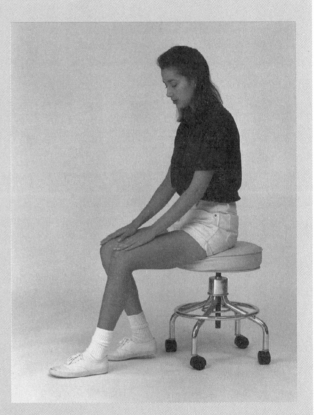

Figure 7-19 Lap stool exercises for hamstring strengthening.

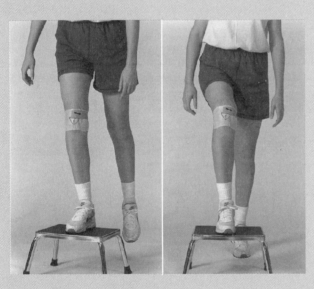

Figure 7-18 Step-ups for the quadriceps.

REHABILITATION PROTOCOL (#2)

Total Knee Arthroplasty CAMPBELL CLINIC

This protocol usually is followed by patients who have a high likelihood of delayed or impaired wound healing (chronic steroid use, diabetes mellitus, etc.).

1 day
- Begin isometric exercises
  Ankle pumps

■ *CPM is not used.*
- Ambulate twice a day with knee immobilizer, walker, and assistance.

3 days
- Begin active ROM exercises and active-assisted ROM exercises if wound is clean and dry.
- Ambulate without knee immobilizer when patient is able to perform 3 straight leg raises in succession without immobilizer.
- Initiate passive ROM exercises on day 3 or 4 for knee flexion and extension.
- Proceed with Campbell Clinic protocol (p. 304).

6 weeks
- Initiate the exercises listed in the accelerated protocol (see p. 308).

■ *Note: The difference between these two protocols is the avoidance of CPM in patients with possible wound healing problems in this protocol.*

Postoperative Exercise Program Total Knee Replacement
GOALS
- To increase the ROM of the knee to full extension and full flexion
- To increase the muscle strength postoperatively of the involved extremity

Quadriceps sets
- Tighten knees, pushing them down into the bed, feeling thigh tighten. Hold for 5 seconds, then relax.
- _____ sets of _____.
- Repeat session _____ times a day.

Straight leg raises
- Lie on back keeping knee straight and foot pointed upward.
- Lift the leg slowly and then return to starting position.
- _____ sets of _____.
- Repeat _____ times a day.

Ankle pumps
- Move foot up and hold, move foot down and hold.
- _____ sets of _____.
- Repeat _____ times a day.

Knee flexion (active-assisted ROM)
- Sitting, slide foot backward as far as possible and then plant operated foot on ground.
- While foot is planted slide knee out over foot and count to 10.
- _____ sets of _____.
- Repeat _____ times a day.

Knee flexion (active-assisted ROM)
- Sitting, gently lower leg to fully flexed position.
- Gently push involved leg back with the good leg until you feel a good stretch.
- _____ sets of _____.
- Repeat session _____ times a day.

Passive knee extension
- Sit with knee propped on a stool so that the knee tends to sag.
- Press hands down on thigh and hold for a count of 10.
- _____ sets of _____.
- Repeat session _____ times a day.

Knee flexion to extension (active ROM)
- Sit with foot as far back as possible, then move foot outward and upward, and then hold for a count of 5.
- _____ sets of _____.
- Repeat session _____ times a day.

Hamstring curls (active ROM)
- Standing, raise foot up behind you and hold for a count of 3.
- _____ sets of _____.
- Repeat session ___ times a day.

Additional exercises:

_____
_____
_____
_____
_____

TABLE 7-4 Recommended Long-Term Activities After Total Replacement of the Hip or Knee   (DE ANDRADE)

Very Good, Highly Recommended	Good, Recommended	Needs Some Skill, Prior Significant Expertise	With Care, Ask Your Doctor	AVOID
Stationary bicycling	Bowling	Bicycling (street)	Aerobic exercise	Baseball
Ballroom dancing	Fencing	Canoeing	Calisthenics	Basketball
Square dancing	Rowing	Horseback riding	Jazz dancing	Football
Golf	Speed walking	Rock climbing		Softball
Stationary (Nordic-Track) skiing	Table tennis	Inline skating		Handball
	Cross-country skiing	Nautilus exercises		Jogging
Swimming		Ice skating		Racquetball/squash
Walking		Downhill skiing		Lacrosse
Weight-lifting			Tennis—doubles	Soccer
			Step machines (for patients with hip replacements; not for those with knee replacements)	Tennis—singles
				Volleyball

Management of Rehabilitation Problems

Recalcitrant Flexion Contracture (Difficulty Obtaining Full Knee Extension)

- Initiate backwards walking.
- Eccentric extension:
  Therapist passively extends the leg and then holds the leg as the patient attempts to lower it slowly.
- With the patient standing, flex and extend the involved knee. Sports cord or rubber bands can be used for resistance.
- Use electrical stimulation and VMO biofeedback for muscle reeducation if problem is active extension.
- Perform passive extension with the patient lying prone with the knee off the table, with and without weight placed across the ankle (see Fig. 5-11, *B*). This should be avoided if contraindicated by the PCL status of the arthroplasty.
- Passive extension also is performed with a towel roll placed under the ankle and the patient pushing downward on the femur (or with weight on top of the femur). (See Fig. 5-11, *A*.)

Delayed Knee Flexion

- Passive stretching into flexion by therapist.
- Wall slides for gravity assistance.
- Stationary bicycle:
  If patient lacks enough motion to bicycle with saddle high, then begin cycling backwards, then forward, until they are able to make a revolution. Typically, this can be done first in a backward fashion.

Recommended Long-Term Activities After Total Joint Replacement

DeAndrade developed an evaluation scale of the activities for patients with total joint replacements. Stress on the replacement should be minimized to avoid excessive wear and tear that would reduce the longevity of the implant. Intensity of the exercise should be adjusted so that it is painless, but still promotes cardiovascular fitness. Running and jumping should be avoided, and shoes should be well cushioned in the heel and insole. Joints should not be placed at the extremes of motion. Activity time should be built up gradually, with frequent rest periods between activity periods. Correct use of walking aids is encouraged to minimize stress on the joint replacement. The first long-term activity undertaken should be walking (Table 7-4).

Bibliography
TOTAL HIP ARTHROPLASTY

Brady LP: Hip pain: don't throw away the cane, *Postgrad Med* 83(8):89, 1988.

Cameron HU: The technique of total hip arthroplasty.

Collis DK: *Total joint arthroplasty*. In Frymoyer JW, editor: *Orthopedic knowledge update, No 4*, 1993, AAOS.

DeAndrade, RJ: Activities after replacement of the hip or knee, *Orthopedic special edition* 2(6):8, 1993.

Horne G, Rutherford A, Schemitsch E: Evaluation of hip pain following cemented total hip arthroplasty, *Orthopedics* 3(4):415, 1990.

Johnson R, Green JR, Charnley J: Pulmonary embolism and its prophylaxis following Charnley total hip replacement, *J Arthroplasty Suppl* 5:21, 1990.

Kakkar VV et al: Heparin and dihydroergotamine prophylaxis against thrombo-embolism of the hip arthroplasty, *J Bone Joint Surg* 67B:538, 1985.

Little JW: Managing dental patients with joint prostheses, *J Am Dent Assoc* 125:1374, 1994.

Pellicci PM: *Total joint arthroplasty.* In Daniel DW, Pellicci PM, Winquist RA, editors: *Orthopedic knowlege update, No 3,* 1990, AAOS.

TOTAL KNEE ARTHROPLASTY

Colwell CW, Morris BA: The influence of continuous passive motion on the results of total knee arthroplasty, *Clin Orthop* 276:225, 1992.

Corsbie WJ, Nichol AC: Aided gait in rheumatoid arthritis following knee arthroplasty, *Arch Phys Med Rehab* 71, April, 1990.

Fox JL, Poss P: The role of manipulation following total knee replacement, *J Bone Joint Surg* 63A:357, 1981.

Kozzin SC, Scott R: Current concepts: unicondylar knee arthroplasty, *J Bone Joint Surg* 71A:145, 1989.

Maloney WJ et al: The influence of continuous passive motion on outcome in total knee arthroplasty, *Clin Orthop* 258:162, 1990.

McInnes J et al: A controlled evaluation of continuous passive motion in patients undergoing total knee arthroplasty, *JAMA* 268:11, 1992.

Morrey BF: Primary osteoarthritis of the knee: a stepwise management plan, *J Musculoskel Med* 79, Sept, 1992.

Ritter MA, Campbell ED: Effect of range of motion on the success of a total knee arthroplasty, *J Arthroplasty* 2:95, 1987.

Ritter MA, Stringer EA: Predictive range of motion after total knee arthroplasty, *Clin Orthop* 143:115, 1979.

Shoji H et al: Factors affecting postoperative flexion in total knee arthroplasty, *Orthopedics* 13:643, 1990.

Steinberg ME, Lotke PA: Postoperative management of total joint replacements, *Orthop Clin North Am* 19(4):19, 1988.

CHAPTER EIGHT

Rehabilitation of Pediatric Patients

WILLIAM C. WARNER, JR, MD

Pediatric orthopaedic patients have different injury patterns and different rehabilitation potentials than do adult orthopaedic patients. When a fracture or injury occurs in a growing child, the dynamic state of growth may be beneficial to the child's rehabilitation or may cause a significant problem. Remodeling of an angulated fracture is a beneficial effect of continued growth; whereas, physeal arrest with shortening and angular deformity is an adverse effect. This must be considered in the treatment and rehabilitation of injuries in children. Since most children want to return to sports or recreational activities as soon as possible, the rehabilitation process occurs naturally, and they will begin using the injured part and try to regain normal function on their own. Although some children require active therapy, rehabilitation is focused more on preventing repeat injury than on regaining function.

In the following section some of the more common pediatric injuries and diseases are described, as well as the expected rehabilitation protocols. Some injuries require an active rehabilitation program, whereas others require only skillful observation.

Clavicular Fractures

Treatment of most clavicular fractures consists of some form of support, such as a figure-eight harness, arm sling, or a Velpeau bandage (Table 8-1). Most clavicle fractures heal uneventfully, although a bony prominence may be seen after fracture healing. Associated neurovascular compromise is very rare.

FRACTURES OF THE MIDDLE THIRD OF THE CLAVICLE

A fracture of the middle portion of the clavicle usually results from a fall on an outstretched hand or shoulder that applies a compressive force between the shoulder and trunk. Direct trauma to the clavicle is a less common mechanism of injury. Pain and swelling are associated with this injury, and radiographs show the typical displacement of a clavicle fracture. The proximal fragment is pulled superiorly by the sternocleidomastoid muscle, and the distal fragment is pulled medially by the subclavius muscle and inferiorly by the pectoralis minor muscle.

TABLE 8-1 **Classification and Incidence of Clavicular Fractures**	
Lateral	9%
Middle	93%
Medial	3%

TABLE 8-2 **Time for Immobilization for Middle Third Clavicular Fractures**	
Age	**Immobilization**
1 to 5 years	1 to 2 weeks
5 to 10 years	2 weeks
≥10 years	2 to 3 weeks

The age of the child determines the amount of time required for immobilization in a figure-eight harness, arm sling, or Velpeau bandage (Table 8-2).

DISTAL CLAVICULAR FRACTURE

Distal clavicular fractures result from a direct blow on the lateral aspect of the shoulder. In children this usually is a sleeve type fracture with the acromioclavicular ligaments remaining attached to a sleeve of periosteum. When the sleeve of periosteum forms new bone, the acromioclavicular joint becomes stable. The displaced bone end may cause a prominence over the distal end of the clavicle, but this tends to remodel with time. Treatment consists of support for the involved extremity for 2 to 3 weeks. A sling usually is all that is needed, but occasionally a figure-eight harness may be used. Surgery rarely is indicated.

MEDIAL CLAVICULAR FRACTURES

Medical clavicular fractures are more likely to be epiphyseal separations, occurring from a fall on an outstretched hand or from a direct blow to the clavicle. Anterior separation is the most common type. This is treated by supporting the involved arm until the fracture has healed. Posterior fracture separation is a more serious injury that may compromise the trachea and neurovascular structures. Closed reduction and possibly open reduction is necessary to treat this injury. A figure-eight harness is used for immobilization for at least 4 to 6 weeks. Anterior fractures tend to redisplace anteriorly, but this is acceptable; residual posterior displacement should not be accepted.

REHABILITATION PROTOCOL

Clavicular Fractures

- Perform active range of motion (ROM) exercises of the hand, wrist, and elbow (daily).
- Perform Codman exercises or gentle pendulum exercises.

- Progress to active abduction, adduction, flexion, extension, internal/external rotation.
- Permit unrestricted activity when fracture is nontender and full shoulder motion is obtained (typically 4 to 5 weeks).

Humeral Fractures

HUMERAL SHAFT FRACTURES

Fractures of the humeral shaft account for 2% of all pediatric fractures; most result from a twisting force or a direct blow to the arm. Most humeral shaft fractures in children can be treated with a Velpeau bandage, a coaptation splint, or a hanging arm cast, although occasionally open reduction and internal fixation are necessary for a floating elbow, multiple trauma, an open fracture, or progressive neurologic loss. Remodeling potential and ROM at the shoulder joint will compensate for a significant amount of residual deformity (see box). (Fig. 8-1). Angulation of up to 40 degrees will remodel significantly in young children; however, as a child becomes more mature, less deformity is acceptable.

Acceptable Alignment of Humeral Shaft Fractures in Children

In children older than 6 years of age, acceptable results can be obtained with the following guidelines:
- 20 degrees of anteroposterior (AP) angulation
- 30 degrees of varus
- 2.5 cm of shortening
- 15 degrees of rotation

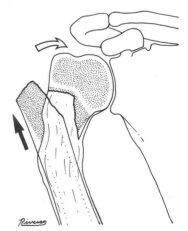

Figure 8-1 Remodeling potential of proximal humeral physeal fracture because of periosteal sleeve. (Redrawn from Ogden JA: *Skeletal injury in the child*, Philadelphia, 1982, Lea & Febiger.)

REHABILITATION PROTOCOL
Humeral Shaft Fractures

Clinical union occurs in 7 to 14 days in neonates, in 4 to 6 weeks in children, and in 6 to 8 weeks in adolescents. After clinical union is apparent, the arm is placed in a sling, and active shoulder and elbow ROM exercises are started. Activities are restricted until full ROM is obtained in the shoulder and elbow and union is evident on radiographs.

Elbow Fractures and Dislocations

SUPRACONDYLAR HUMERAL FRACTURES

Supracondylar humeral fractures account for 60% of all elbow fractures in children between the ages of 3 and 10 years and most commonly result from a fall on an outstretched hand. Approximately 97% of children with supracondylar humeral fractures have extension injuries, and flexion injuries occur in approximately 3%. The mechanism of injury determines the type of fracture and subsequently the treatment. This injury has the potential for significant complications, such as Volkmann contracture, vascular compromise, neuropraxia, and cubitus varus deformity. To alert the orthopaedic surgeon of possible complications and to aid in the treatment, Gartland classified this injury into various types (Tables 8-3 and 8-4).

Technique of closed reduction of supracondylar fractures

Gentle traction is applied to the elbow in the extended position, and counter-traction is applied to the upper arm. The forearm is supinated and the elbow is hyperextended to disengage the fracture fragments. Longitudinal traction is applied and the displacement is corrected in both the medial and lateral planes. Rotational deformity should be corrected at the same time. The elbow is flexed and the thumb is used to push the olecranon forward to reduce the distal fragment. For posteromedial dislocations, the forearm is pronated to correct varus tilt. After this maneuver, the reduction is evaluated by image intensification, and pins are placed percutaneously.

Crossed-pin configuration (Fig. 8-2), one placed laterally and one medially, provides the most stability; however, if the elbow is too swollen to allow easy palpation of the bony landmarks, two parallel lateral pins can be used to stabilize the fracture. After the pins have been placed, the fracture should be stable enough to allow full extension of the arm. At this time, the adequacy of reduction and fixation must be assessed. The most commonly used radiographic measurement is the Baumann angle (Fig. 8-3). The arm is immobilized in a splint with an area cut out to allow easy palpation of the radial artery. A collar-and-cuff sling is applied for support and to prevent the child from externally rotating the arm.

Open reduction of supracondylar fracture is indicated for (1) an open fracture, (2) vascular compromise, and (3) inadequate closed reduction.

TABLE 8-3 Gartland Classification of Supracondylar Humeral Fractures

Type	Description
I	Nondisplaced fracture
II	Displaced or "hinged" fracture with an intact posterior cortex
III	Displaced fracture with no cortical contact (96% displaced posteromedially, 4% displaced posterolaterally)

TABLE 8-4 Treatment of Supracondylar Fractures

Type	Treatment
I	Immobilize in a cast or splint for about 3 weeks. Depending on the home situation, admission to the hospital for 24 hours to observe for neurovascular complications may be necessary.
II	Use closed reduction and casting. If doubt remains about stability, percutaneous pinning and cast or splint immobilization can be performed. The child should be admitted to the hospital for neurovascular checks over 24 hours.
III	Closed reduction and percutaneous pinning, followed by splint immobilization, is the most common treatment method. Pins may be left out of the skin or may be cut at the skin level and left palpable for easy removal in the office. Traction may be used for severely swollen type III fractures; however, this has been associated with a high incidence of malunion. The child should be admitted to the hospital for 24 hours for ice, elevation, and neurovascular checks.

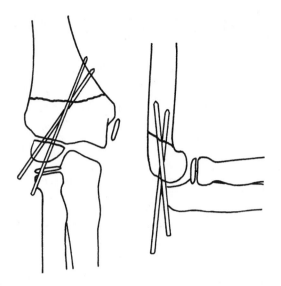

Figure 8-2 Pinning of supracondylar fracture with divergent pins crossing fracture site and opposite cortex.

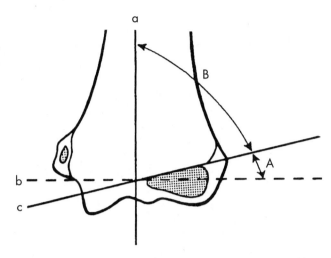

Figure 8-3 Baumann's angle. **A,** Midline diaphysis of humeral shaft. **B,** Line perpendicular to midline. **C,** Line through physis of lateral condyle. Angle A is original Baumann angle. Angle B is more commonly used currently.

Complications

Common complications of supracondylar humeral fractures include Volkmann ischemia, vascular compromise, neurologic impairment, and malreduction of the fracture.

Volkmann ischemic contracture, the most dreaded complication, is caused by swelling about the elbow. If Volkmann ischemic contracture is suspected, tight bandages should be removed immediately, the arm extended, and compartment pressures measured. Fasciotomy and release of tight structures around the elbow may be necessary if compartment pressures remain elevated. Although this complication does not occur frequently, the orthopaedic surgeon should always be aware of the possibility.

Vascular compromise occurs as a result of injury to the brachial artery and requires open reduction and repair of the artery. A vascular surgeon should be consulted to assist in the repair.

Neurologic impairment occurs in about 8% of children with supracondylar humeral fractures. The radial and median nerves are the most commonly injured.

Usually, this is a neuropraxia, and the nerves recover and function returns to normal within several weeks. If neurologic function does not return within 16 weeks, electromyogram (EMG) and nerve conduction studies should be performed.

Cubitus varus, often a difficult complication of supracondylar humerus fractures, was once thought to be caused by growth arrest. Growth arrest from injury to the trochlear physis has been reported, but this is rare. Malreduction, specifically coronal tilting of the fracture site, is now known to be the cause of the unsightly gunstock deformity. Horizontal rotation and anterior angulation predispose the fracture site to tilt into varus. Type II supracondylar fractures with medial comminution and impaction may result in cubitus varus deformity if not recognized and reduced and pinned in the corrected position. If cubitus varus deformity develops, a supracondylar osteotomy can be performed at a later date; however, this complication can be avoided by ensuring that adequate reduction and pinning have been performed.

REHABILITATION PROTOCOL

Supracondylar Fractures

1 week	• See the child in the office and obtain radiographs. If splint immobilization was initially used for swelling, it can be converted to a long arm cast at this time.	3 weeks	• Can remove the pins in the office and place the arm in a posterior splint for another 1 to 2 weeks. Depending on radiographic evidence of healing, the arm may be *Continued*

REHABILITATION PROTOCOL—cont'd

Supracondylar Fractures

3 weeks	placed in a sling and the child may be allowed to begin gentle ROM. For children older than 10 years of age, increasing the length of time of pin immobilization to 4 weeks may be necessary until there is radiographic evidence of callus formation. • Gentle ROM of elbow, wrist, and fingers continues with avoidance of contact sports.	6 weeks	• The child should have regained almost complete ROM. If not, institute an active exercise program under the direction of a physical therapist, focusing on regaining flexion, extension, supination, and pronation. Begin gentle passive ROM and gentle stretching for flexion and extension.
		16 weeks	• Perform EMG and nerve conduction studies if associated nerve deficits are still present.

LATERAL CONDYLAR FRACTURES

Lateral condylar fractures account for 18% to 20% of all distal humeral fractures in children and usually result from a fall on an outstretched hand with the elbow extended. The forearm is forced into varus and the lateral condyle is pulled off, with the extensor mechanism and the lateral ligaments attached to the distal fragment. Another less common mechanism of injury is a valgus stress to the elbow that causes the radial head to push the lateral condyle off the humerus. Because of the attachment of the extensor muscles to the lateral condyle, the fracture fragment may displace and actually rotate (Fig. 8-4), placing the articular cartilage in apposition to the bony fracture surface of the distal humerus.

The classification of lateral condylar fractures as nondisplaced (less than 2 mm of displacement), minimally displaced (2 to 4 mm of displacement and no rotation), or completely displaced (more than 4 mm of displacement, usually with rotation of the distal fragment) is the most useful for determining treatment options (Table 8-5).

Treatment

Treatment recommendations are based on the amount of displacement present (Table 8-6). Nonunion is frequent after lateral condylar fractures, and this possibility must be considered when making treatment decisions.

■ *The pins are left in place under the skin for 6 weeks.*

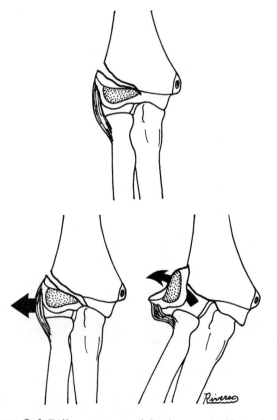

Figure 8-4 Different stages of displacement of lateral condylar fracture: undisplaced, moderately displaced, and completely displaced and rotated. (Redrawn from Jakob R et al: *J Bone Joint Surg* 57B:430, 1975.)

TABLE 8-5 Classifications of Lateral Humeral Condylar Fractures (BADELON ET AL.)

Type	Description
I	Nondisplaced fracture that can be seen on only one radiographic view
II	Fracture with less than 2 mm of displacement
III	Fracture with more than 2 mm of displacement on all views
IV	Completely displaced fracture

TABLE 8-6 **Treatment of Lateral Condylar Fractures**

Type	Treatment
I and II	Nondisplaced and minimally displaced lateral condylar fractures usually can be treated with cast immobilization with the elbow flexed at 90 degrees and the forearm placed in neutral or supination to relax the wrist extensor musculature. At *weekly* office visits, obtain radiographs of the elbow out of plaster to determine if displacement has occurred, and apply a new cast. If loss of reduction is evident, open reduction and pinning are recommended. When there is radiographic evidence of fracture healing, remove the cast and begin general ROM exercises.
II and III	Fractures that are displaced between 2 and 4 mm but are not rotated can be treated with percutaneous pinning or with open reduction and internal fixation. If the fracture is rotated, percutaneous pinning is not an option.
IV	Completely displaced fractures require open reduction through a lateral Kocher J approach. During dissection, the fragment should be approached anteriorly to preserve the posterior blood supply to the fragment. After surgical pinning, the patient usually is immobilized in a cast for 6 weeks. At 6 weeks, remove the cast and pins. If there is concern about loss of motion, the patient can be placed in a removable splint 4 weeks after surgery and started on gentle early active and active-assisted ROM exercises if pin fixation is stable.

REHABILITATION PROTOCOL

Lateral Condylar Fracture—Post surgical

1 to 6 weeks	• Perform active ROM exercises of the shoulder and fingers.		• Pins removed approximately 6 weeks (upon clinical and radiographic evidence of healing).
4 to 6 weeks	• Discontinue immobilization if healing is evident on radiograph, and, if used, remove pins. Begin active ROM exercises, concentrating on flexion and extension of the elbow and pronation and supination of the forearm.	7 to 9 weeks	• Continue exercises for 3 weeks, at the end of which 80% to 90% of motion should be regained. If this has not been achieved, start an active and passive ROM exercise program under the direction of a physical therapist.

MEDIAL CONDYLAR FRACTURES

Medial condylar fractures are rare in younger children and are difficult to diagnose because the medial condyle does not ossify until 9 to 12 years of age. In a young child, an arthrogram may be necessary to determine whether the injury is a true medial condylar fracture or a transcondylar fracture. The medial epicondyle attaches to the medial condyle fracture, along with the ulnar collateral ligament and the common flexor muscles of the forearm. The attachment of the flexor forearm muscles tends to displace the medial condylar fracture and may make the elbow unstable.

Treatment

Medial condylar fractures also are classified according to the amount of displacement (Table 8-7). *Type I* fractures can be treated with immobilization in a pos-

terior splint. Minimally displaced *type II* fractures can be treated with splint or cast immobilization; however, if more than 2 mm of displacement is evident on the radiograph, open reduction and internal fixation are necessary. For *type III* fractures open reduction and internal fixation with smooth pins are used. On the first postoperative day, the child is placed in a posterior splint to allow for swelling. At about 5 to 7 days, the

TABLE 8-7 **Classification of Medial Condylar Fractures   (KILFOYLE)**

Type	Description
I	Greenstick or impacted fracture
II	Minimally displaced fracture
III	Displaced and rotated fracture

splint is converted to a long arm cast, and the arm is immobilized for 4 to 6 weeks. The pins are cut off below the skin, but are left prominent for easy removal in the office. If the pins are not left prominent, surgical removal with the child anesthetized will be necessary. The pins are removed at 4 to 6 weeks after injury. In children younger than 5 years of age with this fracture, pin fixation and immobilization may be necessary for only 3 weeks.

REHABILITATION PROTOCOL
Medial Condylar Fractures

4 to 6 weeks	• Discontinue immobilization. In children younger than 5 years of age, immobilization may be discontinued at 3 weeks. Begin active supination and pronation exercises of the forearm and active flexion and extension exercises.	7 to 9 weeks	• If at the end of 3 weeks of exercise the child has not regained 90% motion, institute an exercise program of active and gentle passive ROM under the direction of a physical therapist.

MEDIAL EPICONDYLAR FRACTURES

Medial epicondylar fractures are the third most common fractures around the elbow in children and account for 5% to 10% of all children's fractures. This injury occurs most commonly in children around the age of 11 years. The mechanism of injury is a valgus stress to the elbow that pulls the medial epicondyle off the distal humerus. Frequently, the ulnar collateral ligament and a portion of the common flexor muscles also are attached to the fragment. Elbow dislocations often accompany these fractures. Residual instability and elbow stiffness are possible complications, and early ROM is essential to avoid a stiff elbow.

■ *A fibrous nonunion with elbow motion is better than a union with a stiff elbow.*

Treatment
Treatment of medial epicondylar fractures ranges from simple immobilization to open reduction and internal fixation with a Kirschner wire or screw.
  Indications for open reduction are:
• Entrapment of the medial epicondylar fracture in the joint with associated elbow dislocation
• Valgus stress instability in the dominant arm of an athlete
• More than 0.5 to 1 cm displacement
• Ulnar nerve dysfunction

REHABILITATION PROTOCOL
Medial Epicondylar Fractures

3 weeks	• Apply a long arm cast with the elbow flexed less than 90 degrees for 3 weeks. After cast removal, start a ROM program, emphasizing active elbow flexion and extension and supination and pronation. If tenderness persists after cast removal, the arm can be supported in a sling for an additional 1 to 2 weeks.	6 weeks	• Begin active and gentle passive ROM exercises under the supervision of a physical therapist if the child has not regained 90% of elbow motion 3 weeks after cast removal. Do not permit full activity (such as contact sports) until the child has symmetric upper extremity strength, full ROM, and a painless elbow.

ELBOW DISLOCATIONS

Elbow dislocations are relatively common in children older than 10 years of age; children younger than 10 years of age usually have associated fractures. When an elbow dislocation occurs in a child, the location of the medial epicondylar fragment must be determined before reduction to avoid entrapment in the joint.

Classification
Dislocations of the elbow are classified according to the direction of the dislocation: posteromedial, posterolateral, anteromedial, or anterolateral. Divergent anteroposterior dislocations and divergent medial and lateral dislocations occur if the proximal radioulnar

joint is disrupted. Also, radioulnar translocation, although rare, can occur.

Treatment

Elbow dislocations are best treated with prompt reduction to avoid neurovascular compromise from the excessive swelling that usually is associated with these injuries. The principles of reduction include longitudinal traction to neutralize the spasms of the biceps and contraction of the brachialis anteriorly and the triceps posteriorly. The traction force should be in line with the humerus. When this is accomplished, a second force is applied to the long axis of the forearm to reduce the dislocation of the proximal ulna and radius, usually from posterior to anterior.

Technique of Reduction of Elbow Dislocation

Several techniques are used, but essentially the dislocated ulna and radius can be pushed or pulled back into place. Sedation is necessary and sometimes general anesthesia may be required if the muscle spasms cannot be overcome adequately. Before reduction is attempted, neurologic and vascular examinations are performed, and the results carefully documented.

For younger children, a **push technique** is used, in which traction is placed on the humerus and the distal forearm, and pressure is applied over the tip of the olecranon, pushing the dislocation back into place. In older children, the **pull technique** is easier. Traction is applied to the arm and the forearm, and the dislocation is reduced by pulling the forearm into the correct position. Treatment of anterior elbow dislocations is similar, and traction is applied along the humerus and the semiflexed elbow. When the spasms of the biceps and the triceps have been overcome, the forearm is reduced by pulling posteriorly.

After the forearm is reduced, radiographs are obtained to ensure that no loose fragments of bone are within the joint. The medial epicondyle and coronoid should be carefully evaluated, and stability of the elbow should be determined.

■ *The ranges of motion in which the elbow is stable after reduction will set the limits for postoperative rehabilitation. This range of motion should be tested and documented.*

REHABILITATION PROTOCOL

Elbow Dislocation

Stable Elbow		**Unstable Elbow**	
1 to 2 weeks	• Ice and elevate for 2 to 3 days. • Apply a posterior splint to allow for swelling to be worn for 5 to 7 days. During this time, encourage active ROM exercises of the fingers and shoulder. Avoid valgus stress to the elbow during shoulder exercises. Once the splint is removed, place the child into a sling and begin active ROM exercises of the elbow; continue for 2 weeks.	1 week	• Determine and document the limits of motion in which the elbow remains stable. Apply a posterior splint with the elbow in 90 degrees of flexion. Ice and elevate for 2 to 3 days. Encourage ROM exercises of the fingers and shoulder during the time in the splint. Avoid valgus stress to the elbow during shoulder exercises.
3 to 6 weeks	• May discontinue the sling at 3 weeks after injury, but continue flexion, extension, pronation, and supination exercises.	2 weeks	• Replace the splint with an upright Bledsoe-type controlled-motion brace, limiting elbow ROM at the points of instability. Perform ROM exercises while wearing the brace.
		3 weeks	• Discontinue the brace to allow full motion, and give the patient a sling for comfort. Continue ROM exercises.
6 to 8 weeks	• Allow the child to return to normal activities if all motion and strength around the elbow has been regained. If limited ROM is noted at the end of this time, refer the child to a physical therapist for a supervised program of active and gentle passive ROM of the elbow.	6 weeks	• The child should have regained enough muscle tone and stability to return to normal daily activities. However, if limited ROM is noted, refer the child to a physical therapist for a supervised program of active and gentle passive ROM of the elbow.

NURSEMAID'S ELBOW

Nursemaid's elbow is common in children younger than 6 years of age, because the radial head, which is still mostly cartilaginous and spheric, allows the annular ligament to be pulled over it and become entrapped between it and the capitellum. As the child matures, the radial head becomes flat and plate-shaped, and displacement of the annular ligament is less likely to occur.

Longitudinal force on the extended elbow with the forearm pronated is the usual mechanism of injury. Often the radial head displaces within the annular ligament, producing a partial tear of the ligament. When the arm is released, the annular ligament becomes trapped between the radius and the capitellum rather than returning to its normal position.

The child holds the elbow in flexion and the forearm in supination, and attempts to move the arm will elicit pain. When the elbow is at rest in this flexed and pronated position, it may not be painful. Radiographs should be obtained to confirm that there is no fracture or other condition that may be causing elbow pain.

Treatment includes reduction and possibly a short period of immobilization in a sling.

Technique of Reduction of Nursemaid's Elbow

With a parent holding the child, the surgeon stabilizes the arm and hand so that the thumb overlies the radial head at the elbow. The other hand manipulates the forearm from full pronation to supination and then back to full pronation. A click usually is felt by the stabilizing hand at the elbow. Reduction sometimes causes a sharp pain, but afterward the child usually begins to use the arm. If the child uses the arm within 10 to 15 minutes after reduction and wants to return to activity, a sling is not necessary.

Recurrent radial head subluxations require that the parents be educated about the causes of this injury and ways to avoid it. Immobilization of the elbow in a cast or splint may be necessary if subluxation has occurred at least three times. As the child matures, the subluxation should resolve and not cause significant problems.

REHABILITATION PROTOCOL

Nursemaid's Elbow

If the elbow is still tender after reduction of the subluxation, a sling may be given to the child to wear for 3 to 5 days. At the end of this time, the child should have regained full ROM and may return to normal activities. The parents should be reminded that preventing this injury is an important aspect of treatment.

Hip Fractures

Fractures of the proximal femur are uncommon in children and account for fewer than 1% of all children's fractures. Generally they result from severe trauma, such as motor vehicle accidents or pedestrian-vehicle accidents. The most common age at which this injury occurs is 8 years. About 25% of children with proximal femoral fractures also have associated injuries that require evaluation and treatment at the same time.

Complications of this injury can be devastating if the physis has been damaged or if the vessels to the femoral head are disrupted. Results of treatment depend largely on the type and extent of the injury, as well as the age of the child.

CLASSIFICATION

The most commonly used classification is that of Delbet, shown in Table 8-8 (Fig. 8-5). This classification is useful not only to assist in making treatment recommendations, but also to alert the treating physician of possible complications, such as avascular necrosis.

TABLE 8-8 **Classification of Hip Fractures in Children (DELBET)**	
Type	**Description**
IA	Transepiphyseal fracture without dislocation of the femoral head
IB	Transepiphyseal fracture with dislocation of the femoral head
II	Transcervical or midneck fracture
III	Cervicotrochanteric or base-of-the-neck fracture
IV	Intertrochanteric fracture

TREATMENT

Type I

Type I fractures account for 7% of proximal femoral fractures and usually occur in younger children. About half of these are dislocated (type IB fractures). Avascular necrosis and premature closure of the physis are frequent complications.

In children aged 0 to 4 years, closed reduction, traction, and cast immobilization can be used. A Pavlik harness may be used for immobilization in children younger than 9 months of age.

In children older than 4 years, traction and closed reduction can be attempted, but if unsuccessful, open reduction and pinning may be required. Smooth pins should be used to avoid injuring the physis. The pins usually are removed at 6 weeks after surgery.

Type II

Fifty percent of proximal femoral fractures are type II. Open reduction and pin fixation is the best method of treatment. Although smooth pins should be used whenever possible, adequate fixation of the fracture should not be compromised.

Type III

Nondisplaced or minimally displaced type III fractures can be treated with abduction casting; however, closed or open reduction and pinning are necessary if the fracture is displaced.

Type IV

Nondisplaced type IV fractures can be treated with casting. If displacement is evident or if displacement occurs after treatment, open reduction and internal fixation are indicated. Open reduction and internal fixation are recommended for adolescent patients with type IV proximal femoral fractures.

COMPLICATIONS

The prognosis of these fractures depends on whether or not avascular necrosis of the proximal femur or femoral head occurs. Ratliff classified avascular necrosis into three types, as shown in Table 8-9 (Fig. 8-6).

The reported frequency of avascular necrosis in the various fracture types is shown in Table 8-10. Other possible complications that may adversely affect the outcome of proximal femoral fractures are nonunion and malunion. If malunion occurs, coxa vara deformity usually results.

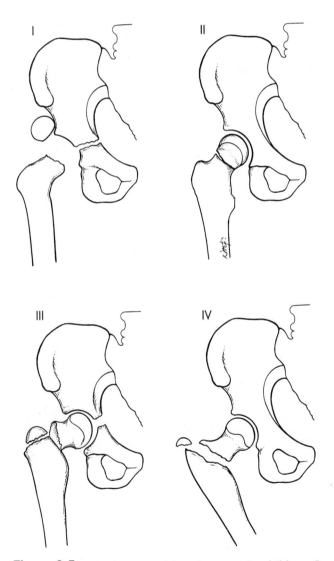

Figure 8-5 Classification of hip fractures in children: I, transepiphyseal, with or without dislocation from the acetabulum; II, transcervical; III, cervicotrochanteric; IV, trochanteric.

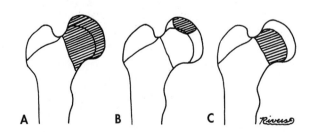

Figure 8-6 Three types of avascular necrosis. **A,** Type I, total head involvement. **B,** Type II, segmental involvement. **C,** Type III involvement from fracture line to physis. (Redrawn from Ratliff AHC: *J Bone Joint Surg* 44B:528, 1962.)

TABLE 8-9 **Classification of Avascular Necrosis (RATLIFF)**

Type	Description
I	Total involvement of the femoral head with disruption of all vessels proximal to the fracture
II	Involvement of only the superior portion of the femoral head with disruption of the lateral ascending artery
III	Proximal metaphyseal involvement with disruption of the endosteal blood supply.

TABLE 8-10 **Frequency of Avascular Necrosis After Hip Fractures in Children**

Type	Frequency
IA	50%
IB	80% to 100%
II	50%
III	25%
IV	14%

REHABILITATION PROTOCOL

Proximal Femoral Fractures

Rehabilitation after a hip fracture in a pediatric patient depends on the type of fracture and the age of the patient. Infants and neonates require no active rehabilitation program. When immobilization is discontinued, hip motion is regained with normal activities such as crawling or walking. In older children, active ROM exercises can be performed to regain hip motion. Protective weight bearing with crutches or a walker may be required for 2 to 3 weeks until full ROM is obtained. After the fracture is completely united and a full range of hip motion is obtained, normal activities are allowed. If internal fixation devices were used to stabilize the fracture, participation in contact sports should be restricted. Activities also should be restricted if any evidence of avascular necrosis is apparent.

FEMORAL SHAFT FRACTURES

Fractures of the shaft of the femur, although common in children, are serious injuries because of the possibility of excessive blood loss and the severity of trauma required to produce this fracture. These fractures usually result from high-energy trauma, such as automobile accidents, and associated injuries often are present.

The most frequent site of femoral shaft fractures is in the area of the normal maximal anterolateral bowing of the diaphysis. Displacement of the fracture fragments is largely determined by the type and location of the injury. Usually the proximal fragment is pulled into flexion by the iliopsoas muscle and abduction of the gluteus medius and minimus muscles. The distal fragment may be drawn proximally by the hamstring and quadriceps muscles and medially by the adductors. A traction treatment program is required to overcome these problems.

Treatment considerations:

- In children between the ages of 3 and 8 years, longitudinal growth is increased in the femur for approximately 1 year.
- Significant remodeling of axial deformities can be expected.
- Only limited remodeling of rotational deformities can be expected.
- Acceptable degrees of varus/valgus and anteroposterior angulation, as well as shortening, depends on the age of the patient (Table 8-11).

TABLE 8-11 **Acceptable Degrees of Valgus/Varus and Anteroposterior Angulation of Femoral Shaft Fractures**

	Varus/Valgus	Anteroposterior Angulation	Shortening
0 to 2 years	30 degrees	30 degrees	15 mm
2 to 5 years	15 degrees	20 degrees	2 mm
6 to 10 years	10 degrees	15 degrees	15 mm
11 years to skeletal maturity	5 degrees	10 degrees	10 mm

Wallace and Hoffman demonstrated that remodeling of femoral fractures occurs because of the Heuter-Volkmann principle. They found that 26% of fracture remodeling takes place at the fracture site and 74% occurs at the physis, and that remodeling at the physis occurs for up to 5 years. Thus, corrective osteotomies for residual angulation should not be attempted for several years to allow maximal remodeling to occur. Wallace et al. determined that 10 to 25 degrees of angulation at the midshaft of the femur will remodel satisfactorily with growth. Union of femoral shaft fractures also depends on the age of the child Table 8-12).

Treatment

Methods of treatment of femoral shaft fractures vary greatly and depend on the skeletal age of the child and the type of fracture. The presence of other fractures, fracture comminution, associated soft tissue injuries, multiple system injuries, head injuries, or spasticity also affect treatment decisions (Table 8-13).

Traction Precautions

Because overgrowth after femoral shaft fractures usually is caused by hyperemia, the fracture fragments should overlap about 1 cm when treated with traction. Radiographs should be obtained initially to confirm adequate alignment in traction and should be repeated every 3 to 4 days.

Once the patient is comfortable and no clinical signs of pain or motion are evident, the child may be placed in a spica cast. The surgeon may opt to wait for radiographic evidence of callus formation, but this usually occurs later than clinical stability.

Pin-site care must be meticulous, and medications such as Valium may be required for control of muscle spasms and pain. After spica cast application, the family must be instructed in proper cast protection and diapering. *The diaper should be inserted **inside** the edges of the cast to keep it dry and prevent soiling, which can result in skin maceration.*

TABLE 8-12 Union of Femoral Shaft Fractures

Younger than 2 years of age	4 to 6 weeks
3 to 8 years of age	6 to 8 weeks
Older than 9 years of age	8 to 12 weeks

TABLE 8-13 Treatment of Femoral Shaft Fractures

Age	Method
• 0 to 2 years of age	Skin traction or modified Bryant's traction until early callus formation is seen, then spica cast immobilization
• 2 to 5 years	90/90 traction or split Russell's-type skeletal traction until early fracture consolidation, then spica cast immobilization
• 5 to 12 years	Treatment in this age group is controversial. The standard method of treatment has been skeletal traction followed by spica cast immobilization. However, because of the lengthy hospitalization that is required and the frequency of angulation after cast immobilization, other methods of treatment have been investigated, including external fixation and flexible intramedullary rod fixation avoiding the growth plates. These have the advantage of holding the fracture in anatomic alignment while allowing the patient to be discharged from the hospital relatively quickly; however, there is increased risk from a surgical standpoint as well as potential problems with overgrowth.
• Older than 12 years	Intramedullary nail fixation, with care not to damage proximal vessels to the femoral head (Fig. 8-7). Other treatment options include traction followed by application of a body cast, external fixation, and flexible intramedullary rods.

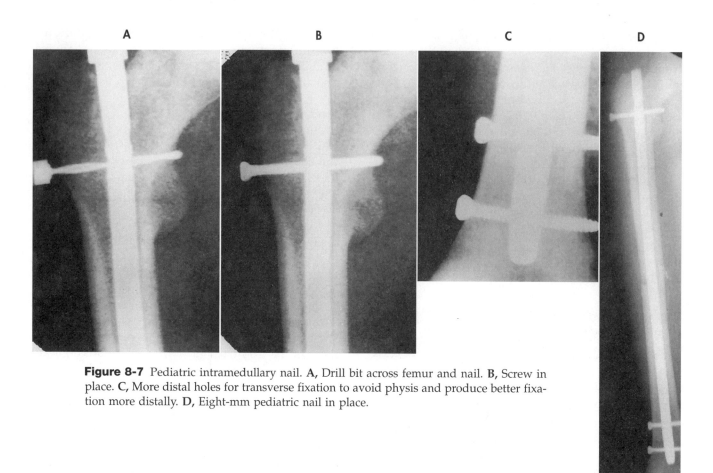

Figure 8-7 Pediatric intramedullary nail. **A,** Drill bit across femur and nail. **B,** Screw in place. **C,** More distal holes for transverse fixation to avoid physis and produce better fixation more distally. **D,** Eight-mm pediatric nail in place.

REHABILITATION PROTOCOL

Femoral Shaft Fractures

Rehabilitation after femoral shaft fracture depends on the age of the patient and the type of treatment used.

- **Treatment with traction and casting.** No special therapy or rehabilitation is required for children aged 0 to 5 years. After the cast is removed, allow a return to activities at the child's own pace. Almost all of the normal motion of the hip and knee is regained within 3 to 4 weeks after cast removal. The child may limp for 4 to 6 weeks, but this usually resolves gradually as the child returns to normal activities.

In children aged 5 to 12 years, instruction in active ROM exercises of the knee and hip may be beneficial after cast removal. Crutch ambulation can be used for 1 to 2 weeks, until the child regains some hip and knee motion. Children in this age group also may limp for 4 to 6 weeks after cast removal, and parents should be warned to expect this. The limp usually resolves over time as the child resumes normal activities.

- **Treatment with external fixation.** Non–weight-bearing crutch ambulation can be allowed immediately, progressing to partial weight bearing when callus formation around the fracture is evident. Pin sites are cleaned daily with hydrogen peroxide and cotton-tipped swabs. Encourage active motion of the knee and hip.

Crutches are used for 6 weeks after fracture union and fixator removal. Allow touchdown weight bearing only to protect the femur from fracture through the pin holes.

Motion of the hip and knee should be nearly normal 6 weeks after fixator removal. A slight limp may be present, but this usually resolves with resumption of normal activities.

- **Treatment with locked intramedullary nailing.** Allow early touchdown weight bearing on crutches. Perform active straight leg raising exercises and active ROM exercises of the knee and hip. The fracture usually heals within 3 months, and unrestricted ambulation can be allowed at that time. At 1 year from injury, the intramedullary rod can be removed, after which crutches are used for 6 weeks to minimize the risk of fracture through the screw holes.

Tibial Fractures

TIBIAL EMINENCE FRACTURES

Tibial eminence fractures usually involve the medial aspect of the tibial eminence. Although uncommon, these fractures may occur after a fall that results in forced valgus and external rotation of the tibia on the femur. Because the attachment and the midsubstance of the anterior cruciate ligament are stronger than the epiphyseal cancellous bone, a fracture of the tibial eminence usually results. A partial tear of the anterior cruciate ligament with some elongation of the fibers may be associated with this injury. Occasionally, a tear of the medial collateral ligament also occurs.

Classification and Treatment

The system of Myers and McKeever is useful in recommending treatment modalities (Fig. 8-8) (Tables 8-14 and 8-15).

Complications

Lack of knee extension is a frequent complication of tibial eminence fractures. Incomplete reduction and changes in the size or shape of the tibial eminence after fracture union have been noted to block extension. An increase in blood flow during healing that causes enlargement of the tibial eminence also has been suggested as a cause of limited extension of the knee. Even after solid union, a measurable increase in anterior drawer test may be noted; however, clinical signs or symptoms of an anterior cruciate–deficient knee are rarely reported.

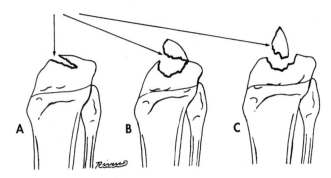

Figure 8-8 Fractures of intercondylar eminence of tibia. **A,** Type I. **B,** Type II. **C,** Type III. (Redrawn from Roberts JM: *Fractures and dislocations of the knee.* In Rockwood CA Jr, Wilkins KE, King RE, editors: *Fractures in children,* Philadelphia, 1984, JB Lippincott.)

TABLE 8-15 **Treatment of Tibial Eminence Fractures**

Type	Treatment
I	Cast immobilization (6 weeks) with the knee in almost full extension
II	Aspiration of the knee joint and casting with the knee in full extension to reduce anterior displacement. Anterior displacement less than 1 to 2 mm on radiograph is acceptable, and the patient can be treated in a cast for 6 weeks. If reduction is unacceptable, arthroscopic or open reduction is necessary.
III	Arthroscopic reduction and fixation or open reduction and fixation of the fracture into the fracture bed. Frequently, the anterior horn of the lateral meniscus prevents reduction, and this should be dealt with at the time of reduction. Fixation is obtained by passing sutures through the ligament and the displaced fracture fragment and through drill holes in the epiphysis. A Herbert screw, cannulated screws, or Kirschner wires also can be used for fracture fixation. Care must be taken not to damage the physis, which may cause growth arrest of the proximal tibia.

TABLE 8-14 **Classification of Tibial Eminence Fractures**

Type	Description
I	Nondisplaced fracture
II	Fracture elevated from the anterior fracture bed but with a posterior hinge
III	Completely separated and displaced fracture

REHABILITATION PROTOCOL

Tibial Eminence Fractures

During the 6 weeks of cast immobilization, encourage straight leg raising exercises. After cast removal, begin active flexion and extension exercises to regain knee motion. Crutch ambulation may be required until full knee motion is obtained. After full knee motion is obtained, begin further strengthening exercises of atrophied quadriceps and hamstring muscles and continue until the thigh circumference is within 1 cm of that of the uninjured leg. Full activities are then allowed.

TIBIAL TUBEROSITY FRACTURES

Tibial tuberosity fractures usually result from forced flexion of the knee against isometric contraction of the quadriceps. This injury is most common in children between the ages of 13 and 16 years, because the tibial tuberosity is weaker and more vulnerable to fracture during this time. This fracture also has been noted to occur in patients who have Osgood-Schlatter disease.

Classification

Watson-Jones classified this fracture into three types (Table 8-16).

Treatment

Treatment recommendations for nondisplaced types I and II fractures include immobilization in a cylinder or long leg cast with the knee in extension, usually for 8 weeks. All displaced types I and II fractures and all type III fractures require open reduction and internal fixation with a cannulated cancellous screw (Fig. 8-9), followed by application of a long leg or a cylinder cast that is worn for 6 to 8 weeks until the fracture heals.

TABLE 8-16 **Watson-Jones Classification of Tibial Tuberosity Fractures**	
Type	**Description**
I	Fracture through a small distal portion of the tibial tuberosity before the secondary ossification and epiphyseal ossification centers have joined.
II	Fracture after the tuberosity ossification centers have joined; the fracture line divides the tuberosity from the proximal tibial plateau.
III	Fracture extending from the tibial tuberosity through the primary ossification center into the joint.

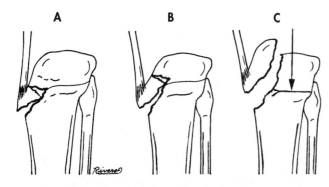

A   B   C

Figure 8-9 Types of avulsion fracture of tibial tuberosity. **A,** Type I, through secondary ossification center. **B,** Type II, at junction of primary and secondary ossification centers. **C,** Type III, across primary ossification center (Salter-Harris type III) with physis near closing posteriorly. (Redrawn from Roberts JM: *Fractures and dislocations of the knee.* In Rockwood CA Jr, Wilkins KE, King RE, editors: *Fractures in children,* Philadelphia, 1984, JB Lippincott.)

REHABILITATION PROTOCOL

Tibial Tuberosity Fractures

1 to 6 weeks	• During the time in the cast, start active quadriceps exercises if fixation is secure. If fixation is not secure, delay exercising until healing around the fracture site is apparent.	9 to 12 weeks	• Full ROM of the knee should be obtained 3 to 4 weeks after cast removal. Complete knee motion and nearly normal thigh circumference should be present before return to full activity is allowed.
6 to 8 weeks	• After cast removal, begin active ROM exercises of the knee and strengthening exercises of the quadriceps and hamstring muscles. Crutch ambulation may be continued until full knee motion is regained.		

TIBIAL SHAFT FRACTURES

Fractures of the tibia and fibula are common in children and may result from indirect or direct forces. Indirect forces, such as a rotational injury to the lower extremity, are the most common causes of these fractures and often result in oblique- or spiral-type fractures. Fractures resulting from direct blows usually are transverse or comminuted.

Because of the increased risk of compartment syndrome and neurovascular compromise after tibial fractures, thorough examination of the extremity is necessary at the time of injury and during early treatment.

Treatment

Nondisplaced tibial shaft fractures can be treated with cast immobilization. If the fracture is minimally displaced, reduction and casting can be done in an outpatient setting with the patient sedated. However, if significant displacement is evident, reduction and application of a long leg cast should be performed with the patient under general anesthesia.

The time of cast immobilization depends on the age of the patient and the type of fracture. Nondisplaced fractures in children younger than 5 years of age usually heal within 4 to 6 weeks. Displaced fractures in adolescents may require 3 months of cast immobilization.

Before treatment is started, the parents should be forewarned about the possibility of angular deformity that may occur after certain types of tibial fractures.

■ *Children between the ages of 4 and 6 years often develop posttraumatic tibial valga after proximal tibial fractures, and distal tibial fractures tend to drift into varus.*

The amount of acceptable lower extremity angulation depends on the age of the child (Table 8-17).

TABLE 8-17 **Acceptable Ranges of Lower Extremity Angulation**

Lower Extremity Angulation	Acceptable Ranges of Normal	
	< 8 Years	> 8 Years
Varus/valgus	8 degrees	5 degrees
Recurvatum	15 degrees	10 degrees
Anterior angulation	8 degrees	5 degrees
Shortening	10 mm	5 mm
Rotation	5 degrees	5 degrees

REHABILITATION PROTOCOL
Tibial Shaft Fractures

Most children with tibial shaft fractures do not require a prescribed therapy program. For several weeks after cast removal, they may limp or walk with the leg externally rotated, but approximately 6 to 8 weeks after injury, ambulation without a detectable limp should be possible. If restricted motion is still present after that time, an active physical therapy program can be instituted.

Ankle Fractures

Most ankle fractures in children are Salter-Harris type II injuries that can be treated with closed reduction and casting. Salter-Harris type II fractures that cannot be adequately reduced and Salter-Harris types III and IV fractures usually require open reduction and some type of internal fixation to hold the fracture in good alignment. Other fractures of the ankle include juvenile Tillaux fractures (Fig. 8-10) and triplane fractures.

Juvenile Tillaux fractures occur from an external rotation or abduction type of injury in which the anterolateral portion of the epiphysis is pulled off by the anteroinferior tibiofibular ligament. Because this is an intraarticular injury, only 2 mm of displacement is acceptable. Fractures with less than 2 mm of displacement can be treated in a long leg cast with the

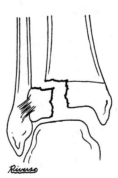

Figure 8-10 Tillaux fracture. (Redrawn from Weber BG, Sussenbach F: *Malleolar fractures.* In Weber BG, Brunner C, Freuler F: *Treatment of fractures in children and adolescents,* New York, 1980, Springer-Verlag.)

ankle and foot internally rotated. However, if more than 2 mm of displacement is present, open reduction and internal fixation are required.

Triplane fractures occur in three planes—transverse, coronal, and saggital—hence, its name. Several fracture patterns and variations have been described, and two, three, or four fragments may be present. The epiphyseal fracture occurs in the saggital plane. The physeal separation, which often is not seen, but is in-

ferred from the position of the fragment, occurs in the transverse plane. The metaphyseal fracture occurs in the coronal plane and is apparent on a lateral radiograph. Triplane fractures usually require open reduction and internal fixation with intrafragmentary screw fixation for anatomic reduction. After reduction, the patient can be immobilized with touchdown weight bearing in either a long leg or short leg cast for 6 to 8 weeks, depending on the stability of fixation.

REHABILITATION PROTOCOL
Ankle Fractures

After immobilization is removed, begin active ROM exercises, focusing on dorsiflexion and plantar flexion of the ankle, and inversion and eversion of the hindfoot. When motion has been regained, a home muscle-strengthening program using a Theraband is begun. Muscle strengthening is focused on the plantar flexor, dorsiflexor, invertor, and evertor musculature. During this time, start proprioceptive exercises using a BAPS board. Unrestricted activity is allowed when full range of ankle motion, proprioception, and muscle strength have been regained. The length of rehabilitation varies, but most patients can return to full activity after 4 to 6 weeks of rehabilitation.

Bibliography

Alburger PD, Weidner PL, Betz RR: Supracondylar fractures of the humerus in children, *J Pediatr Orthop* 12:16, 1992.

Armstrong PF: Serious fractures and joint injuries involving the foot and ankle, *Instr Course Lect* 41:413, 1992.

Aronson J, Tursky EA: External fixation of femur fractures in children, *J Pediatr Orthop* 12:157, 1992.

Badelon O, Bensahel H, Mazda K, Vie P: Lateral humeral condylar fractures in children: a report of 47 cases, *J Pediatr Orthop* 8:31, 1988.

Beatty E et al: Wrist and hand skeletal injuries in children, *Hand Clin* 6:723, 1990.

Beaty JH: Fractures and dislocations about the elbow in children, *Instr Course Lect* 41:373, 1992.

Beaty JH: Fractures of the proximal humerus and shaft in children, *Instr Course Lect* 41:369, 1992.

Bond SJ, Gotschall CS, Eichelberger MR: Predictors of abdominal injury in children with pelvic fracture, *J Trauma* 31:1169, 1991.

Boyd DW, Aronson DD: Supracondylar fractures of the humerus: a prospective study of percutaneous pinning, *J Pediatr Orthop* 12:789, 1992.

Briggs TWR, Orr MM, Lightowler CDR: Isolated tibial fractures in children, *Injury* 23:308, 1992.

Buckley SL et al: Open fractures of the tibia in children, *J Bone Joint Surg* 72A:1462, 1990.

Campbell RM: Operative treatment of fractures and dislocations of the hand and wrist region in children, *Orthop Clin North Am* 21:217, 1990.

Celiker O, Pestilci FI, Tuzuner M: Supracondylar fractures of the humerus in children: analysis of the results in 142 patients, *J Orthop Trauma* 4:265, 1990.

Crawford AH: Operative treatment of spine fractures in children, *Orthop Clin North Am* 21:325, 1990.

Curtis RJ Jr: Operative management of children's fractures of the shoulder region, *Orthop Clin North Am* 21:315, 1990.

D'souza S, Vaishya R, Klenerman L: Management of radial neck fractures in children: a retrospective analysis of one hundred patients, *J Pediatr Orthop* 13:232, 1993.

Davison BL, Weinstein SL: Hip fractures in children: a long-term follow-up study, *J Pediatr Orthop* 12:355, 1992.

France J, Strong M: Deformity and function in supracondylar fractures of the humerus in children variously treated by closed reduction and splinting, traction, and percutaneous pinning, *J Pediatr Orthop* 12:494, 1992.

Gartland JJ: Management of supracondylar fractures of the humerus in children, *Surg Gynecol Obstet* 109:145, 1959.

Graves SC, Canale ST: Fractures of the olecranon in children: long-term follow-up, *J Pediatr Orthop* 13:239, 1993.

Hansen ST: Internal fixation of children's fractures of the lower extremity, *Orthop Clin North Am* 21:353, 1990.

Hope PG, Cole WG: Open fractures of the tibia in children, *J Bone Joint Surg* 74B:546, 1992.

Johnson FG: Pediatric Lisfranc injury: bunk bed fracture, *AJR* 137:1041, 1981.

Kasser JR: Femur fractures in children, *Instr Course Lect* 41:403, 1992.

Kasser JR: Percutaneous pinning of supracondylar fractures of the humerus in children. *Instr Course Lect* 41:385, 1992.

Kendall NS, Hsu SYC, Chan K-M: Fracture of the tibial spine in adults and children: a review of 31 cases, *J Bone Joint Surg* 74B:848, 1992.

Kilfoyle FM: Fractures of the medial condyle and epicondyle of the elbow in children. *Clin Orthop* 41:43, 1965.

Kling TF Jr: Operative treatment of ankle fractures in children, *Orthop Clin North Am* 21:381, 1990.

Larsen CL, Kiær T, Lindequist S: Fractures of the proximal humerus in children: nine-year follow-up of 64 unoperated cases, *Acta Orthop Scand* 61:255, 1990.

Loder RT, Bookout C: Fracture patterns in battered children, *J Orthop Trauma* 5:428, 1991.

Meyers MH, McKeever FM: Fracture of the intercondylar eminence of the tibia, *J Bone Joint Surg* 41A:209, 1959.

Moseley CF: Occult fractures, *Instr Course Lect* 41:361, 1992.

Nierenberg G et al: Pelvic fractures in children: a follow-up in 20 children treated conservatively, *J Pediatr Orthop* 13(part B):140, 1993.

Ratliff AHC: Complications after fractures of the femoral neck in children, *J Bone Joint Surg* 44B:528, 1962.

Reeves RB, Ballard RI, Hughes JL: Internal fixation versus traction and casting of adolescent femoral shaft fractures, *J Pediatr Orthop* 10:591, 1990.

Roy DR, Crawford AH: Operative management of fractures of the shaft of the radius and ulna, *Orthop Clin North Am* 21:245, 1990.

Rumball K, Jarvis J: Seat-belt injuries of the spine in young children, *J Bone Joint Surg* 74B:571, 1992.

Salter RB, Best TN: Pathogenesis of progressive valgus de-formity following fractures of the proximal metaphyseal region of the tibia in young children, *Instr Course Lect* 41:409, 1992.

Schlesinger I, Wedge JH: Percutaneous reduction and fixation of displaced juvenile Tillaux fractures: a new surgical technique, *J Pediatr Orthop* 13:389, 1993.

Wallace ME, Hoffman EB: Remodeling of angular defomity after femoral shaft fractures in children, *J Bone Joint Surg* 74B:765, 1992.

Watson-Jones R: *Fractures and joint injuries,* Baltimore, 1957, Williams & Wilkins.

Wiley JJ, Baxter MP: Tibial spine fractures in children, *Clin Orthop* 225:54, 1990.

Wilkins KE: The operative management of supracondylar fractures, *Orthop Clin North Am* 21:269, 1990.

Willis RB et al: Long-term follow-up of anterior tibial eminence fractures, *J Pediatr Orthop* 13:361, 1993.

Wozasek GE et al: Trauma involving the proximal tibial epiphysis, *Arch Orthop Trauma* 110:301, 1991.

CHAPTER NINE

Reflex Sympathetic Dystrophy

SUSAN W. STRALKA, PT

Reflex sympathetic dystrophy syndrome (RSDS) is a common disorder that has been reported to occur after 5% of all injuries. According to information from the Reflex Sympathetic Dystrophy Syndrome Association, this disorder affects millions of people in the United States.

RSDS has been reported to occur after inflammatory disorders, surgery, immobilization, frostbite, burns, drugs, and malignancies, but traumatic accidental injury appears to be the most common precursor of this syndrome. Common orthopaedic injuries that precede RSDS include sprains; dislocations; fractures (usually of the hands, feet, or wrists); traumatic amputation or crush injuries of fingers, hands, or wrists; contusions; and even minor cuts. Interestingly, no known correlation exists between the severity of the injury and the incidence of RSDS.

In recent years, RSDS has been recognized with increasing frequency in children. Pillemer and Micheli reported 20 children with RSDS after injuries sustained during organized sports activities. These authors believe that the stress of the sports activity may have perpetuated the RSDS in these children. In Lankford's series, the most common precipitating events were knee surgeries in which sensory or somatic nerves were traumatized, wrist fractures, and crush injuries of the hand. Other studies by Gersh, Doury, and Wyndell, however, indicate that a precipitating event usually is not identified in 30% to 50% of patients.

Many authors believe that RSDS is underreported, and that a substantial number of cases remain undiagnosed or misdiagnosed in both children and adults. In a study of 70 patients by Wilder et al., the average interval between the onset of symptoms and the visit to the physician was 10 days, but the average time until RSDS was diagnosed was 12 months.

Typical Symptoms of RSDS

- Diffuse, burning pain
- Cutaneous hypersensitivity
- Allodynia (pain from a stimulus that does not normally provoke pain)
- Edema
- Hyperhidrosis
- Hypohidrosis
- Dystrophic changes of the involved tissue, such as atrophy of the fat pad, taut and shiny skin, loss of skin wrinkling, and stiffness
- Vasomotor instability
- Bone resorption
- Decreased motor function

Clinical Variants

According to Payne, reflex sympathetic dystrophy syndrome is a generic term used to describe a cluster of symptoms and signs that occur after injury to bone, soft tissue, and nerves. Descriptions of this syndrome have appeared in the literature under an array of names, including Sudeck's atrophy, shoulder-hand syndrome, posttraumatic pain syndrome, sympathalgia, chronic traumatic edema, algodystrophy, and major and minor causalgia.

In 1864 Mitchell used the term causalgia to describe the syndrome that occurs after nerve injury. Some authors now believe that causalgia should be considered a special type of RSDS. A subcommittee of the International Association for the Study of Pain Taxonomy describe causalgia as a syndrome of sustained burning pain after a traumatic nerve injury combined with vasomotor, pseudomotor, and later trophic changes that differs from RSDS because of its association with peripheral nerve injuries. Common features of trauma associated with causalgia involve tearing or stretching of a nerve or avulsion of the brachial plexus roots, surgical retraction of bone and soft tissue, intramuscular injections, and even venipuncture. In more than 80% of patients with causalgia, the pain begins within a few hours to 1 week after injury.

Classification

Because of the confusion regarding the many names and forms of RSDS, classification was attempted. Lankford and Thompson categorized the following forms of RSDS according to precipitating causes, severity, and location:
- Minor causalgia following sensory nerve injury
- Minor traumatic dystrophy following minor non–nerve trauma
- Shoulder-hand syndrome
- Major traumatic dystrophy following major soft tissue or bony injury without nerve trauma
- Major causalgia, usually involving a high-velocity wound to a major mixed nerve

Bonica classified this disorder by differentiating between sympathetic maintained pain (SMP), with two groups—causalgia and RSDS—and sympathetic independent pain (SIP). More recently, Jänig proposed three groups of RSDS: (1) algodystrophy, the full-blown syndrome; (2) sympathetic dystrophy (RSDS) without pain; and (3) SMP, in which pain is the only manifestation of RSDS.

Clinical Course

RSDS represents a spectrum of clinical signs and symptoms, although patients do not exhibit the same signs and symptoms in sequence. The *acute stage* of RSDS begins at the time of injury and often is characterized by burning or aching pain that is spontaneous and may or may not be associated with hyperpathia. The *second stage,* the dystrophic stage, begins 3 months after injury. The *third stage* is the atrophic stage (see box).

It recently has been recognized that RSDS is an on-

RSDS Staging

Stage 1 (Acute or Traumatic Stage—Onset Immediate or Delayed)
Early Signs (First to Third Week of Onset)
Soft, puffy edema
Acute, intractable pain
Hyperesthesia
Limited range of motion in affected part
Muscular spasm
Hyperthermia

Later Signs (Normally Within 3 to 6 Weeks of Onset)
Hair and nail growth
Hyperhidrosis
Cold, clammy, and cyanotic skin (three C's)
Osteoporosis (Sudeck's atrophy)

Stage 2 (Dystrophic Stage—Usually Within 2 to 6 Months of Onset)
Decrease in spontaneous pain
Brawny edema
Taut, shiny, cyanotic skin (skin wrinkles lost)
Hyperhidrosis
Hyperesthesia
Hypothermia
Progressive joint stiffness and loss of motion
Atrophy of the subcutaneous tissue (fat pads on fingers and toes)
Atrophy of muscle
Hyperemia of flexor creases
Hair and nail growth
Diffuse osteoporosis

Stage 3 (Atrophic Stage—Usually Within 6 to 9 Months of Onset)
Dissemination of pain (less acute as this stage progresses)
Muscular and bony atrophy
Thickening of fascia
Soft tissue atrophy
Joint ankylosis
Atrophic, cool, glossy, and taut skin (cyanosis is gone)

going vasomotor-instability problem in which vasodilation, vasoconstriction, or both may be present.

■ *The most prominent clinical feature in RSDS is pain that is disproportionate to the severity of the injury.*

The clinical course of pain and dystrophy is not related to the degree of injury, to the age of the patient, or to associated soft tissue injury, and it does not follow any dermatomic pattern, spreading both proximally and distally. The prognosis and duration of pain are variable. Researchers report that pain persists for longer than 6 months in 85% of patients and longer than a year in 25%. We concur with Payne and other authorities who advocate early, aggressive treatment of pain with the use of sympathetic blocks. Decreasing pain allows early therapy and rehabilitation that appears to prevent progression to endstage RSDS, although this has not been proven.

Lankford and Thompson described the vicious cycle of RSDS, in which advanced sympathetic reflexes are put into play because of an abnormal feedback mechanism that occurs in the internuncial pool (Fig. 9-1). Because of acute pain, the patient refuses to move the affected area and stiffness ensues, progressively worsening throughout the course of the disease. The patient's immobility and decreased muscle use result in a decrease in lymphatic drainage, causing stagnation in capillary permeability, thereby increasing carbon dioxide levels, vasodilatation, and ultimately edema. The entire cycle causes the serofibrinous precipitate from the edema to organize and form adhesions. The longer edema is allowed to persist, the greater a complicating factor it becomes. Peacock et al stress that edema reduction is important, because

edema decreases motion and causes remodeling of collagen in a shortened position. Mackin recommends early movement and edema control to lessen the severity of RSDS. However, all aspects of this vicious cycle, such as pain, edema, fibrosis, osseous demineralization, sudomotor and temperature changes, trophic changes, and vasomotor instability, must be considered in the treatment regimen to obtain the best clinical results.

Bone demineralization is present early, but the mechanisms of this process are not clearly understood. One theory is that after injury to a limb or extremity, loss of vascular tone or persistent vasodilatation assists in rapid bone resorption. Another explanation is that poor blood flow allows a low pH to develop, thereby promoting localized demineralization. Arnstein and Kozin et al. reported that bone demineralization occurred in 30% to 70% of patients with RSDS.

■ *Early weight bearing is indicated to maintain mineralization of bone.*

Most RSDS patients describe burning or shooting pain that often is exacerbated by light touch. They may describe their pain as throbbing, deep aching, cramping, searing, or increased pressure. Controlling acute pain is important in the treatment of RSDS, because uninterrupted pain may lead to the following:

• Loss of muscle tone, strength, endurance
• Loss of joint mobility
• Loss of bone minerals
• Contracture of joints
• Reduction in blood flow
• Changes in hair, nails, sweating
• Changes in cutaneous sensitivity
• Changes in kinesthesia
• Changes in attitude and wellness

Psychologic Ramifications

Lankford and Thompson were the first to recognize that certain personality types had a predisposition for developing RSDS, and Mullins referred to "a certain diathesis." Weiss et al believe that hypersympathetic body characteristics are important psychogenic factors in the development of this syndrome. Amadio asserted that although an injury may trigger the onset of RSDS, anger and other psychologic factors are the principle underlying causes of pain dysfunction and can hinder recovery. Bernstein et al., after psychologic testing of children with RSDS, found that they were accepting of responsibility beyond their years and often had difficulty expressing anger. Interestingly, a number of his patients with RSDS had family conflict, which the syndrome enabled them to avoid.

Gersh postulated that hyperarousal of the sympathetic nervous system manifests in the patient's hy-

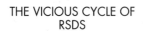

THE VICIOUS CYCLE OF
RSDS

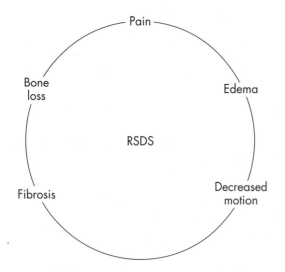

Figure 9-1 The vicious cycle of RSDS.

peremotional temperament and causes an overly anxious response to stress. Numerous authors have reported that the psychopathology of an anxiety state or even repressed anxiety increases autonomic arousal and increases the intensity and frequency of afferent and efferent simulation. Schwartzmann and McLellan stated that anxiety increases sympathetic discharge, which exacerbates the pain.

Because patients with RSDS or causalgia often remain undiagnosed or are misdiagnosed, the acute pain often becomes chronic, and major depression usually ensues. Formerly, these patients were believed to be psychoneurotic or hysterical, and their symptoms were believed to be purely psychogenetic; however, Bonica pointed out that in most patients the psychoneurotic clinical picture resolved immediately after the pain was relieved, and patients resumed a normal life. He believed this to be a clear indication that the change in personality is the result rather than the cause of an unendurable disorder. Other psychologic studies of RSDS support Bonica's statement.

The Minnesota Multiphasic Personality Inventory Test (MMPI) often is used to identify somatiform disorders. According to Zucchinin et al and Grunert et al, the MMPI generally shows increased hypochondriasis, hysteria, and depression in patients with RSDS.

Rehabilitation

Successful rehabilitation of patients with RSDS requires a combination of disciplines: an interested physician, a knowledgeable anesthesiologist, a supportive counselor or psychologist, and an interested therapist. Individuals treating patients with RSDS must be not only technically capable, but also sensitive and compassionate. The success of treatment depends as much on the attitude of the therapist as on technical skill. In establishing a therapeutic program for the treatment of RSDS, all health care professionals must be involved in the reduction of sympathetic arousal and vasomotor dysregulation. Because of vasomotor instability, the clinician should attempt to determine the physiologic status of the limb according to vasomotor tone. When vasomotor tone is identified, a treatment program should be chosen that will not exacerbate it.

PHARMACOLOGIC MANAGEMENT

Drug therapy for RSDS may include tricyclic antidepressants, nonsteroidal antiinflammatory drugs (NSAIDs), corticosteroids, and anticonvulsants, depending on the clinical dystrophic or atrophic changes that are present. Dystonia with difficulty in initiating movement or with increased tone must be pharmaco-

logically managed with anticonvulsants, or motor planning activation will be affected.

Tricyclic antidepressants often are used as adjuvant analgesics in the management of neuropathic pain. The mechanism of action involves blockage of serotonin reuptake in the central nervous system, thereby augmenting the antinociceptive actions of the descending inhibitory pain modulating pathways. The analgesic effect appears to be independent of the antidepressant effect. It has been reported that antidepressants ameliorate the pain/depression cycle and also have proved useful in assisting patients to rest throughout the night so that they maintain a normal sleep cycle. Wyndell emphasized the importance of the sleep cycle, stating that without a normal sleep pattern, hyperirritability of the musculoskeletal system and exacerbation of the painful symptoms occur.

Neumann found NSAIDs to be effective in reducing pain and inflammation associated with RSDS, and many authors advocate the use of NSAIDs or dose packs of Depo-Medrol at the early signs of stiffness to assist in decreasing the fibrotic reaction. The recognition of neurotransmitting substances that mediate peripheral inflammation and the identification of low-grade inflammatory changes support the early use of medication, sympathetic blocks, and therapy. In a few patients, however, early intervention does not halt or slow the fibrotic process. Definitive reasons for this remain unclear. One theory is that trauma, immobility, and stiffness, in association with the autonomic regulation dysfunction, result in vasospasms of the small arterioles and veins, causing edema; thus, the outflow from capillaries of plasma and fibrin result in ischemic tissue. The process of tissue ischemia and fibrin deposits certainly are contributing factors in the development of stiffness.

TRANSCUTANEOUS ELECTRICAL NERVE STIMULATION (TENS)

In treating patients with RSDS, it is important to choose a method that allows long-term use. TENS is a treatment modality that has proved successful in controlling both acute and chronic pain and may be used indefinitely. TENS is used for pain control in many orthopaedic problems, and several research studies have shown clinical efficacy of TENS in patients with RSDS. Finney treated 70 patients with RSDS and monitored vasomotor normalization and pain relief with low-frequency TENS. The best response was in stages 1 and 2, the cold phases, in which temperature increases simultaneously showed pain decreases. Omer and Thomas believe that the best results with TENS are obtained when it is initiated within 3 months of onset of pain. Leo reported a 10-year-old child with lower extremity RSDS pain who was totally asymptomatic after the use of low-rate, high-amplitude TENS. Mannheimer and Lampe reported the successful use of conventional TENS for patients with Colles fractures who developed RSDS. Kaada used TENS successfully to modulate abnormal sympathetic activity in six patients with decreased skin temperature and ischemic pain. Casale and Tiengo reported one patient in whom the use of TENS relieved pain and allowed performance of a rehabilitation program.

OTHER MODALITIES

Continuous passive motion (CPM) devices may be effective for improving range of motion (ROM), but these devices should not be substituted for active motion and should be used only when the patient is resting. It is important to use CPM only through a pain-free ROM; if motion is painful, CPM should be discontinued or the ROM should be adjusted. Some authors have suggested that CPM may improve periarticular and cartilage nutrition.

Allodynia, or a painful response to nonpainful stimuli, can be treated with a desensitization program that is used throughout the day. The program should be outlined carefully for the patient to avoid increasing symptoms. *Fluidotherapy* can be used in the clinic to allow neutral warmth, desensitizing, and active motion. The patient is then responsible for using different tactile stimulation throughout the day.

The use of *superficial and deep heating* has been effective in pain reduction. According to Michlovitz, the physiologic effects of *ultrasound* cause a tissue temperature rise that increases collagen tissue extensibility. Changes in nerve conduction velocity, increased pain threshold, and changes the contractile activity of skeletal muscle, as well as blood flow, also occur. Research has shown that increasing the tissue temperature to 40° to 45° C and applying a stretch increases the length of tissue. This modality often is used to gain tissue extensibility in the treatment of stiffness and decreased ROM associated with RSDS. Clinical statements with progress-note documentation have been used as empirical evidence of pain control, but few experimental studies are available.

Active stress loading through weight bearing and distraction has been shown to be effective in diminishing pain and resolving vasomotor instability.

Autogenic temperature regulation and *biofeedback* are useful pain-reduction strategies. Grunert et al. reported that a combination of thermal biofeedback, relaxation training, and supportive psychotherapy helps patients control their symptoms.

Splinting may be effective if it does not exacerbate symptoms. *Dynamic and static splinting* should be used, but should not take the place of active move-ment and active functional activities. The use of low-load prolonged stress by static progressive splinting and serial casting or splints can be used after the symptoms have decreased in intensity.

Procedures for edema control should include elevation of the extremity, which decreases hydrostatic pressure and assists in lymphatic drainage. A combination of elevation, retrograde massage, and active exercise may decrease edema, as well as decrease stiffness. The use of *intermittent compression* for short periods also has been recommended, as has the use of *high-volt pulsed direct current (HVPDC)*.

Treatment protocols with documentation of clinical efficacy for RSDS are unknown. The following guidelines are outlines for developing a treatment protocol (see box). Proper evaluation is essential to determine the physiologic status of the involved extremity.

Regardless of the treatment protocol followed and the skill of the therapist, the vicious cycle can be broken only by treating each component of the cycle: pain, cutaneous hypersensitivity, vasomotor instability, edema, decreased motion, fibrosis, bone loss, and emotional aspects.

■ *Emphasis on any one component may temporarily improve that particular parameter, but the cycle will recur unless all components are corrected.*

Any unrecognized and untreated underlying pathologic condition also will result in recurrence of the syndrome. Thus, the importance of identifying an inciting lesion cannot be overemphasized.

CLINICAL CONSIDERATIONS

Treatment of RSDS is directed toward restoring normal function, and treatment must be individualized. Health care professionals working with this difficult disorder should use a team approach, if possible, for the best outcome. The therapist must always evaluate the physiologic status of the involved part, decide on the appropriate treatment regimen, and continually monitor the clinical outcome.

Guidelines for Treatment of RSDS

Establishment of patient rapport and referral to counseling as needed
Stress control
Pain control
Edema control
Stiffness control
Desensitization
Weight bearing
Motor-planning activities
Functional activities
Work reintegration

TABLE 9-1 **Case Study Number One**				
	Clinical Problems	**Treatment**	**Rationale**	**Clinical Efficacy Test**
Initial visit	Pain (burning)	TENS	Reduces pain	Visual analog scale
	Allodynia (hypersensitivity)	Fluidotherapy	Desensitizes	Visual analog scale
	Edema	Active exercise with Theraband	Reduces edema Muscle pumping action	Volumeter
	Inability to bear weight	BAPS board Gymnastic ball	Increases proprioception Inhibits pain	Scale and balance system
	Decreased ROM	Theraband	Proprioceptive input to aid in pain control	Goniometric measurements
Home program		TENS as needed for pain control 24 hours/day		
		Elevation (24-hour control, as possible)		
		Ankle exercises and weight bearing		
		Desensitizing with five different texture materials		
		Retrograde massage as tolerated		
		Physical therapy continued three times a week		
2 weeks		Initial nerve block Elavil begun	Following nerve block, hypersensitivity decreased and edema was resolving	
		Coban wraps added to foot	Patient was able to bear more weight and could ambulate with crutches for short periods. ROM was improved and less painful.	
		Weight bearing in Jacuzzi		
		Intermittent sock and shoe wear		
6 weeks		Second nerve block	Symptoms decreased for 38 hours before returning, but with much less intensity than original presentation.	
		Above protocol continued		
		Added additional weight bearing		
14 weeks		Third nerve block	Patient began ambulating with full weight bearing without crutches.	
		Elavil discontinued		
		Advanced weight bearing program on Stairmaster		
		Plyometrics added		
		Motor planning activities		
17 weeks		Discharged from physical therapy	Running on treadmill, Stairmaster activities, was able to resume all activities of daily living with only occasional pain	

TABLE 9-2 Case Study Number Two

	Clinical Problems	Treatment	Rationale	Clinical Efficacy Test
Initial visit	Pain	TENS	Assist in regulating blood flow	Thermistor measurements
	Cold intolerance	Biofeedback		
	Allodynia	Fluidotherapy	Desensitizing	Visual analog scale and material testing
	Stiffness	Ultrasound, exercise	Pain relief, alters viscoelastic properties, increased motion	Goniometric measurements
	Edema	Active stress loading retrograde massage	Pain relief, edema reduction	Volumetric measurements
Home program		TENS as needed for pain control 24 hours/day		
		Elevation (24 hours/day)		
		Active stress loading, 6 to 8 times/day		
		Retrograde massage		
		Splint wear at night		
3 weeks		First nerve block	Following nerve block, burning ischemic pain decreased. Patient was able to bear more weight in active stress loading. Temperature was normalized, ROM improved	
		Elavil started		
		Circumferential desensitizing in corn and flour		
		Baltimore Therapeutic Equipment Company (BTE) work simulator baseline measurements established		
4 weeks		Second nerve block	Symptoms continued to resolve. (Patient lived long distance from physical therapy facility; therefore, he was seen once a week.	
9 weeks		Third nerve block	Follow-up Baltimore Therapeutic Equipment Company (BTE) work simulator measurements obtained. Significant improvement seen.	
		Baltimore Therapeutic Equipment Company (BTE) work simulator exercises		
		Coordination activities		
11 weeks		Discharged from physical therapy	Patient continued home program.	

An area that cannot be overlooked in the treatment of patients with RSDS is the level of decreased activities, such as fitness and wellness. The patient must be evaluated, and an appropriate exercise program must be established, such as an aquatic or low-impact aerobics program. The symptoms may last indefinitely, and the clinician should instruct the patient to join an RSDS support group, which is known to be helpful to both the patient and the family.

Measurements to establish baseline values assist in monitoring progression and resolution of the condition and provide a guide to therapy (see box).

Case Studies

NUMBER ONE

History

A 9-year-old female sustained an inversion sprain to her right ankle. She was treated in the emergency room for a grade 1 ankle sprain and was given crutches for weight bearing to tolerance, a compression ankle wrap, and instructions for home ice and elevation. One week after injury she returned to see her orthopaedist and was referred to physical therapy. Physical evaluation revealed a hypersensitive foot and

Documentation of Clinical Efficacy

Pain	Visual analog scale
	Grading pain on joint palpation
	McGill pain questionnaire
Edema	Volumetric measurements
Skin temperature	Thermography
	Skin thermistors
	Biofeedback
Range of motion	Goniometric measurements
Weight-bearing status	Scales
	Balance system
Functional activity	Task-performance activities
	Work simulators

ankle, limited ROM, coldness to touch, discoloration and a mottled appearance on the dorsum of the foot, an inability to bear weight, and complaints of burning, shooting pain in the foot and toes (Table 9-1, p. 339).

NUMBER TWO

History

A 41-year-old attorney fell at home, sustaining a fracture of the right distal radius. The fracture was reduced on the day of injury and was pinned several days later. At 6 weeks, he had a carpal tunnel release because of persistent problems. Because of immediate postoperative complaints, he sought a second opinion. His chief complaints were severe, burning pain, extremity swelling, waxy skin, moderate edema, stiffness, and cold intolerance. Clinical signs and symptoms, as well as a positive bone scan, were conclusive for RSDS (Table 9-2, p. 339).

Bibliography

Akeson et al: Collagen cross-linking alterations in joint contractures: changes in the reducible cross-links in periarticular connective tissue collagen after nine weeks of immobilization, *Connect Tissue Res* 5:15, 1977.

Amadio PC: Current concepts review pain dysfunction syndromes, *J Bone Joint Surg* 70A:944, 1988.

Arnstein A: Regional osteoporosis, *Orthop Clin North Am* 3:58, 1972.

Bernstein BH, Singsen B, Kent JT, et al: Reflex neurovascular dystrophy in childhood, *J Pediatr* 93:211, 1978.

Bonica JJ: Causalgia and other reflex sympathetic dystrophies, In Bonica JJ, editor: *Management of pain*, ed 2, Philadelphia, 1990, Lea & Febiger.

Bonica JJ: Sympathetic nerve blocks for pain: *diagnosis and Therapy, vol 1*, New York, 1980, Breon Laboratories.

Casale R, Tiengo M: Flexion withdrawal reflex: a link between pain and mobility. In Tiengo M et al, editors: *Advances in pain research and therapy, vol 10*, New York, 1987, Raven.

Doury P: Algodystrophy: reflex sympathetic dystrophy syndrome, *Clin Rheumatol* 7:173, 1988.

Finney JW, Mallams JT, Pearce KB, Munger G: Low-frequency transcutaneous nerve stimulation in reflex sympathetic dystrophy syndrome, *J Neurol Orthop Med Surg* 12:270, 1991.

Frank C: Normal ligament properties and ligament healing, *Clin Orthop* 196:15, 1985.

Gersh MR: Reflex sympathetic dystrophy syndrome; a model for the multidisciplinary management for patients with pain, *Phys Ther Prac* 2:34, 1993.

Griffin JW et al: Reduction of chronic posttraumatic hand edema: a comparison of high-voltage pulsed current, intermittent pneumatic compression, and placebo treatments, *Phys Ther* 70:279, 1990.

Grunert BK, Devine CA, Sanger JR, et al: Thermal self-regulation for pain control in reflex sympathetic dystrophy syndrome, *J Hand Surg* 15A:615, 1990.

Hollister L: Tri-cyclic antidepressants, *N Engl J Med* 60:321, 1978.

Horowitz SH: Iatrogenic causalgia: classification, clinical findings, and legal ramifications, *Arch Neurol* 41:821, 1984.

Jänig W: Pathophysiological mechanism operating in reflex sympathetic dystrophy. In Sicuteri F (ed): *Advances in pain research and therapy*, Vol 20, New York, 1992, Raven Press.

Kaada B: Vasodilation induced by transcutaneous electrical nerve stimulation in peripheral ischemia (Raynaud's phenomenon and diabetic polyneuropathy), *Eur Heart J* 3:303, 1982.

Kozin et al: Bone scintigraphy in reflex sympathetic dystrophy syndrome, *Radiology* 138:437, 1981.

Lankford LL: Reflex sympathetic dystrophy. In Hunter JM et al, editors: *Rehabilitation of the hand*, ed 3, St. Louis, 1990, Mosby–Year Book.

Lankford LL, Thompson JE: Reflex sympathetic dystrophy, upper and lower extremity; diagnosis and management, *Instr Course Lect* 26:163, 1977.

Lemahieu, RA, Van Laere C, Verbruggen LA: Reflex sympathetic dystrophy: an underreported syndrome in children? *Eur J Pediatr* 147:47, 1988.

Leo KC: Use of electrical stimulation at acupuncture points for treatment of RSDS in a child, *Phys Ther* 63:957, 1983.

Levine DZ: Burning pain in an extremity: breaking the destructive cycle of reflex sympathetic dystrophy, *Postgrad Med* 90:175, 1991.

Lichtenstein L: *Diseases of bone and joints*, ed 2, St. Louis, 1990, CV Mosby.

Mackin EJ: Prevention of complications in hand therapy, *Hand Clin* 2(2):429, 1986.

Mannheimer JS, Lampe GN: Clinical transcutaneous electrical nerve stimulation. Philadelphia 1984, In FA Davis.

Michlovitz S: Thermal agents in Rehabilitation. Philadelphia, 1986, FA Davis.

Mitchell SW, Moorehouse GR, Keen WW: *Gunshot wounds and other injuries of nerves*, Philadelphia, 1864, Lippincott.

Mullins P: Management of common chronic pain problems in the hand, *Phys Ther* 69:1050, 1989.

Neumann MM: Nonsurgical management of pain secondary to peripheral nerve injuries, *Orthop Clin North Am* 19:165, 1988.

Olsson GL, Arner S, Hirsch G: Reflex sympathetic dystrophy in children. In Tyler DC, Krane EJ, editors: *Advances in pain research therapy, vol 15*, New York, 1986, Raven.

Omer GE Jr, Thomas SR: The management of chronic pain syndromes in the upper extremity, *Clin Orthop* 104:37, 1974.

Payne R: Neuropathic pain syndromes, with special reference to causalgia and reflex sympathetic dystrophy syndrome, *Clin J Pain* 2:59, 1986.

Payne R: Reflex sympathetic dystrophy syndrome: diagnosis and treatment, *Clin J Pain* 5:107, 1979.

Peacock EE Jr, Maden JW, Trier WC: Some studies on the treatment of burned hand, *Ann Surg* 171:903, 1970.

Pillemer FG, Micheli LJ: Psychological considerations in youth sports, *Clin Sports Med* 7:679, 1988.

Reflex Sympathetic Dystrophy Syndrome Association of America (RSDSA) Haddonfield, New Jersey.

Schwartzmann RJ, McLellan TL: Reflex sympathetic dystrophy: a review, *Arch Neurol* 44:555, 1987.

Stanton RP et al: Original research. Reflex sympathetic dystrophy syndrome: an orthopedic perspective, *Orthopedics* 16:773, 1993.

Watson HK, Carlson L: Treatment of reflex sympathetic dystrophy of the hand with an active "stress loading" program, *J Hand Surg* 12A(2, pt 1):779, 1987.

Weiss L, Alfano A, Bardfell P, et al: Prognostic value of triple-phased bone-scanning for reflex sympathetic dystrophy syndrome in hemiplegia, *Arch Phys Med Rehab* 74:716, 1993.

Wilder RT et al: Reflex sympathetic dystrophy in children. Clinical characteristics and follow-up of seventy patients, *J Bone Joint Surg* 74A:910, 1992.

Wyndell H: Reflex sympathetic dystrophy. In May Jr JW, Littler JW, editors: *Plastic surgery, vol 7*, The Hand, Part 1, Philadelphia, 1990, WB Saunders.

Zucchini M, Alberti G, Moretti MP: Algodystrophy and related psychological features, *Funct Neurol* 4:153, 1984.

CHAPTER TEN

Foot Orthoses

ROBERT DONATELLI, PT
JILL BRASEL, PT
S. BRENT BROTZMAN, MD

Classification of Orthoses

Foot orthoses are of three kinds: (1) biomechanical, (2) accommodative, and (3) rehabilitation posting.

BIOMECHANICAL ORTHOSES

■ *The role of a biomechanical orthosis is to control excessive and potentially harmful subtalar and midtarsal joint movement.*

Biomechanical orthoses alter the position or mechanics of the foot during *weight bearing.* They can control the rate and/or the amount of harmful subtalar joint (STJ) and midtarsal joint motion, but are used primarily to control excessive pronation caused by excessive forefoot varus and/or rearfoot varus. The amount of control of pronation appears to be inversely related to the rigidity of the orthotic device. The maximum pronation velocity may be decreased by using either soft or semirigid materials. Today most biomechanical orthotics are semirigid. Rigid (e.g., Rohadur) orthotics seldom are used because of their rigidity, narrow profile, and lack of cushioning for "overuse" types of situations.

Biomechanical orthoses may influence submaximal exercise economy after a breaking-in period. In runners, the primary benefit of a foot orthosis appears to be injury prevention.

The *stance phase* is the phase that can be altered with biomechanical orthotics.

ACCOMMODATIVE ORTHOSES

Any orthotic device that does not attempt to establish foot function around the STJ neutral position, thus allowing the foot to compensate for forefoot and/or rearfoot deformities, is an accommodative orthosis. Accommodative orthotics simply cushion or more evenly distribute pressure under the foot. Examples include molds, arch supports, soft tissue supplemental devices made from casts not taken in STJ neutral position, or impressions constructed of materials incapable of controlling foot function around STJ neutral.

Soft tissue supplements—a subcategory of accommodative orthoses—are soft, resilient, protective devices that can be placed in a shoe or added to an orthotic device to protect bony prominences (Fig. 10-1). They improve shock absorption, relieve pressure-intolerant areas, and reduce plantar surface shearing. Materials such as Plastizote, Spenco, and viscoelastic may be used to cushion painful areas or bony prominences on the plantar aspect of the foot.

Occasionally a soft tissue supplement is used as a biomechanical orthosis for mild imbalances or as a

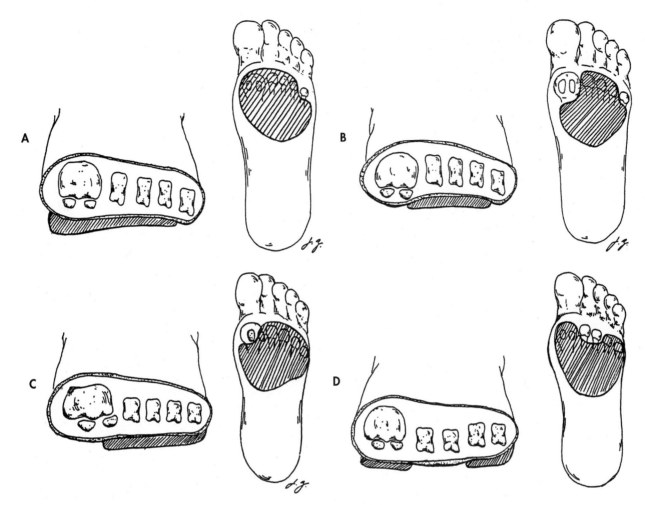

Figure 10-1 A, Accommodative padding to protect the fifth metatarsal. **B,** Accommodative padding to protect the first and fifth metatarsal heads. **C,** Accommodative padding to protect the first metatarsal head. **D,** Accommodative padding to protect the second and third metatarsal heads. (From Donatelli R: *Biomechanics of the foot and ankle*, FA Davis.)

temporary biomechanical orthosis to determine if a permanent orthosis will be beneficial.

REHABILITATION POSTING ORTHOSES

Rehabilitation posting orthoses are specialized devices and are discussed in the section on rehabilitation (p. 365).

Subtalar Neutral

Much of the literature dealing with orthotics describes the foot in a subtalar neutral (STN) position (Fig. 10-2).

■ *Subtalar neutral is the position of the foot in which the subtalar joint, talonavicular joint, and calcaneocuboid joint are all in a congruous relationship. From this subtalar neutral position the foot may function properly in gait.*

The importance of obtaining the STN position is that from this position, the static positions of the forefoot and hindfoot in a particular patient can be determined (such as hindfoot varus and forefoot varus).

■ *In the subtalar neutral position, foot deformities can be measured and determined.*

DETERMINING STN

STN is located by palpating either side of the talonavicular joint, and then centering the navicular on the talus (Fig. 10-3). Once the talonavicular position is congruous (STN) the static positions of forefoot and rearfoot can be estimated.

STN can be palpated with the patient either standing or, more commonly, prone with the posterior surface of the calcaneus aligned with the frontal plane of the body (Fig. 10-4). With the patient prone, STN is determined by palpating with the inside hand (thumb

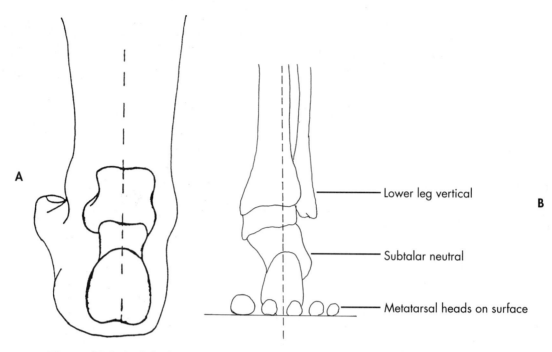

Figure 10-2 **A,** Subtalar neutral position. In the neutral or vertical position of the STJ, a vertical line would bisect both the talus and calcaneus. **B,** Subtalar neutral. (**A** from Donatelli R: *The biomechanics of the foot and ankle,* Philadelphia, 1990, FA Davis.)

Lower leg vertical

Subtalar neutral

Metatarsal heads on surface

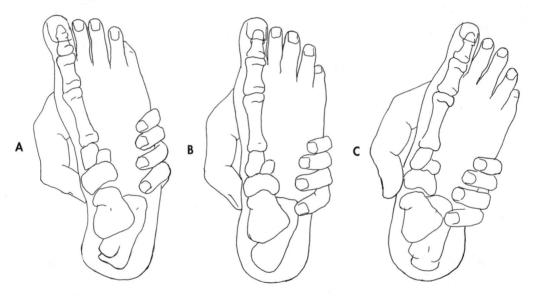

Figure 10-3 **A,** Palpation of the relationship between the navicular and talus (incongruous). **B,** A congruous talonavicular joint. **C,** An incongruous talonavicular joint.

and index finger) and moving the joint by grasping the fourth and fifth metatarsal heads with the other hand until the STN position is found. Some techniques of locating STN require dorsiflexing the foot to load the midtarsal joints, but this results in a common error: the forefoot is moved in valgus rather than dorsiflexion. The forefoot must be moved precisely so that the true position of the forefoot is found relative to the neutral position of the STJ (Fig. 10-4).

The patient may also stand during gentle palpation with the thumb and index finger on either side of talonavicular joint; the patient should then actively invert and evert the foot until the talus feels equidistant between the palpating digits. This also can be achieved by passively moving the foot until a neutral position is achieved.

Both forefoot and rearfoot positions are determined with the foot in STN (Fig. 10-5).

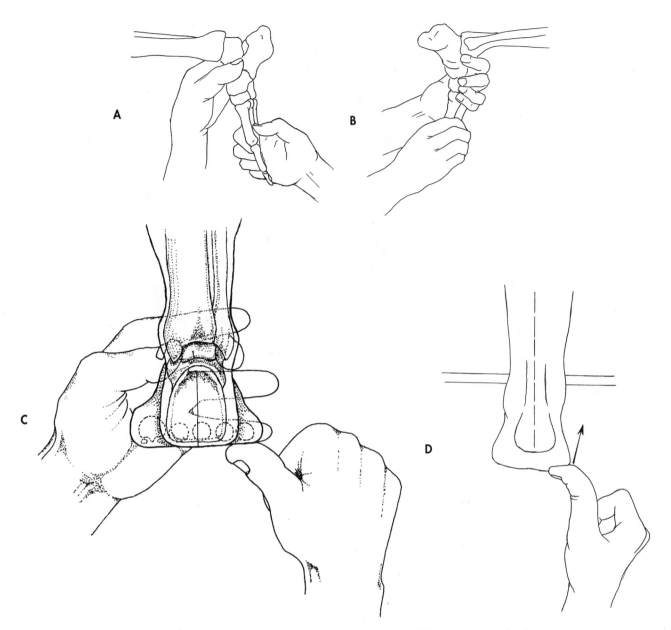

Figure 10-4 **A** and **B,** Prone assessment of subtalar neutral. The examiner maintains congruency of the talus and navicular. This is referred to as the neutral position of the subtalar joint. The examiner then firmly locks the fourth and fifth metatarsals, thereby locking the lateral column. **C,** Parameters for norm. The patient rests in a prone position as the examiner maintains the head of the talus directly behind the navicular. This illustration demonstrates ideal alignment of the leg, rearfoot, forefoot, and metatarsal head. **D,** Prone examination of the subtalar neutral. (C from Michaud TC: *Foot orthoses,* Baltimore, 1993, Williams & Wilkins.)

Biomechanics and Movement

Basic motions of the joints in the foot may be described in three planes or around three axes. Rotation in the sagittal plane (X axis) is defined as dorsiflexion and plantar flexion. Rotation in the frontal plane (Y axis) is defined as inversion and eversion. Rotation in the transverse plane (Z axis) is defined as internal and external rotation (adduction/abduction) (Fig. 10-6). Motion of the subtalar, talonavicular, and calcaneocuboid joints occur in all three planes simultaneously. These complex motions, which refer to the positioning of the entire foot (rather than an individual joint), are referred to as supination and pronation (Fig. 10-7).

Pronation (Fig. 10-8) (open kinetic chain or non–weight bearing) includes dorsiflexion, eversion, and

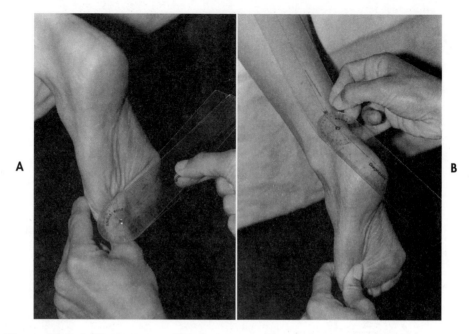

Figure 10-5 **A,** Measurement of forefoot varus with subtalar joint in neutral position. **B,** Measurement of rearfoot varus in subtalar joint neutral.

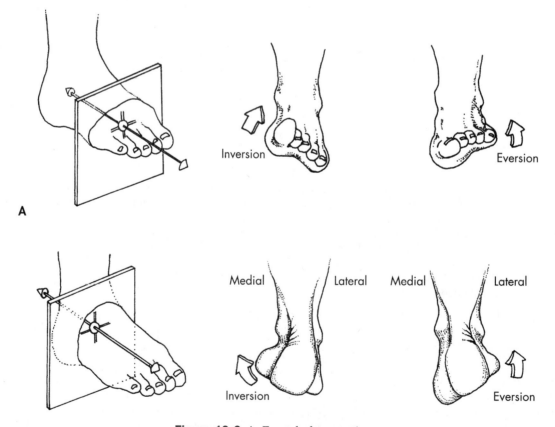

Figure 10-6 A, Frontal plane motions.

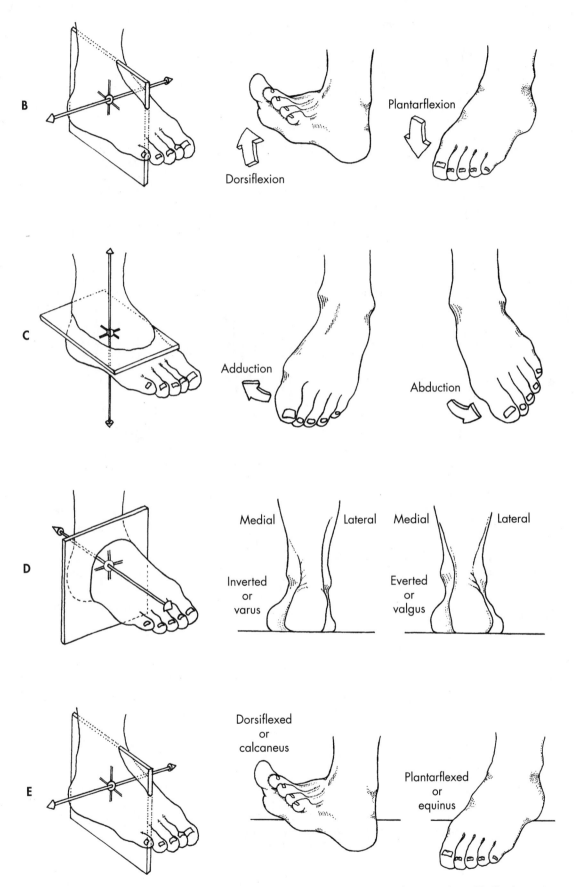

Figure 10-6—cont'd B, Sagittal plane motions. **C,** Transverse plane motions. **D,** Static frontal plane positions. **E,** Static sagittal plane positions.   *Continued.*

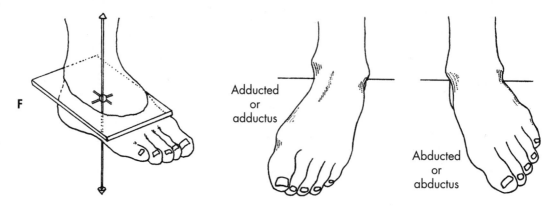

Figure 10-6—cont'd F, Static transverse plane positions. (*A* through *F* from Michaud TC: *Foot orthoses,* Baltimore, 1993, Williams & Wilkins.)

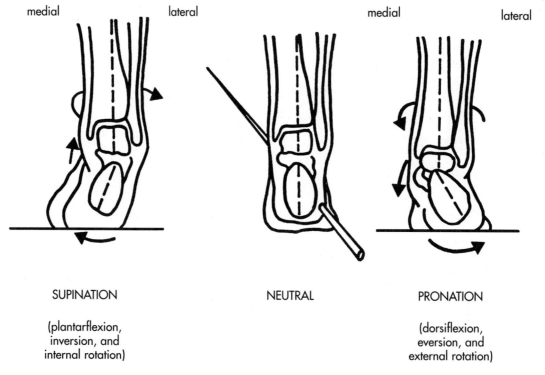

medial   lateral   medial   lateral

SUPINATION   NEUTRAL   PRONATION

(plantarflexion,
inversion, and
internal rotation)

(dorsiflexion,
eversion, and
external rotation)

Figure 10-7 Supination (plantar flexion, inversion and internal rotation) and pronation (dorsiflexion, eversion and external rotation). (From McPoil T: *J Orthop Sports Phys Ther* 7:69, 1985.)

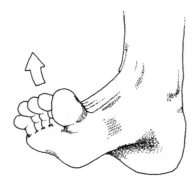

Figure 10-8 Pronation: abduction, dorsiflexion and eversion. (From Michaud TC: *Foot orthoses,* Baltimore, 1993, Williams & Wilkins.)

external rotation (abduction). During the stance phase of gait, pronation is normal when it occurs immediately after foot contact (shock absorption) and through the first 25% of the stance phase of gait. Pronation is abnormal when it occurs excessively throughout the stance phase of gait or when the duration of the pronation movement is greater than 50% of the stance phase of gait (Fig. 10-9).

Supination (Fig. 10-10) involves plantar flexion, inversion, and internal rotation (adduction). Supination is normal during gait and is a necessary component occurring from heel-rise to toe-off (push-off) and as the heel strikes the ground from the swing phase. Supination becomes dysfunctional when it is excessive at heel contact and continues throughout the stance phase of gait. A plantar-flexed rigid first ray or a foot with forefoot valgus along with rigid rearfoot (hindfoot) varus are factors that lead to dysfunctional supination during the gait cycle.

Because the lower extremity responds to foot and ankle movement during gait, internal rotation of the leg occurs during pronation and external rotation of the leg occurs during supination.

Gait Cycle

Many terminologies are used to describe three basic phases of weight-bearing gait, also called stance phase (Fig. 10-11).

HEEL-STRIKE TO FOOT-FLAT

The foot has been supinated during swing phase and is supinated when heel-strike occurs. *It begins to pronate immediately to absorb shock,* adapt to the terrain, and attenuate rotary forces. The calcaneus rapidly everts, placing the calcaneocuboid and talonavicular joints in position to allow more *flexibility* of the midfoot, and shock absorption at ground contact. Maximum pronation occurs at the end of foot-flat phase or after approximately 25% of the stance phase has occurred. During the remaining 75% of the stance phase, the foot is preparing for push-off by becoming a rigid lever. Thus, if pronation occurs beyond this initial 25% of the stance phase, a rigid lever for push-off may not be achieved. An unstable foot at push-off can result in progressive soft tissue microtrauma and pathologic conditions of the foot.

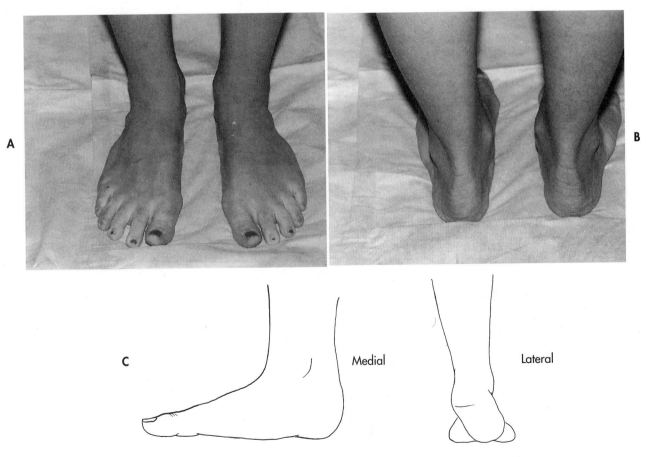

Figure 10-9 A and B, Pronation. C, Flexible flat-foot—pronation during weight bearing.

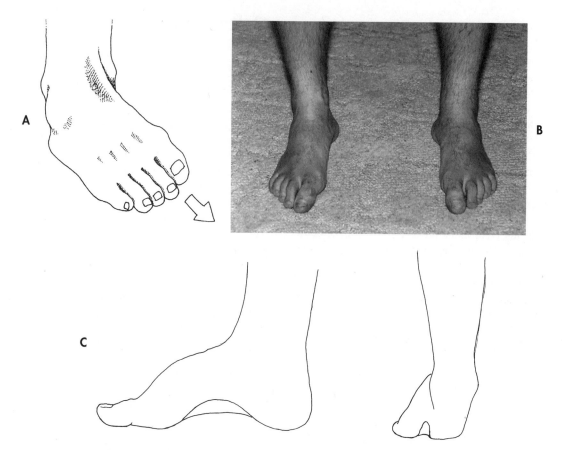

Figure 10-10 **A,** Supination—adduction, plantar flexion, and inversion. **B,** Supination of foot—cavus type of deformity. **C,** Supinated (cavus) foot type during weight bearing. (*A* from Michaud TC: *Foot orthoses,* Baltimore, 1993, Williams & Wilkins.)

MIDSTANCE—FOOT-FLAT TO HEEL-RISE

This is the transition from pronation to supination as the foot begins moving into supination and the posterior tibialis muscle begins to concentrically contract to resupinate the foot. The foot should be pronated at midstance. When this fails to occur, the foot remains supinated, which does not allow the shock-absorbing mechanisms of pronation to occur; nor can the foot adapt to uneven terrain. This may make inversion ankle sprain more likely.

PUSH-OFF—HEEL-OFF TO TOE-OFF

During push-off, the foot is supinated and the plantar fascia tightens as the great toe dorsiflexes (windlass mechanism) (Fig. 10-12). The foot becomes a *rigid lever* to aid in push-off. When the foot is supinated, it has much less flexibility (rigid lever). Much more flexibility is present at the midfoot and forefoot when the foot is pronated. As mentioned above, the deleterious effects of excessive pronation often occur during the push-off phase of gait, when the foot needs to become a stabilizer or rigid lever.

Muscle function is less efficient when pronation occurs too rapidly or during the wrong period of the gait cycle. The posterior and anterior tibialis muscles, extensor digitorum and extensor hallucis longus, and the gastrocnemius and soleus muscles function as decelerators of pronation and control movement. When the foot is pronating excessively, these muscles may develop overuse symptoms because of the lengthened position in which they are forced to function. Conversely, when pronation fails to occur, the foot remains supinated during stance. Excessive activity and/or overstretching of the peroneus longus and brevis may occur. Ankle sprains and peroneal tendonitis may result from lack of control of the supinators at heel contact and overactivity of the first ray plantar flexor (peroneus longus) (Table 10-1).

Forefoot Position

Forefoot position is measured with the foot held in STN (see Fig. 10-8, *A*). The position of the forefoot relative to the rearfoot determines whether the forefoot is in valgus, varus, or neutral position.

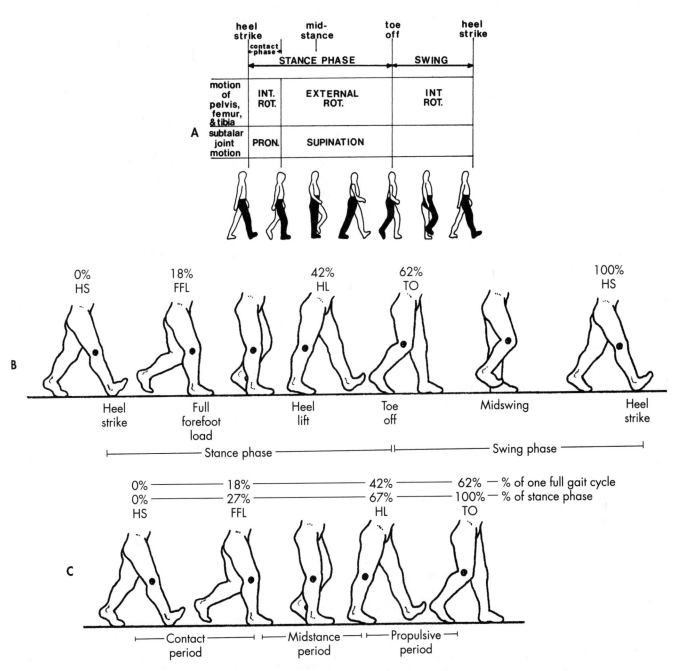

Figure 10-11 A, Gait cycle: transverse plane of motion of the lower extremity during the walking cycle. **B,** Gait cycle of the right leg. Stance phase begins at heel-strike and ends when the great toe leaves the ground. Swing phase continues until the heel again strikes the ground. The length of stride, which refers to the distance between successive ipsilateral heel strikes, is approximately 0.8 times a person's body height, and the average cadence is approximately 115 steps/minute (slightly lower for men and higher for women). It should be emphasized that there is marked individual variation in stride length and cadence, as each person seems to choose a gait pattern that is metabolically more efficient. **C,** The various periods of stance phase. HS, heel-strike; FFL, full forefoot load; TO, toe-off. (*A* from McPoil TG: *J Orthop Sports Phys Ther* 7:69:1985; *B* and *C* from Michaud TC: *Foot orthoses,* Baltimore, 1993, Williams & Wilkins.)

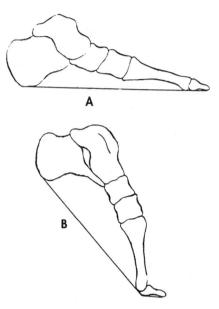

Figure 10-12 The windlass effect. **A,** Plantar aponeurosis slack position. **B,** Tightening of the plantar aponeurosis in push-off. (From Donatelli R: *J Orthop Sports Phys Ther* 7(5):92.)

Forefoot varus is an inverted position of the forefoot in relationship to the rearfoot with the subtalar joint in neutral position. The medial border (first metatarsal) is **higher** than the lateral border (fifth metatarsal) (Fig. 10-13, *A*). Forefoot varus is reported to be the most common forefoot deformity associated with symptoms of foot and ankle pain for which biomechanical foot orthoses are prescribed.

Several etiologies for forefoot varus have been proposed; most commonly forefoot varus is believed to be an osseous foot deformity due to insufficient valgus rotation of the head and neck of the talus during fetal development. Malposition of the calcaneocuboid joint may also be responsible for the varus attitude of the forefoot.

■ *Patients with low arches (flexible flat feet, pronators) in weight bearing often exhibit forefoot varus when the foot is held in STN (see Fig. 10-9)*

Forefoot varus in itself is not destructive to the foot. However, to permit the medial forefoot to contact the ground, the forefoot varus may be compensated for by rearfoot subtalar pronation (eversion) (Fig. 10-13, *B*). Excessive and prolonged subtalar pronation during the gait cycle is deleterious (Fig. 10-13, *B*, Fig. 10-14, and box). Although this abnormal STJ compensatory pronation does allow the varus forefoot to contact the ground, it results in "unlocking" the foot, thus creating hypermobility and loss of the rigid lever from midstance through push-off (Fig. 10-15).

In addition to the increased amount of pronation, forefoot varus may lead to increased speed of pronation (from midstance to push-off), thus increasing the

TABLE 10-1 **Muscle Function During Stance Phase of Gait**	
Muscle	**Heel Contact to Weight Acceptance**
Anterior tibialis	**Eccentric:** control pronation of subtalar joint, decelerate plantar flexion
Extensor hallucis longus Extensor digitorum	**Eccentric:** decelerate plantar flexion and posterior shear of tibia on talus
Posterior tibialis Soleus Gastrocnemius	**Eccentric:** decelerate pronation of subtalar joint and internal rotation of tibia
	Midstance
Posterior tibialis Soleus Flexor hallucis longus Flexor digitorum longus	**Eccentric:** decelerate forward movement of tibia
Posterior tibialis Soleus Gastrocnemius	**Concentric:** supinate subtalar and midtarsal joints
	Push-off and Propulsion
Peroneus longus Abductor hallucis Peroneus brevis	**Concentric:** plantar-flex first ray **Antagonistic:** to supinators of subtalar and midtarsal joints
Flexor digitorum longus	**Concentric:** stabilize toes against ground
Extensor hallucis longus and brevis	**Concentric:** stabilize first metatarsophalangeal joint
Abductor hallucis Abductor digiti quinti Flexor hallucis brevis Flexor digitorum brevis Extensor digitorum brevis Interossei, lumbricals	**Concentric:** stabilize midtarsal and forefoot, raise medial arch of foot in push-off

From Donatelli R: *Biomechanics of the foot and ankle,* 2 ed, Philadelphia, 1995, F.A. Davis.

eccentric work requirements of the anterior and posterior tibialis and the flexor digitorum longus and brevis muscles as they assist in lowering the medial forefoot to reach the ground. If pronation is excessive and prolonged beyond the initial 25% of the stance phase, a rigid lever is never fully achieved, thus producing excessive stress and microtrauma during walking or running. Lutter reported that abnormal pronation accounted for 56% of foot problems experienced by runners.

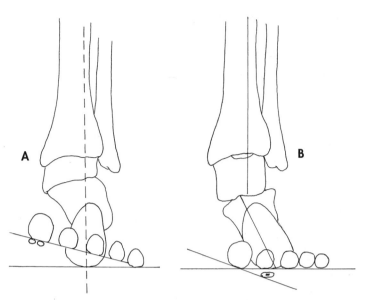

Figure 10-13 A, Forefoot varus. Medial ray (first ray) "higher" than lateral ray (fifth ray). **B,** Compensated forefoot varus. Rearfoot has compensated by everting (rearfoot pronation) to allow the foot to become plantigrade. This compensatory pronation is deleterious.

Possible Associated Problems
COMPENSATED FOREFOOT VARUS

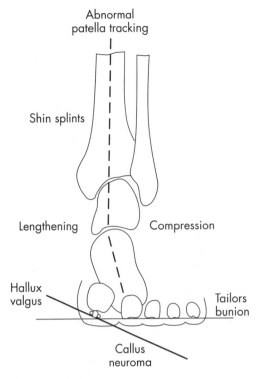

Figure 10-14 Compensated forefoot varus: possible associated problems.

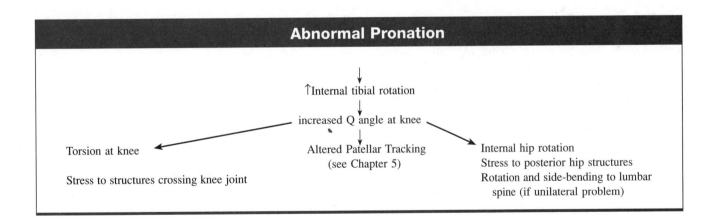

With excessive pronation, the posterior tibial tendon works eccentrically during stance to help control excessive pronation of the foot, often becoming overloaded and/or inflamed. Sinus tarsi pain may result from lateral impingement as a consequence of excessive pronation. Patients with flat feet usually push off on the inside of the hallux, causing keratoses and placing valgus stresses across the hallux, possibly contrib-

uting to the development of hallux valgus (prehallux foot).

In patients with compensated forefoot varus (via hindfoot pronation), the first ray is unstable and does not contribute to propulsion, which may lead to transfer metatarsalgia or second-metatarsal stress fractures.

Treatment of compensated forefoot varus consists of a medial forefoot post to prevent pronatory com-

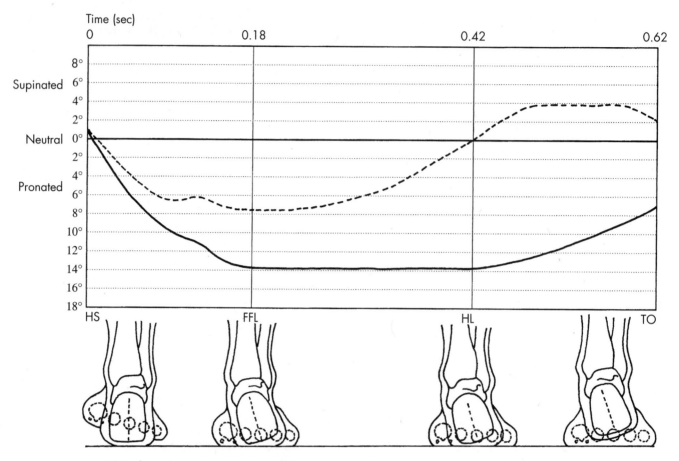

Figure 10-15 Stance phase motions with a forefoot varus deformity *(solid line).* HS, heel-strike; FFL, full forefoot load; HL, heel lift; TO, toe-off. (From Michaud TC: *Foot orthoses,* Baltimore, 1993, Williams & Wilkins.)

pensation of the STJ (see Fig. 10-13). This allows the foot to enter the propulsive period with all of the articulations fixed and stable.

■ *In summary, compensated forefoot varus (via hindfoot eversion) resembles a pes planus or flat foot. Posteriorly the calcaneus is everted. Medially the longitudinal arch is lessened. Stress is often concentrated under the plantar aspect of the second and third metatarsals. Multiple musculotendinous problems, as described above, may develop as a result of compensation to obtain a plantigrade foot.*

With *forefoot valgus,* the lateral border (fifth metatarsal) is higher than the medial border (first metatarsal). The forefoot is everted in relation to the rearfoot with the STJ in neutral position. Two structural types of forefoot valgus exist: in one, all the metatarsal heads are everted (Fig. 10-16, *A*), whereas in the other, only the first metatarsal head is plantar flexed while the second through fifth heads are in a neutral or varus position in relation to the rearfoot in STN position (Fig. 10-16, *B*). The plantar-flexed first ray may be rigid (the first ray is *fixed* below the plane of the lesser metatarsals) (Fig. 10-17, *C*), *flexible* (the plantar-flexed first ray can be easily moved above its resting level

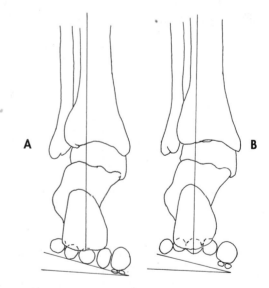

Figure 10-16 A, Total valgus—all metatarsal heads are everted. **B,** Plantar-flexed first ray only.

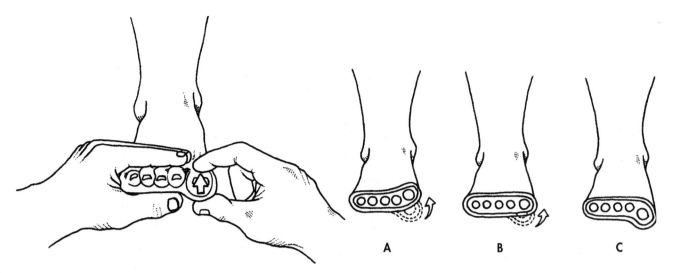

Figure 10-17 Categorization of the plantar-flexed first rays. The first ray is maximally dorsiflexed as the lesser metatarsals are held stationary. If the first ray can dorsiflex above the common transverse plane of the lesser metatarsals *(A)*, it is referred to as the **flexible** deformity. If it dorsiflexes to the same level as the lesser metatarsals *(B)*, it is referred to as a **semiflexible** deformity. If it is unable to reach the common transverse plane of the lesser metatarsals *(C)*, it is referred to as a rigid deformity. (From Michaud TC: *Foot orthoses*, Baltimore, 1993, Williams & Wilkins.)

with a dorsally applied force at the first metatarsal) (Fig. 10-17, *A*), or *semirigid* (the first ray can be moved dorsally but not past the other rays) (Fig. 10-17, *B*).

■ *Forefoot valgus is often associated with high arches or cavus feet. The foot deformity is commonly referred to as a cavovarus foot or a pes cavus deformity. Careful evaluation usually reveals a plantar-flexed first ray with other rays neutral.*

During stance, the subtalar joint compensates (inverts) to allow the lateral border of the forefoot to contact the ground (Fig. 10-18, *C*), creating a supinatory position of the foot. As a result of this abnormal supination during stance, the foot's function to absorb shock and adapt to uneven surfaces is less available because these functions occur due to pronation (Fig. 10-19). This rigid foot is more prone to stress injuries over the fifth ray or under the first metatarsal head (Fig. 10-19); recurrent lateral ankle sprains; and peroneal tendonitis, a condition that develops secondary to overuse of the peroneal tendons, which must work eccentrically to control supination from a lengthened position.

Orthotic treatment of forefoot valgus is discussed on p. 363.

Forefoot Mobility

Inversion and eversion of the forefoot occur around the longitudinal axis of the midtarsal joint, and may be assessed by grasping the forefoot (metatarsals) and

moving it into inversion and eversion. The rearfoot is held to prevent compensations.

Excessive inversion of the forefoot may indicate instability of the midtarsal joint and is often associated with forefoot varus. Excessive inversion is defined as a position of the forefoot that is parallel to the lower leg. Neutral position is when the forefoot is perpendicular to the lower leg.

Abduction and adduction of the forefoot occur around the transfer axis of the midtarsal joint. Twenty degrees of adduction and 10 degrees of abduction are normal. Rigid metatarsus adductus deformities are associated with pes cavus.

Rearfoot Position

Rearfoot varus is defined as the sum of subtalar varus and tibial varum. The calcaneus (rearfoot) is in a position of inversion with the STJ in neutral. Three to 4 degrees of inversion is considered to be within the limits of normal. Beyond this, STJ compensation (excessive eversion) during weight bearing may be required to get the medial calcaneal border to the ground (i.e., plantigrade) after heel strike.

Rearfoot valgus is a position of calcaneal eversion with the STJ in neutral. In STN, this deformity is quite rare. *Usually rearfoot valgus is a result of compensation for forefoot varus* (see compensatory mechanisms of forefoot varus).

The most common *combined deformity* is a combi-

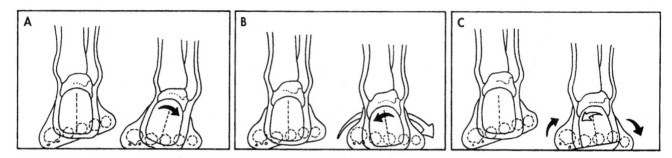

Figure 10-18 Patterns of compensation for forefoot valgus deformity. If the forefoot deformity is rigid *(A)*, the subtalar joint must supinate in order to bring the lateral plantar forefoot to the ground. When a flexible forefoot valgus is present *(B)*, the plantar forefoot is able to make ground contact without affecting subtalar motions, as long as the range of forefoot inversion is large enough to compensate for the forefoot valgus deformity. However, if the size of the deformity exceeds the range of inversion available around the longitudinal midtarsal joint axis (as in *C*), the forefoot, in its attempt to make ground contact, will invert its full range around the longitudinal midtarsal joint axis (note the central metatarsals), then continue to compensate via pronation (dorsiflexion and inversion) around the first ray axis and supination (plantar flexion and inversion) around the fifth ray axis (arrows in *C*).

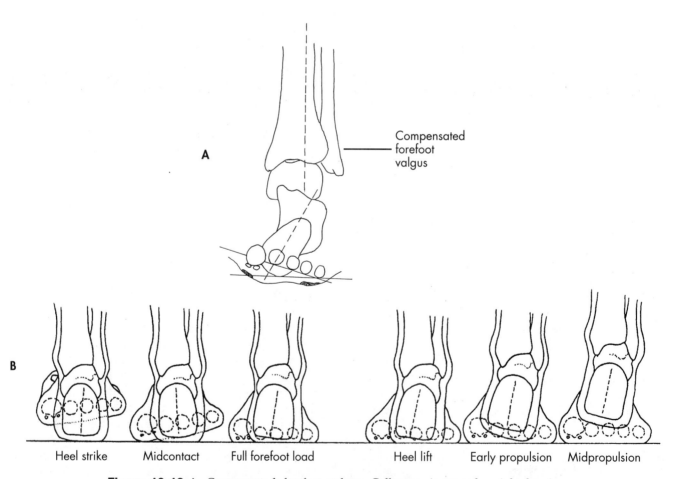

Figure 10-19 A, Compensated forefoot valgus. Callouses, increased weight bearing, stress injuries over the first and fifth metatarsals. **B,** Foot motions with a rigid forefoot valgus (posterior view of the right foot). Note the rearfoot compensation (rearfoot varus). (**B** from Michaud TC: *Foot Orthoses*, Baltimore, 1993, Williams & Wilkins.)

nation of forefoot and rearfoot varus in a pronator. Many late pronators (pronation past stance) exhibit (1) isolated forefoot varus or (2) rearfoot varus plus flexible plantar-flexed first ray and neutral or varus forefoot (2 to 5 rays).

A supinator (one who does not pronate during the gait cycle) may have a combination of forefoot valgus and rearfoot varus, a rigid plantar-flexed first ray and rearfoot varus, a semirigid plantar-flexed first ray and rearfoot varus, or forefoot and rearfoot valgus (rare).

Rearfoot equinus (restricted ankle dorsiflexion) has a variety of causes, but all result in a common pattern of compensation by the foot. During foot-flat to toe-off in normal gait, the foot dorsiflexes as the body passes over it. With rearfoot equinus, three alterations in gait may occur because of restricted ankle dorsiflexion: (1) Most commonly, the foot pronates excessively to allow further dorsiflexion. With excessive pronation, the forefoot bears more weight and the plantar ligaments of the longitudinal arch are overstressed. Se-

vere calcaneal pronation (eversion) may cause sinus tarsi pain from impingement laterally. (2) The patient walks on the toes and never places the foot flat on the ground. (3) The knee hyperextends to allow the foot to reach foot flat.

Mild problems that are symptomatic only with distance running and not with normal gait, may be successfully treated with heel lifts or stretching of the gastrocnemius and soleus complex (Fig. 10-20).

Evaluation for Orthoses

The evaluation should determine if any forefoot or rearfoot deformities are present during non–weight bearing and if compensations occur during the gait cycle or with weight bearing alone. Evaluation should also reveal muscular tightness or weakness; leg-length discrepancies (functional or anatomic); callous formation, yielding information on weight-bearing areas;

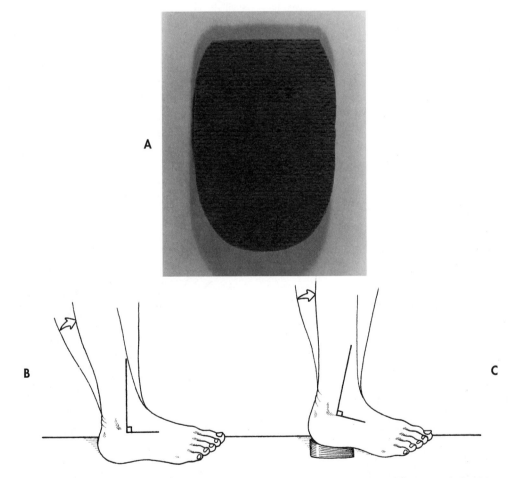

Figure 10-20 A, Heel lift. **B,** The foot is unable to dorsiflex the ankle beyond the 90-degree mark, and the subtalar and midtarsal joints will most likely compensate for this deformity by pronating during the late stance phase. **C,** Note how the addition of a heel lift allows this foot to move safely into its propulsive period. (*B* and *C* from Michaud TC: *Foot orthoses,* Baltimore, 1993, Williams & Wilkins.)

and areas of pain or tenderness. The patient's history is a very important component of the evaluation process. Because orthoses are only one tool in the treatment of lower extremity dysfunction, assessment of other factors is required to provide a comprehensive, effective treatment program.

The following evaluation form was designed to include a thorough biomechanical assessment, patient's history, and musculoskeletal examination (see box).

Fabrication of Orthoses

■ *A biomechanical orthosis attempts to place the foot closer to STJ neutral position to decrease the necessity for STJ compensations during gait.*

Shock absorption is an important component of an orthosis. For a supinator, it may be the primary goal of the orthosis. Even excessive pronators may need shock absorption to decrease stresses on inflamed tissues or joints. In this case a semirigid orthosis is indicated. In addition to medial or lateral forefoot and rearfoot posting, metatarsal bars or pads, first ray extensions, first ray cut-outs, 2-to-5 bar posts, 1-to-4 bar posts, various relief cut-outs, and heel lifts can be fabricated in an orthosis.

Temporary posting is one method of evaluating the effectiveness of an orthotic device. Forefoot and rearfoot postings are placed on a one-dimensional material and are worn for 1 to 2 weeks. If effective, a permanent pair of orthoses will be fabricated (Fig. 10-21). Casting in STN and sending to a laboratory for fabri-

cation, with an evaluation form, requires 1 to 2 weeks. In-house systems allow an STN mold or blank to be made and posting to be added accordingly (Fig. 10-22). With in-house systems, such as Foot Technology, Inc., an STN mold is formed and a great deal of intrinsic posting can be achieved through finishing materials of different densities; if further posting is necessary, extrinsic forefoot and/or rearfoot posts may be added. *Extrinsic posting* is that which is added to the outer shell of the orthotic device to add medial or lateral support (Fig. 10-23). *Intrinsic posting* is the amount of medial or lateral control capture by the STN position in which the cast or impression is made. Included are the materials added within the shell of the orthotic device to achieve the neutral position of the foot (Fig. 10-24).

REARFOOT POSTING (DONATELLI)

A rearfoot post alters the position of the subtalar joint (STJ) from heel-strike to foot-flat. The effect of rearfoot posting on the biomechanics of the STJ is not completely understood. Smith et al. reported that semirigid orthotics reduce the rate and amount of calcaneal eversion during running. Cavanaugh, Nigg et al., and Clarke et al. demonstrated that a rearfoot medial post significantly reduces maximum calcaneal eversion. Others have found no significant change in maximum eversion with medial posting.

Root et al. recommend that the STJ be posted in a "neutral" position. A minimum of 4 degrees of pronation is needed directly after heel-strike to allow proper shock absorption. Thus, the rearfoot post should al-

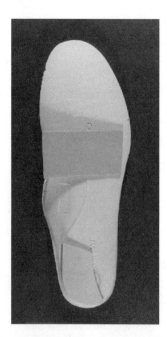

Figure 10-21 Example of temporary posting. Medial 4 degree rearfoot and forefoot posts added to insole of shoe.

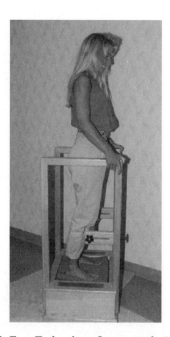

Figure 10-22 Foot Technology System technique for attaining an STN mold for fabricating biomechanical orthoses.

Static and Dynamic Evaluation
The Campbell Clinic Physical Therapy Foot Orthotic Patient Evaluation

Patient _____ Date _____

Physician _____ PT _____ Account no. _____

Patient information: Age _____ Shoe size _____

Patient's history:

_____

_____

Heel pain: How long have you been having pain? _____

Does your heel hurt when you first get up in the morning? _____

If yes, does it get better when you have walked on it a little while? _____

Surgery: yes or no   Date: _____

Areas of pain/dysfunction R/L: _____ Palpation/tenderness _____

Prone observation _____

_____

Draw callous formation

Flexibility

L/R   L/R

Forefoot: Varus _____   First ray: Does patient have flex, semirigid, or rigid? _____

Valgus _____   _____

Inver/ever _____   _____

Add/abd _____   _____

Rearfoot: STN _____   _____

Position of RF when STJ is neutral, (I.E., degrees of inversion or eversion)

G-SOL KE/KF _____

ROM: Inversion _____   Great toe first MTP _____

Eversion _____   Hip IR/ER _____

Upright: LLD: yes or no _____

MMT

L/R   L/R

1. Anterior tibialis _____   6. Flexor dig 1,2,3,4,5 _____

2. Extensor hallicus longus _____   7. Abductor hallicus _____

3. Posterior tibialis _____   8. Peroneus longus _____

4. Extensor digitorum _____   9. Peroneus brevis _____

5. Extensor dig 1,2,3,4 _____   10. Gastrocnemius and soleus _____

Unilateral balance timed (seconds) _____

Stand: STN (falls in from neutral or out—this may not reveal true dysfunction) _____

Knees _____

Hips _____

Calcaneus _____

Gait analysis

NL gait:

HS: Begin in supinated position _____

FF: (stance) roll into pronation _____

PO: back toward supinated calcaneal _____

Position is important _____

Assessment: _____

_____

Plan (orthotic RX/exercise RX/pain scale/formal PT): _____

_____

Special order: yes or no

Follow-up: Dates:

Signature: _____

Registered physical therapist

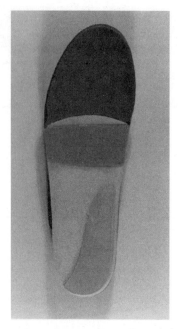

Figure 10-23 Extrinsic posting added to orthosis.

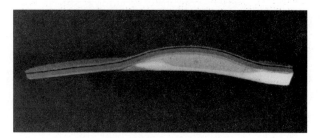

Figure 10-24 Intrinsic posting.

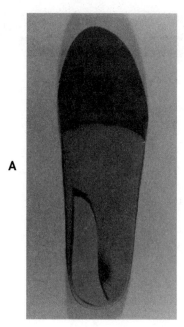

A

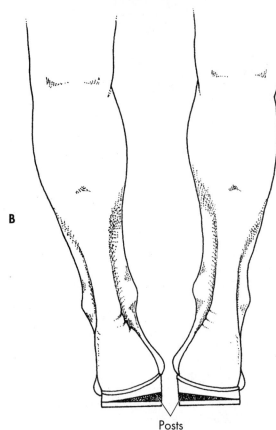

B

Figure 10-25 A, Medial rearfoot posts. (Examples are extrinsic, but often they are fabricated intrinsically.) **B,** The rearfoot varus post. (From Michaud TC: *Foot orthoses*, Baltimore, 1993, Williams & Wilkins.)

low the STJ to hit near neutral and control, but not eliminate, pronation from heel-strike to foot-flat. **Neutral** is determined by calculating the ration of subtalar inversion to eversion and is defined as one third of the total STJ motion from the fully everted position.

If the calcaneus is excessively everted at heel-strike, the STJ is pronated. A rearfoot medial post (varus post) inverts the calcaneus closer to neutral to allow more normal (not excessive) pronation from heel-strike to foot-flat (Fig. 10-25). The maximum amount of rearfoot posting is usually 5 to 6 degrees, because subtalar motion should be controlled but not eliminated.

Conversely, a rearfoot lateral post (valgus post) is used in conditions where the STJ is excessively supinated (inverted) at heel-strike. A lateral rearfoot post can be used only if the calcaneus has the available eversion range of motion (ROM) to be placed into a less inverted position during weight bearing. A minimum of 4 degrees eversion from the calcaneal perpendicular position is a safe guideline before rearfoot valgus posting is attempted. In some patients, the supinated foot will have a rigid rearfoot varus (inverted)

Permanent orthotic prescription*

Therapist Information
Name _____
Address _____

Patient Information
Name _____
Address _____
Occupation/Activity _____
Age __ Height __ Weight __
Shoe size ____ Sex _____

Orthotic Type
____ Rohadur (we seldom use)
____ Sports
____ Semirigid
____ Accommodative
____ Children (gait plate, Roberts Whitman, etc.)

Posting Instructions
Forefoot: ____ extrinsic ____ intrinsic
Left ____ •varus ____ •valgus
Right ____ •varus ____ •valgus

Rearfoot:
Left ____ •varus ____ •valgus
Right ____ •varus ____ •valgus

Heel Lift:
Left ____ inch
Right ____ inch

Covers/Extensions:
____ Spenco
____ Leather
____ PPT
____ Vinyl

Special Instructions:
_____
_____
_____

*A generic prescription form for casted orthotics. Format will vary depending on the laboratory used.

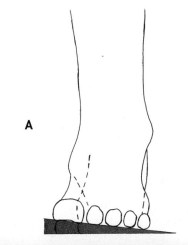

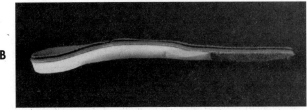

Figure 10-26 A, Forefoot medial post for forefoot varus. **B,** Forefoot varus (medial post).

foot" during the foot-flat and push-off phases of gait. This reduces the need for the STJ pronatory compensation. A forefoot post is indicated when the forefoot deformity leads to problems during the propulsive phase of stance (late pronation).

Forefoot valgus deformity should be supported by a lateral post. A forefoot valgus deformity is, by definition, an everted position of the forefoot in relation to the rearfoot with the STJ in neutral position. The compensation for forefoot valgus is to roll into excessive forefoot inversion and cause the STJ also to invert (supinate) to allow the fifth ray to touch the ground. The lateral posting "brings the ground" to the outside of the foot, decreasing the need for the excessive compensatory supination of the STJ, which could lead to abnormal supination.

A conservative approach to orthotic prescription for a patient with a forefoot valgus deformity and a supination compensation at the STJ is as follows:
• Post the forefoot valgus first, 60% to 70% of the forefoot valgus deformity, and reevaluate the patient's symptoms in 1 week.
• Post the rearfoot in valgus a maximum of 4 degrees only if the calcaneus can passively move into 4 degrees of eversion from the perpendicular position.

PLANTAR-FLEXED FIRST RAY

For a semirigid or rigid deformity, a post is placed under rays 2 through 5 to more evenly distribute weight

and cannot be actively or passively moved toward neutral. This is one reason it is important to measure available calcaneal inversion and eversion during an orthotic evaluation.

FOREFOOT POSTING

Forefoot posts are used for three deformities: forefoot varus, forefoot valgus, and semirigid or rigid plantar-flexed first ray.

Forefoot varus deformity should be supported by a medial post (Fig. 10-26). A forefoot varus post supports the deformity by "bringing the ground up to the bearing (Fig. 10-27). Often a first ray cut-out is combined with a 2-to-5 bar post (Fig. 10-28), because semi-rigid or rigid plantar flexed first ray often leads to increased weight bearing by the first metatarsal head, inducing symptomatic sesamoids (medial or lateral) or increasing stress on the great toe flexor tendons. We have found the dancer pad by HAPAD, a soft tissue supplement, to provide excellent relief of the plantar flexed first ray (Fig. 10-29).

FLEXIBLE DEFORMITY FIRST RAY

A foot with this deformity must be evaluated to determine if a forefoot post is necessary and which type is indicated. Often, a foot with a flexible plantar-flexed first ray without evidence of excessive weight bearing under the first ray may have a forefoot varus when all the rays are in the same plane, and medial forefoot posting may be helpful. Full correction is not necessary. The size of the forefoot post is limited by shoe constraints and the patient's tolerance. Donatelli found in a review of 80 patients that the average forefoot varus deformity was 8.5 degrees. The average forefoot varus post prescribed corrected 62% of the abnormality.

In patients with 10 degrees of forefoot varus, a 6-degree medial post was used. In patients with 8.5 degrees of forefoot varus, a 5-degree post was used (62% correction). In patients with 6 degrees or less of forefoot varus, a forefoot post corrected 90% to 100% of the deformity.

Recent Advances

Johanson et al. demonstrated, through the use of two-dimensional motion analysis of rearfoot movement during the stance phase of gait, that maximal control of rearfoot frontal plane pronation was accomplished by varus posting of the forefoot and rearfoot. Rearfoot posting alone also demonstrated a significant amount of rearfoot pronation control during the stance phase of gait. The subjects used in the study demonstrated a forefoot varus deformity of 8 degrees or more, and the eversion ROM of the STJ was a minimum of 8 degrees. The amount of posting for the orthotics was determined by the forefoot varus measurement. Sixty percent of the forefoot varus measurement was used for the forefoot post, and 50% was used for the rearfoot post. For example, 10 degrees forefoot varus equals 6 mm forefoot varus post and 5 mm rearfoot varus post.

Eng and Plerrynowski, with the use of a three-dimensional motion analysis system, demonstrated that soft foot orthotics that support forefoot varus and calcaneal valgus can result in changes in transverse

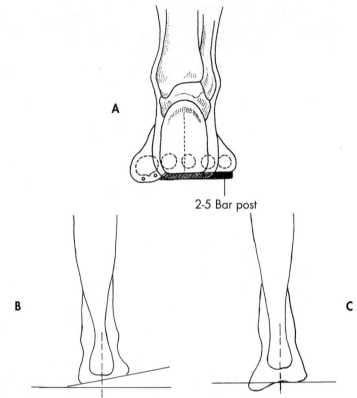

2-5 Bar post

Figure 10-27 A, The 2-to-5 bar post. A forefoot bar post (a bar post represents an unangled forefoot post) is situated beneath the distal shafts of the second through the fifth metatarsals. The portion of the bar post that would normally extend beneath the distal first metatarsal shaft is "cut out" to allow the first metatarsal head to rest in its plantar position (hence the name 2-to-5 bar post). The thickness of the bar post is determined by the distance between the first metatarsal head and the common transverse plane of the lesser metatarsals; the post is of sufficient height so that the first metatarsal head makes ground contact and the sagittal bisection of the rearfoot is vertical. As with all forefoot posts, shoe fit is the limiting factor, and a bar post larger than 10 mm is often difficult to tolerate. It should be noted that different laboratories use different terms to describe the 2-to-5 bar post. Because the plantar-flexed first ray deformity behaves almost identically to a forefoot valgus deformity (particularly when the plantar-flexed first ray is rigid), many laboratories refer to the 2-to-5 bar post as a forefoot valgus post with a first ray cut-out. The degree of posting necessary to accommodate the first metatarsal head is determined by measuring the degree of forefoot valgus between the first and fifth metatarsal heads and the plantar calcaneus. (The foot should be maintained in its neutral position during this measurement.) Although it is more accurate to refer to this addition as a 2-to-5 bar post (as long as the second through fifth metatarsals are neither in valgus or varus), either approach is fine, and it is really just a matter of semantics. **B** and **C,** Plantar-flexed forefoot deformities. **B,** Valgus. **C,** Plantar-flexed first ray. (*A* from Michaud TC: *Foot orthoses,* Baltimore, 1993, Williams & Wilkins.)

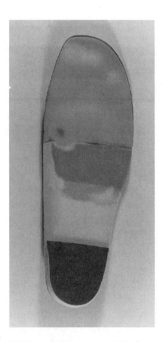

Figure 10-28 2-to-5 bar post with first ray cut out.

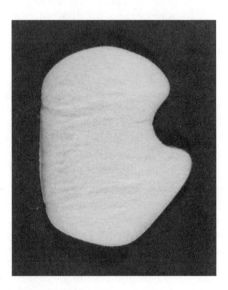

Figure 10-29 Dancer HAPAD to relieve pressure under the first metatarsal head.

and frontal plane movement of the foot and knee. The degree of posting was determined by calcaneal valgus and forefoot varus. The hindfoot varus posting ranged from 2 to 4 degrees and the forefoot varus posting ranged from 4 to 6 degrees.

Other Posting Principles

In painful foot lesions, such as metatarsal head lesions, posting usually is not tolerated. Softer materials, metatarsal pads, or relief cut-outs are used instead.

Posting is contraindicated for an insensate foot. Accommodative orthoses should be used instead.

The rearfoot should always be posted with the forefoot, generally a 2:1 (forefoot:rearfoot) relationship (e.g., 4-degree forefoot post and 2-degree rearfoot post).

REHABILITATION POSTING

A post may be added to encourage ROM, either medially or laterally. This usually is placed at the rearfoot, and often is helpful after prolonged immobilization or traumatic injury with resultant decreased mobility of the STJ. For example, if a patient has limited rearfoot eversion, a rearfoot lateral post may be used to add a prolonged stretch from inversion toward eversion.

Temporary heel lifts may be added to orthoses or onto shoes to decrease stress on the Achilles tendon and plantar fascia during treatment of Achilles tendonitis and plantar fasciitis. A stretching program would be in effect simultaneously.

Permanent heel lifts are used to correct anatomic leg-length differences, decreased ankle-joint dorsiflexion, or chronic resistant plantar heel pain. Heel lifts decrease the need for compensatory subtalar pronation due to tight Achilles tendon. The maximum amount tolerated is 5 to 6 mm.

Summary

The ability to place the foot in STN and evaluate deformity in this position is the cornerstone of proper evaluation and treatment of foot deformity. A sound working knowledge of foot biomechanics, gait cycle components, structural evaluation, and posting principles is required to assess requirements adequately and prescribe appropriate orthotics. We use many of the troubleshooting tips in Table 10-2 for problems with orthotics.

TABLE 10-2 Specific Problems: Probable Causes and Corrective Actions

Location of Discomfort	Possible Causes and Rationale	Corrective Action
Bunion pain increases with use of orthotic.	a. Large rearfoot/forefoot varus post lifting the medial forefoot (and bunion) into shoe gear	a. Reevaluate the need for posting. If the post angles are correct, have the laboratory grind the posts to the shell. This lowers the overall height of the orthotic without affecting function. Another method of treatment is to have a cobbler stretch the leather over the bunion or switch to a shoe with a wider toe box.
Sesamoid pain continues despite use of orthotic.	a. Not enough rearfoot control; the patient continues to pronate excessively, thereby compressing the sesamoids.	a. Consider increasing post angles and/or using a more controlling orthotic. To control propulsive period pronation, the rearfoot posts may be placed beneath the distal edge of the orthotic, and the soles of the shoes may be cut to allow for low-gear push-off.
Sesamoid pain develops with orthotic.	a. Orthotic too long b. Large forefoot valgus post causing forefoot to slide medially	a. Return to laboratory for adjustment or simply taper the distal edge in office. b. Reevaluate need for post. If the post is correct, use Spenco top to prevent slippage.
Distal end of orthotic extension (particularly those that end at sulcus)	a. Overly sensitive soft tissues	a. Have patient wear thick socks until the soft tissues can accommodate the extension or simply taper the plantar surface of the extension. Another consideration is to have the patient rest a flat Spenco insert over the orthotic. (This also serves to cushion the toes.)
Dorsal fifth metatarsal head	a. Large forefoot valgus post lifting lateral forefoot into shoe gear b. A large forefoot varus post causing the patient to slide laterally off the orthotic, jamming the fifth metatarsal head into the shoe c. Incorrect use of a curve-lasted shoe in patient with rectus foot type	a. Have cobbler stretch shoe over fifth metatarsal head (especially if a tailor's bunion is present). b. Reevaluate post angles: if correct, consider adding Spenco top cover to prevent slippage or have patient insert felt strip under tongue of shoe. c. Switch to straight-lasted shoe.
Dorsal first metatarsophalangeal joint pain and/or first interphalangeal joint pain develops with orthotic.	a. Incorrect use of a forefoot varus post. The posting material prevents the normal plantarflexion motions of the first metatarsal necessary for a full range of hallux dorsiflexion. The interphalangeal joint may be injured as it hyperextends to compensate for the limited metatarsophalangeal joint motion. b. Incorrect use of Morton's extension, which also limits the plantarflectory movements of the first metatarsal c. Cast was taken with forefoot supinated.	a. Reevaluate need for forefoot varus post. b. Reevaluate need for Morton's extension. c. Recast patient.

TABLE 10-2 **Specific Problems: Probable Causes and Corrective Actions—cont'd**

Location of Discomfort	Possible Causes and Rationale	Corrective Action
Interdigital neuritis continues despite use of orthotic.	a. Investigate possible pathologic condition in tarsal tunnel or spine (particularly if the interdigital pain is bilateral). b. Patient continues to wear tight-fitting shoes or overly flexible shoes that allow for a range of digital dorsiflexion that tractions the interdigital nerve against the transverse ligament.	a. Order appropriate diagnostic tests. b. Switch to shoes with a more spacious toe box and stiffer soles that lessen the range of digital dorsiflexion. Also, subtle changes in the position of metatarsal pad may have a dramatic effect on reducing interdigital pain.
Medial arch pain develops with orthotic.	a. Rearfoot varus posting is too high. b. Inadequate strength, flexibility, and/or proprioception c. Incorrect choice of material (particularly if rigid shell is used for rigid foot type) d. Full arch height used with equinus foot type: as the midtarsals attempt to compensate for limited ankle dorsiflexion, the plantar medial arch is compressed into the orthotic. e. Negative impression is taken with the STJ supinated.	a. Reevaluate need for posting. Consider softer posting material. b. Increase frequency of treatments and/or home rehabilitation procedures. c. Consider changing materials or add soft top cover to present orthotic. d. Add temporary bilateral heel lifts, have laboratory lower the medial longitudinal arch, and/or use softer materials. e. Have laboratory lower arch. Consider recasting patient.
Medial border of orthotic digging into soft tissues	a. Laboratory error: failure to lower arch for equinus foot type b. Inadequate shoe gear: patient rolling over orthotic c. Inadequate levels of proprioception and/or muscle strength d. Overweight patient with a severe genu valgum deformity	a. Have laboratory lower arch, add bilateral heel lifts, and/or use softer orthotics. b. Change shoe gear and/or remake orthotic with medial flange. c. Correct with appropriate rehabilitation techniques. d. Remake orthotic with medial flange, reinforce shoe gear, strengthen intrinsic musculature.
Plantar fascial/medial arch discomfort continues despite use of orthotic	a. Too little control or tissues too inflamed to tolerate a functional orthotic b. Inadequate strength/flexibility and/or proprioception c. Incorrect diagnosis of mechanical foot pain. The seronegative spondylo-arthropathies often produce symptoms at the medial tuberosity of the calcaneus.	a. Consider using more functional orthotic and/or use low-dye taping procedures with orthotic. b. Increase frequency of treatment and/or home rehabilitation procedures. c. Request appropriate laboratory tests.
Plantar first metatarsal shaft pain at distal end of orthotic	a. Large rearfoot/forefoot varus post lifting medial orthotic into first metatarsal b. Laboratory error, the medial distal edge of device too long	a. Reevaluate need for posting: if correct, have patient wear thick pair of socks until soft tissues accommodate new stress or send to laboratory and add a compressible post to sulcus. (This distributes weight off the metatarsal necks onto the metatarsal heads.) b. Return to laboratory for adjustment (or just grind edge down in office).

Continued

Location of Discomfort	Possible Causes and Rationale	Corrective Action
Tissues over metatarsal pad become uncomfortable	a. Normal part of break-in as tissues accommodate new stresses b. Metatarsal pads too large or poorly positioned, creating bowstring effect on central band of plantar fascia.	a. Proceed more slowly with break-in and/or wear thick pair of socks. b. Return to laboratory for smaller and/or softer pads or for repositioning.
Tarsometatarsal pain after using balance for lesion beneath a painful metatarsal head	a. Normal part of break-in b. Balance too deep, allowing for excessive plantar flexion of involved metatarsal head (thereby straining the proximal tarsometatarsal articulation).	a. Proceed more slowly with break-in. b. Have laboratory partially fill balance, remove if necessary.
Medial, posterior, and/or lateral heel pain at edge of heel cup	a. If the laboratory does not allow for sufficient displacement of calcaneal fat pad when modifying the positive model of a non–weight-bearing impression, the edge of the orthotic heel seat will become a source of chronic irritation as it digs into the displacing soft tissues. Also, shoes with inadequate heel counters may allow for excessive displacement of the fat pad and may therefore be a source of chronic discomfort at the edge of the orthotic.	a. Initially, make sure the shoe's heel counter is firm and snug (consider adding felt to the inside of heel counter) and feather the edge of heel seat at point of irritation. If necessary, return to laboratory for modification (always pinpoint the painful area by marking the edge) and consider requesting a deeper heel seat to allow for improved containment of the fat pad.
Plantar-lateral surface of calcaneus	a. This is frequently a normal part of the break-in process, as a rearfoot varus post will redistribute a greater percentage of ventrical forces toward the lateral heel.	a. Proceed more slowly through break-in. If discomfort continues, reevaluate need for rearfoot posting or use softer material for shell or post.
Plantar-medial surface of calcaneus	a. Too little control. (The patient continues to pronate excessively, jamming the medial condyle into orthotic.) b. Too much control (Overposting with rearfoot varus wedge will compress and irritate the medial plantar heel.) c. Heel height of orthotic is shifting weight to the forefoot, thereby stressing plantar fascia and, in turn, its origin on the medial tuberosity.	a. Increase post angle, check shoe gear, strengthen gastrocnemius/soleus and tibialis posterior. b. Reevaluate post angle; consider softer posting material. c. Test by having patient walk on toes for 30 seconds: if heel symptoms increase, remove heel lifts and grind the rearfoot posts into the shells.
Lateral heel pain at edge of heel cup	a. Patient slides off orthotic because of large varus post.	a. Reevaluate need for post. Consider adding Spenco cover to prevent slippage. Also, check fit of heel counter.
Achilles tendonitis develops or continues, despite use of the orthotic.	a. Orthotic under- or overposted with resultant misalignment of rearfoot and leg b. Failure to lower medial arch for equinus foot type; this increases workload on the Achilles tendon as midtarsal compensation is disallowed.	a. Reevaluate post angles. b. Lower medial arch of orthotic, add bilateral heel lifts, and/or use softer orthotics.
Soleus strain develops with orthotic.	a. Incorrect use of forefoot valgus post: the faulty post is prematurely locking the midtarsal joint prior to heel lift, thereby preventing the rearfoot from inverting to its vertical position. The soleus muscle is constantly strained as it attempts to bring the rearfoot to vertical by lifting the entire medial foot up and over the oversized forefoot valgus post.	a. Remove post and stretch soleus.

TABLE 10-2 **Specific Problems: Probable Causes and Corrective Actions—cont'd**

Location of Discomfort	Possible Causes and Rationale	Corrective Action
Medial tibial stress reaction continues despite use of orthotic.	a. Too little control	a. Reevaluate post angles, orthotic selection (consider more controlling orthotic), shoe gear, and casting technique. (Consider neutral position technique.)
	b. Inadequate strength, flexibility, and/or proprioception	b. Reevaluate treatment program.
	c. Problem not mechanical, rule out vascular disorder.	c. Reevaluate patient; consider referral if necessary.
Peroneous longus and/or brevis discomfort develops with orthotic.	a. Normal part of break-in as peroneals attempt to accommodate rearfoot varus post.	a. Slow down break-in and incorporate peroneal stretches.
	b. Excessive rearfoot varus post straining peroneus brevis as it attempts to bring the subtalar joint back to its neutral position	b. Reevaluate post angles.
	c. Incorrect use of forefoot varus post: the faulty post inverts forefoot during late midstance, thereby unlocking the midtarsal joint. Peroneus longus, by virtue of its insertion into the base of the first metatarsal, attempts to stabilize the midtarsals by forcefully plantar flexing the first metatarsal (which would evert the forefoot and lock the midtarsal joint). However, resistance from the post prevents this action and is thereby responsible for chronically straining this muscle.	c. Remove post.
Medial knee (typically a pes anserine bursitis) and/or retropatellar discomfort continue despite use of orthotic.	a. Too little control; the subtalar joint continues to pronate excessively. This most frequently results from use of an overly flexible shell with a hypermobile foot type and/or inadequate shoe gear.	a. Reevaluate post angles. Consider a more controlling orthotic and check shoe gear (especially the fit of the heel counter).
High-impact symptoms continue, despite use of orthotic.	a. Inadequate posting of rigid forefoot valgus/plantar-flexed first ray, allowing for continued supinatory compensation by the STJ	a. Increase post angles as needed and consider adding shock-absorbing material beneath the heel.
High-impact symptoms develop with orthotic: typically, lateral knee pain (a diffuse bony ache) and/or chronic sacroiliac instability.	a. Normal part of break-in as tissues attempt to accommodate new stresses	a. Proceed more slowly with break-in.
	b. Too much control: the orthotic is disallowing the amount of subtalar pronation necessary to absorb shock. This may result from excessive rearfoot/forefoot varus posting, faulty casting technique (especially if STJ was supinated), and/or incorrect choice of materials, e.g., a rigid orthotic was used to treat a rigid foot type.	b. Reevaluate post angles, consider having lab lower the medial arch (or recast), and/or switch to a softer orthotic.

*Modified from Langer S: *Langer Biomechanics Newsletter,* 14(2):4, 1987.

Bibliography

Axe MJ, Ray RL: Orthotic treatment of sesamoid pain, *Am J Sports Med* 16:411, 1988.

Bates PT et al: Foot orthotic devices to modify selected aspects of lower extremity mechanics, *Am J Sports Med* 7:338, 1979.

Blake RL, Denton JA: Functional foot orthoses for athletic injuries, *J Am Podiatr Med Assoc* 75:359, 1985.

Clarke TE, Frederick EC, Hamill CL: The effects of shoe design parameters on rearfoot control in running, *Med Sci Sports Exerc* 15:376, 1983.

Clement DB: A survey of overuse running injuries, *Phys Sports Med* 9:47, 1981.

D'Ambrosia RD: Orthotic devices in running injuries, *Clin Sports Med* 4:611, 1985.

Donatelli R: Abnormal biomechanics of the foot and ankle, *J Orthop Sports Phys Ther* 9:11, 1987.

Donatelli R: *The biomechanics of the foot and ankle,* Philadelphia, 1990, FA Davis.

Donatelli R et al: Biomechanical foot orthotics: a retrospective study, *J Orthop Sports Phys Ther* 10:205, 1988.

Donatelli R, Wooden MJ, editors: *Orthopaedic physical therapy,* New York, 1989, Churchill Livingstone.

Doxey GE: Clinical use and fabrication of molded thermoplastic foot orthotic devices, *Phys Ther* 65:1679, 1985.

Eng JJ, Plerynowski MR: Evaluation of soft foot orthoses in the treatment of patellofemoral pain syndrome, *Phys Ther* 73:62, 1993.

Graves SC, Badwey TH, Graves KO: Biomechanics and orthotics of the foot in athletes, *Oper Tech Sports Med* 2:2, 1994.

Jahss MH: *Disorders of the foot and ankle: medical and surgical management,* ed 2, Philadelphia, 1991, WB Saunders.

Johanson MA et al: Effects of three different posting methods on controlling abnormal subtalar pronation, *Phys Ther* 74(2):149, 1994.

Lockard MA: Foot orthoses, *Phys Ther* 68:1866, 1988.

Lutter LD: Running athletes in office practice, *Foot Ankle* 3:153, 1982.

Mann RA: Biomechanical approach to the treatment of foot problems, *Foot Ankle* 2:205, 1982.

Marshall RN: Foot mechanics and joggers' injuries, *NZ Med J* 88:288, 1978.

McPoil TG Jr: The foot and ankle: biomechanical evaluation and treatment. In Gould J, editor: *Orthopaedic and sports physical therapy,* ed 2, St. Louis, 1990, Mosby–Year Book.

McPoil TG, Knecht HG: Biomechanics of the foot in walking: a functional approach, *J Orthop Sports Phys Ther* 7:69, 1985.

Nigg BM, Morlock M: The influence of lateral heel flare of running shoes on pronation and impact forces, *Med Sci Sports Exerc* 19:294, 1987.

Root ML, Orien WP, Weed JN: *Clinical biomechanics. Normal and abnormal function of the foot, vol 2,* Los Angeles, 1977, Clinical Biomechanics.

Tiberio D: Pathomechanics of structural foot deformities, *Phys Ther* 68:1840, 1988.

CHAPTER ELEVEN

Low Back Disorders

ARTHUR H. WHITE, MD
S. BRENT BROTZMAN, MD

Rehabilitation Rationale

The accurate, objective study of low back pain, its natural history, and effective treatment is difficult because of the multiple factors involved, such as the favorable natural history of low back pain, regardless of treatment, the presence of secondary gain in Western societies, and the methodologic problems in setting up studies.

Low back disability appears to have dramatically increased in Western society over the last 30 years. Waddell concluded, however, that this is not indicative of an increase in injuries or in the occurrence of low back pain, but rather of an increase in work loss, sick certification, compensation, and long-term disability award.

ACUTE BACK PAIN

Acute back pain is common, affecting between 70% and 85% of adults at some point in their lives. Back complaints are second only to upper respiratory conditions as a cause of work absenteeism. An estimated 1.3 billion days a year are lost from work because of back pain. The usual onset of low back pain is in the third decade of life, with the peak prevalence during the fifth decade.

Some risk factors have become evident. Nondisabling low back pain is three times more common in pregnant women than in their nonparous counterparts. Cigarette smoking has been found to be a possible risk factor for low back pain, as well as low back pain with concomitant sciatica due to lumbar disc herniation. Occupational risk factors associated with an increased risk of developing acute low back pain or delayed recovery include (1) employees' perceptions of their jobs as boring, dissatisfying, or repetitious, (2) an unpleasant or noisy work environment, (3) perception of poor social support in the work environment with regard to employer/employee interaction, and (4) the employer's perception of the employee as less competent.

Eighty percent to 90% of patients with acute low back pain episodes recover in about 6 weeks, regardless of the administration or type of treatment. Nearly 60% of patients return to work within 1 week. In patients whose symptoms of chronic back pain result in continued work loss, the likelihood of returning to work 6 months after an episode is 50%, by 1 year 20%, and at 2 years the probability of return approaches 0%. The return-to-work rate is significantly diminished with the presence of a lawyer or threatened legal action. The rate of recurrence after an acute low back pain episode ranges from 40% to 85%.

CHRONIC BACK PAIN

Currently, it is estimated that 5.2 million people in the United States are chronically disabled because of low back pain (half permanently, half temporarily). This group of patients produces 80% to 90% of the costs of low back pain. Chronic disability has been associated with psychosocial dysfunction, multiple painful conditions (e.g., headache), and psychosocial profiles indicative of depression, hysteria, and hypochondriasis, on various cross-sectional surveys. In the Boeing study, Spengler et al. showed HY and HS scales on the Minnesota Multiphasic Personality Inventory (MMPI) were predictive of later disability; however, a predictive risk model did not demonstrate this predictive value.

Chronic pain is a completely different clinical syndrome than acute pain. Chronic pain, chronic disability, and chronic illness behavior, in contrast to acute pain, become increasingly dissociated from their original physical basis. Instead, they become increasingly associated with emotional distress, depression, failed treatment, and adoption of a sick role. Once a patient reaches the physician, medical assessment and treatment of low back pain appears to be influenced more by the patient's illness behavior and distress than the actual physical disorder.

SCIATICA, DISC HERNIATION

Surgery for sciatica has been shown to hasten the initial recovery (demonstrated by return to work and reduction of symptoms), but has minimal influence on the risk of recurrence, ultimate functional status, or residual symptoms. In cross-sectional studies that demonstrate a lifetime incidence of 40% of sciatica, the lifetime incidence of lumbar disc surgery ranges from 1% to 2%.

Maigne et al. prospectively followed the natural history of 48 patients with lumbar disc herniations treated by conservative means. The disc herniations were evaluated by serial CT scans. Follow-up revealed that most herniations spontaneously decreased in size with conservative treatment. The largest herniations had the greatest tendency to decrease in size. Nine of the herniations decreased by at least 25%, eight between 50% and 75%, and 31 between 75% to 100%; several completely disappeared.

Evaluation

RADIOGRAPHIC EVALUATION

Eight controlled studies and two reviews have shown little, if any, relationship between clinical symptoms and degenerative changes on lumbar radiographs. Radiographs of patients with acute low back pain of in-

sidious onset (no history of trauma) typically yield little additional information. Liang and Komaroff, as well as Deyo and Diehl, outlined the indications for radiographic evaluation of patients with acute low back pain (Table 11-1).

PHYSICAL EXAMINATION

Physical examination of a patient with low back pain is essential to establish the clinical diagnosis (see box), to plan diagnostic testing, and to initiate appropriate treatment.

TABLE 11-1 Indications for Spinal Radiographs in Patients with Acute Low Back Pain

Indication	Significance
Age greater than 50 years	Risk of tumor, severe degeneration
History of trauma	Fracture likely
History of osteoporosis	Compression fracture
Known primary cancer	Spinal metastasis
Unrelenting pain at rest	Spinal cancer or infection
Unexplained weight loss	Spinal cancer or infection
History of corticosteroids	Increased risk of spinal infection
Organ recipient	
AIDS	
Diabetes mellitus	
Drug abuse	
Alcohol abuse	Increased risk of spinal fracture
Findings suggestive of spondylolysis	
Neurologic deficit	Rule out bony, tumor, or infectious cause

From Frymoyer JW, Nachemson A: *Natural history of low back disorders.* In Frymoyer JW, editor: The adult spine: principles and practice, New York, 1991, Raven Press.

Common Causes of Low Back Pain

- Musculoskeletal strain
- Vertebral compression fracture
- Spinal stenosis
- Ruptured intervertebral disc (HNP)
- Spondylolysis/spondylolisthesis
- Hip pathology
- Sacroiliac joint pathology
- Renal pathology
- Vertebral osteomyelitis/epidural abscess
- Tumor
- Aneurysm

Patients should be examined standing, sitting, and lying prone and supine. In addition to the usual observation, palpation, measurements, and muscle testing, several special diagnostic maneuvers are helpful for patients with low back pain.

The *straight leg raise* (Lasègue sign) is a well-known and generally accepted test of disc protrusion. Although it may suggest disc herniation and/or sciatic nerve irritation, it is not diagnostic alone. With the patient supine, each leg is passively raised to approximately 90 degrees (unless limited by pain). At the point of pain, the foot is gently dorsiflexed; this further stretches the sciatic nerve and should worsen the pain. A lack of response indicates that the patient's problem may not affect the lumbar roots.

A variation of this test is to straighten out the leg as the patient sits on the examining table for examination of the knee and foot. Patients with a true abnormality will lean back as the leg is straightened to relieve pressure on the nerve, or will not allow the leg to be straightened at all. In some patients, raising the uninvolved leg causes discomfort on the involved side. This is referred to as the "crossed straight leg raising sign," and is further evidence of a protruding disc or other space-occupying lesion.

Sacroiliac joint evaluation is performed with the patient supine. The examiner's thumbs are placed on the anterior-superior iliac spines with the hands on the iliac crest, and compression is applied toward the midline. If the patient complains of pain around the sacroiliac joints, this may indicate a pathologic condition in that area. The sacroiliac joints should also be palpated. Compression rarely evokes pain in patients whose pathologic condition lies elsewhere.

Patrick test, or the *figure-four test*, is performed to identify pathologic conditions both of the hips and the sacroiliac joints. With the patient supine, the foot of the involved side is placed on the opposite knee. If this position elicits inguinal pain, a pathologic condition in the hip or surrounding muscles may be present. To stress the sacroiliac joint, the examiner places one hand on the patient's knee and the other hand on the anterior-superior iliac spine of the opposite side, then presses as if opening a book.

Burns test is performed by having the patient kneel on a chair and try to touch the floor. The kneeling position relieves stress on the lower back and tension on the sciatic nerve. Even patients with disc herniation and sciatica usually can perform this test; the malingerer, on the other hand, will probably claim to be unable to perform this maneuver because it causes too much pain.

Response to *disc pressure* is an important indication of an acute herniated disc (HNP). Patients with HNP are typically most comfortable in a recumbent position, less comfortable standing, and least comfortable sitting. Nachemson's intradiscal pressure studies in living subjects suggest the reason for this: intradiscal pressure increases progressively from supine, standing, and sitting postures. Side-lying also has a notable increase in intradiscal pressure.

Nachemson's studies showed that active extension of the back in the prone position increases intradiscal pressure (Fig. 11-1), and *McKenzie* emphasizes *passive* back extension in his exercise regimen (Fig. 11-2). Extension allows the viscoelastic disc to "milk forward" (Fig. 11-3, *B*), but prevents any free (extruded) disc fragment from migrating anteriorly (Fig. 11-3, *D*). Increased nerve-root pressure by constriction at the intervertebral foramen may increase radicular pain. Any radicular pain increase with extension is a contraindication to extension therapy, but an initial increase in localized back pain only with extension therapy is not a contraindication and, in fact, may be expected.

Williams flexion exercises have been used for both low back pain and HNP (Fig. 11-4). Nachemson's demonstration that Williams' first exercise increased intradiscal pressure to 210% over standing appears to contradict the use of these exercises in patients with HNP. In fact, three of the six exercises in the Williams regimen were found to increase intradiscal pressures significantly.

Treatment

The goals of treatment of acute low back pain are shown in the box. Most patients with low back pain can be successfully treated with conservative measures. The most commonly used treatment methods are bed rest and exercise.

BED REST

Bed rest is the most frequently used treatment for low back pain. The traditional rationale for bed rest is twofold: (1) many patients with mechanical low back pain, as well as those with HNP, report symptomatic relief in the supine position, and (2) measurements indicate that intradiscal pressure is minimized in the supine

---

Goals of Treatment of Acute Low Back Pain

- Alleviate pain
- Promote healing of injured tissue
- Relieve muscle spasm
- Restore normal range of motion (ROM), spinal mechanics, and muscle function
- Educate patient to prevent further episodes
- Return patient to activities of daily living/workplace

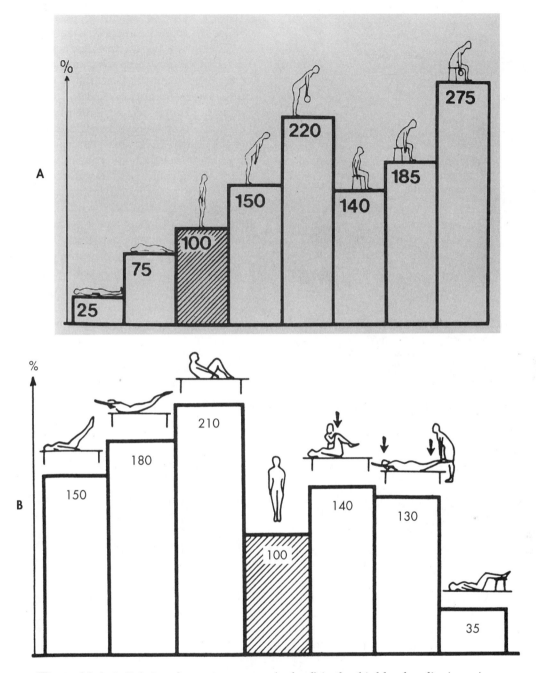

Figure 11-1 **A**, Relative change in pressure (or load) in the third lumbar disc in various positions in living subjects. **B**, Relative change in pressure (or load) in the third lumbar disc in various muscle-strengthening exercises in living subjects. (From Nachemson A: *The lumbar spine, an orthopaedic challenge*, Spine 1:59, 1976.)

position. However, nearly 50% of patients with back pain report only minimal relief with bed rest, and intradiscal pressure rises to 75% of that in the standing position when patients simply roll onto their side.

Comparison of 2 days of bed rest to 7 days of bed rest in outpatient-clinic patients with acute low back pain revealed equally prompt pain resolution and return of function, but those given the shorter bed rest recommendation returned to work 45% sooner (3.1 versus 5.6 days). Thus, it appears that in patients with

no neuromotor deficits, 2 days of bed rest are as effective as longer periods. A similar study compared 4 days of bed rest to no bed rest in 270 patients. Those with no bed rest returned to their usual activities 42% faster than those with 4 days of bed rest. Gilbert et al. found no statistically significant differences between bed rest, exercise, and no treatment, although the results tended to favor early mobilization.

■ *These studies suggest that although bed rest may provide some symptomatic relief for patients with acute low back*

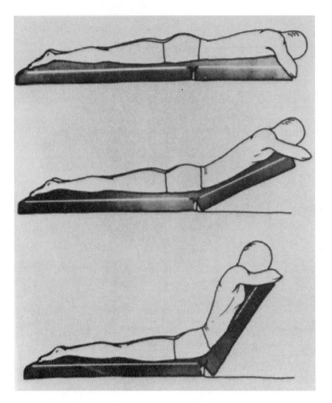

Figure 11-2 Passive extension using table. (From Kopp JR et al: *Clin Orthop* 202:211, 1986.)

pain, a brief period (if any) should be sufficient. Bed rest does not appear to alter the natural history of recovery.

Bed rest also has medical and social side effects. According to Deyo, these may include perception of severe illness (even myocardial infarction does not require a week of strict bed rest); economic loss (absenteeism is strongly related to bed rest); muscle atrophy (1% to 1.5% per day); cardiopulmonary deconditioning (15% in 10 days); and acute complications such as thromboembolism, bone mineral loss, hypercalcemia, and hypercalciuria. To prevent deconditioning, many experts now recommend at least a brief daily ambulation for patients with HNP, with or without neurologic deficit, after 3 days of bed rest. Several studies have demonstrated improved disc nutrition with motion.

Compliance is also a problem. Most patients sit to read or watch television, raising intradiscal pressure to a level higher than that in a standing position.

EXERCISE PROGRAMS

Several exercise programs have been developed for acute low back pain. These include those designed by McKenzie (mainly extension exercises), Williams, Aston, Heller, and Feldenkreis, and other lumbar stabilization programs, stretching regimens, and aerobic conditioning programs.

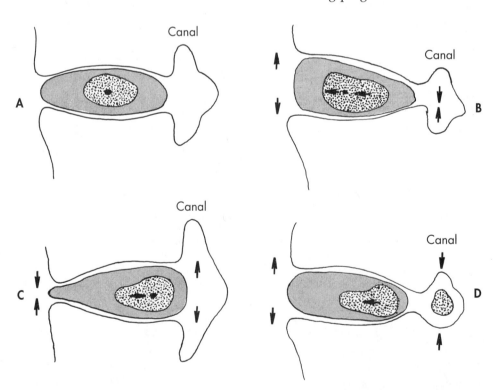

Figure 11-3 A, The nucleus pulposus with spine in neutral. **B,** The nucleus pulposus with the spine in extension. **C,** The nucleus pulposus with the spine in flexion. **D,** Extension with extruded fragment. The fragment cannot return through the incompetent anulus fibrosus and, as a consequence, must share the narrowed foramen with nerve root, increasing symptoms. (Redrawn from McKenzie RA: *The lumbar spine: mechanical diagnosis in therapy,* Waidanae, NZ, 1981, Spinal.)

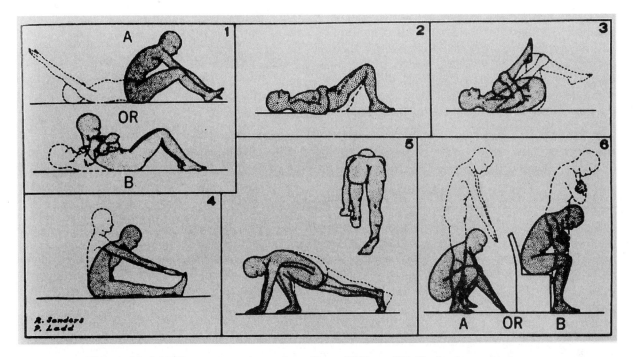

Figure 11-4 Williams postural exercises. (From Williams PC: *The lumbosacral spine, emphasizing conservative management*, New York, 1965, McGraw-Hill.)

McKenzie Technique

The McKenzie technique is one of the most popular of the many conservative care programs. It is a method of diagnosis and treatment based on movement patterns of the spine. For any spinal condition, certain movements aggravate the pain and other movements relieve the pain. Because the McKenzie method works best for acute back pain that responds to lumbar extension, mobilization, and exercises, the technique has been erroneously labeled an extension exercise program. McKenzie, in fact, advocates position and movement patterns, flexion or extension, that best relieve the patient's symptoms.

McKenzie's method is complex and much has been written explaining its theoretical basis. In his text, *The Lumbar Spine: Mechanical Diagnosis and Therapy*, he classifies low back pain based on spinal movement patterns, positions, and pain responses, and describes a postural syndrome, derangement, and dysfunction. Each classification has a specific treatment that includes education and some form of postural correction. A basic explanation of the method is as follows. Some stages of the lumbar degenerative cascade create symptoms because of pathoanatomic abnormalities, which can be positively altered by spinal positioning. This hypothesis has led to several forms of spinal manipulation, including chiropractic and osteopathy. The McKenzie technique is a more passive form of spinal manipulation in which the patient produces the motion, position, and forces that improve the condition. Examples of pathoanatomic alterations include a tear in the anulus and acute facet arthritis. Repeated

lumbar extension may reduce edema and nuclear migration in an anular tear or may realign a facet joint in such a way as to reduce inflammation and painful stimuli. Through trial and error, the position and exercise program that best relieve the patient's symptoms can be found.

Cyclic ROM exercises (usually in passive extension) are the cornerstone of the McKenzie program. These repetitive exercises "centralize" pain, and certain postures prevent end-range stress. Lumbar flexion exercises may be added later, when the patient has full spinal ROM.

Treatment is based on evaluation of pain location and maneuvers that change the pain location from referred to centralized. Once identified, the direction of exercise and movement (such as extension) is used for treatment. Centralization, as McKenzie uses the term, refers to a rapid change in perceived location of pain from a distal or peripheral location to a proximal or central one. Donelson et al. reported centralization of asymmetric or radiating pain in 87% of patients during the first 48 hours of care.

For a movement to eventually centralize pain, it must be performed repetitively, because the initial movement often aggravates or intensifies the pain. Centralization also occurs more rapidly if the initial movements are performed passively to end range. Centralization most frequently occurs as a result of extension movement, occasionally from lateral movements, and only rarely with flexion.

McKenzie reported that 98% of patients with symptoms for less than 4 weeks who experienced centralization during their initial assessment had excellent or good results; 77% of patients with subacute symptoms (4 to 12 weeks) had excellent or good results if their pain centralized initially.

The great value of this program is that it gives patients an understanding of their condition and responsibility for maintaining proper alignment and func-tion. Disadvantages are that the program requires active, willing participation of the patient, who must have the ability to centralize the pain; better results are obtained for patients with acute pain than for those with chronic pain, and the complex regimen requires a therapist trained in McKenzie's techniques to obtain the best results.

REHABILITATION PROTOCOL

Acute Low Back Pain MCKENZIE

McKenzie recommends implementation of this protocol by a therapist with specialized training in the McKenzie method to ensure proper recognition and correct implementation of treatment in response to the patient's clinical relief derived from specific maneuvers. To determine which exercises produce centralization, the physical therapist tests the patient with a standardized series of lumbar movements, such as flexion, extension, lateral bending, rotation, and side-gliding (a combination of lateral bending and rotation). Once the therapist identifies the movement (usually extension or lateral bending) that decreases peripheral symptoms, the patient is taught to perform an individualized exercise program in that direction of movement. The movement is performed repetitively to the passive end range. Maneuvers that "peripheralize" or exacerbate symptoms are discontinued.

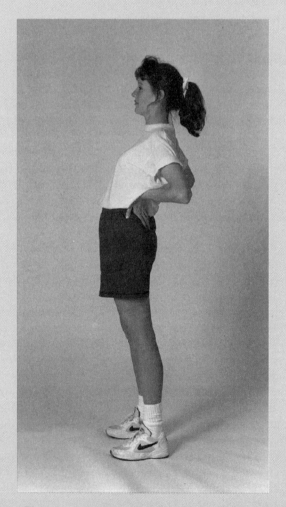

Figure 11-5 Extension in a standing posture.

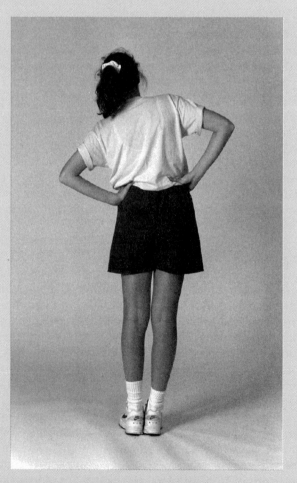

Figure 11-6 Side-gliding.

REHABILITATION PROTOCOL—cont'd

Repeat End-Range Movements While Standing
Back bending (extension) (Fig. 11-5):
The patient stands upright with feet slightly apart (A). Place the hands on the small of the back with fingers pointing backward. The patient then bends backward (from the waist) as far as possible, using the hands as a fulcrum (B). Keep the knees straight. Hold this position for 1 to 2 seconds, then the patient returns to the starting position. This exercise incorporates the effect of gravity because it is performed in an upright position.
- Side gliding (Fig. 11-6),
- Forward bending (lumbar flexion)

Recumbent End-Range Movements
- Passive extension while prone (Fig. 11-7):
  In this exercise, the patient lies face down, with hands positioned under the shoulders (A), then pushes up by slowly extending the elbows (B) while keeping the pelvis, hips, and legs relaxed (this allows the back to sag). Maintain this position for 1 to 2 seconds, then the patient slowly lowers the upper body to the floor. This exercise eliminates the loading effects of gravity because it is performed prone.
- Knees-to-chest while supine (Fig. 11-8):
  The patient lies supine, with knees flexed and feet flat on the floor or bed (A). Patient places the hands around the knees (B) and slowly pulls both knees up toward the chest as far as possible (C). This position is maintained for 1 to 2 seconds, then the patient slowly lowers the feet back to the starting position. The patient must not raise the head while performing this exercise or straighten the legs while lowering them.

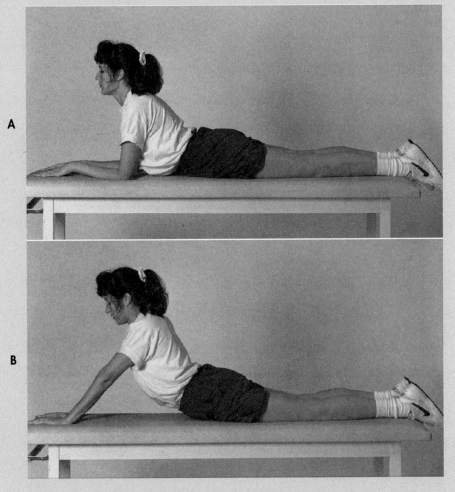

Figure 11-7 Passive extension while prone.

Continued

Acute Low Back Pain MCKENZIE

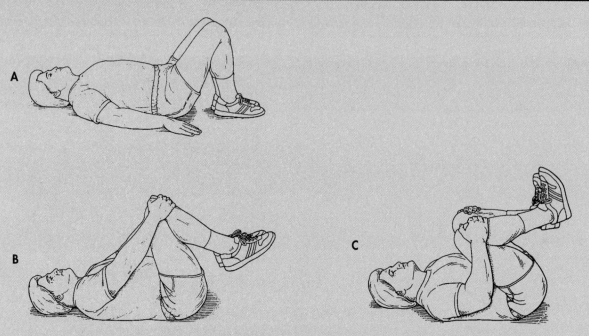

Figure 11-8 Knees-to-chest while supine. (From Dimaggio A, Mooney V: The McKenzie program: exercise effective against back pain, *J Musculo Med* p. 63, Dec 1987.)

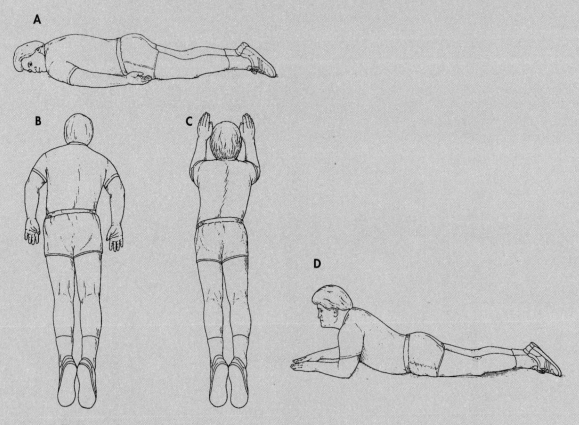

Figure 11-9 Lateral movement with extension. (From Dimaggio A, Mooney V: The McKenzie program: exercise effective against back pain, *J Musculo Med* p. 63, Dec 1987.)

REHABILITATION PROTOCOL—cont'd

• Prone lateral shifting of hips off midline (Fig. 11-9) (patients with unilateral symptoms):
The patient lies face down, arms at sides *(A)*, moves hips away from the side of pain and maintains this position for a few seconds *(B)*. With the hips off center, the patient then places the elbows under the shoulders and leans on the forearms *(C and D)*; the patient relaxes in this position for 3 or 4 minutes. The patient can then perform the maneuver "extension while lying prone," keeping the hips off center

• Flexion while sitting (Fig. 11-10):
The patient sits on the edge of a steady chair or stool, with legs apart and hands resting on knees *(A)*. The patient bends forward from the waist to touch the floor with the hands. The patient holds this position for 1 to 2 seconds and then slowly returns to upright. Once able to bend forward comfortably, the patient can hold onto the ankles and pull self further down *(B)*.

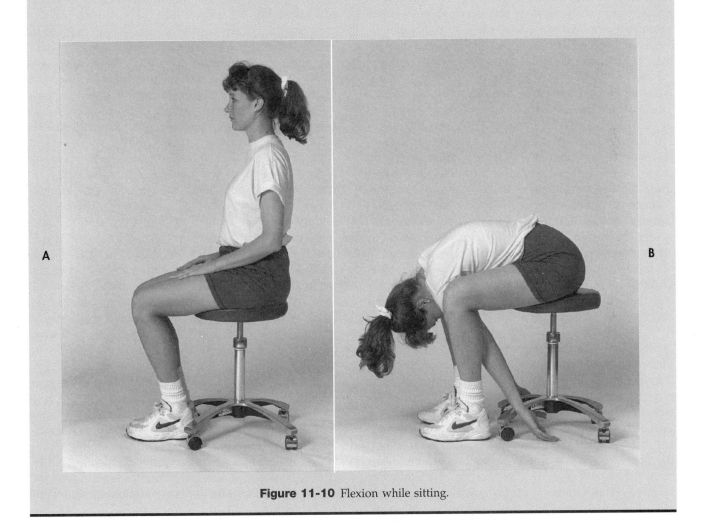

Figure 11-10 Flexion while sitting.

Each movement is taken to its end range repetitively as long as distal pain continues to diminish. McKenzie stresses the importance of taking the movements to the end range permitted by the patient to accurately observe changes in the pain pattern. If distal symptoms worsen, that specific movement is discontinued. Pain location from these maneuvers are carefully observed and recorded.

Based on the clinical response to centralization, the patient is taught to perform home spinal exercises in that direction of movement (usually extension). For example, for a patient with acute pain, the self-care exercise program may include prone extension for a few seconds at a time, with sets of 10 repetitions performed every hour or two. The patient is also taught modified resting positions (for sitting, standing, and lying) and work postures that will maintain central-ization and avoid peripheralization.

Most patients have centralization of pain in the first 2 days or sooner. Treatment outcomes in "centralizers" are typically good.

McKenzie classified lumbar movements that have the potential to centralize symptoms into extension, flexion, lateral bending, rotation, and side-gliding (combination of lateral bending and rotation). These may be used individually or in combination to diminish the peripheral pain. Gravity-elimination (prone) versus gravity-assisted (standing) symptom reduction further increases the number of lumbar-movement combinations that the therapist must understand and possibly use in an effort to centralize symptoms. The result is that more than 40 different exercise regimens are available, and application of the appropriate regimen may require complex customization.

Williams Flexion Exercises (see Fig. 11-4)
The goals of this isometric flexion regimen, developed in the 1930s, are to (1) widen the intervertebral foramina and facet joint to reduce nerve compression, (2) stretch hip flexors and back extensors, (3) strengthen abdominal and gluteal muscles, and (4) reduce "posterior fixation" of the lumbosacral junction. A concern with this method is that certain flexion maneuvers increase intradiscal pressure, possibly aggravating herniated or bulging discs. According to Nachemson, Williams' first exercise increases intradiscal pressure to 210% over that in a standing posture. Three of the six exercises increase intradiscal pressure, and these three are contraindicated for patients with acute herniated disc.

Lumbar Stabilization Programs
There is no evidence that early return to activity increases the likelihood of recurrences. On the contrary, physically fit individuals have fewer and shorter attacks of low back pain and are more tolerant of pain. With a better understanding of spinal biomechanics, specific activities and positions that increase loads on the spine can be avoided. Numerous studies have shown that patients with low back pain can perform selected activities almost normally without increasing pain. Body mechanics that avoid painful positions are called cautious or preventative body mechanics. Body mechanics that attempt to overcome the condition with muscular effort and knowledge of body positions has led to the field of stabilization training.

Back schools, which gained prominence in the 1970s, gave education and training in cautious or pre-

ventative body mechanics for routine daily activities, but they did not provide techniques for heavy laborers or for high-performance athletes, who require dynamic, ballistic body mechanics for high-level activities. Practitioners with backgrounds in martial arts or sports training, and some therapists with European influences in training, developed stabilization training primarily for these patients.

The basic premise of stabilization training is that an individual with back pain (considered an unstable condition) can be taught to stabilize the painful pathologic condition through muscular development and movement patterns that allow painless return to a higher-than-normal level of functional activities. Stabilization training incorporates almost all aspects of conservative treatment: education, body mechanics, manual therapy, the McKenzie technique, Williams' exercises, yoga, martial arts, work hardening, and functional restoration. The techniques of stabilization training have been extensively demonstrated in many texts and videotapes, and the techniques are used by many therapists who treat high-performance athletes with back problems.

The main goal of the lumbar stabilization program is to build musculature that stabilizes the torso, with co-contraction of abdominal muscles to provide a corseting effect on the lumbar spine. This concept is centered on the assumption that an injured lumbar motion segment may create a weak link in the kinetic chain, with subsequent predisposition to reinjury. This program is used in conjunction with other methods aimed at controlling acute pain (such as nonsteroidal antiinflammatory medication). Emphasis is on positioning the spine in a nonpainful orientation, termed the *neutral spine.* Stretching and ROM exercises are then completed daily in this configuration. Supervision by an appropriately oriented trainer is advised.

The *second phase* of treatment consists of active joint mobilization methods, including extension exercises in prone and standing positions, and alternating midrange flexion extension in a four-point stance. Simple curl-ups for abdominal muscle strengthening is progressed to dynamic abdominal raising. This includes "dead bug" exercises, using alternate arm and leg movements while supine. Diagonal curl-ups and incline board work are performed.

Progression to aerobic exercise, exercise with a ball, and weight training may be added (see box). The program endpoint is determined by *maximal functional improvement,* the point beyond which no further improvement in function will result from additional exercise.

Exercise Training in the Lumbar Stabilization Program

Soft Tissue Flexibility
- Hamstring musculotendinous unit
- Quadriceps musculotendinous unit
- Iliopsoas musculotendinous unit
- Gastrocnemius-soleus musculotendinous unit
- External and internal hip rotators

Joint Mobility
- Lumbar spine segmental mobility
  Extension
  Flexion (unloaded)
- Hip range of motion
- Thoracic segmental mobility

Stabilization Program
- Finding neutral position
  Standing
  Sitting
  Jumping
  Prone
- Prone gluteal squeezes
  With arm raises
  With alternate arm raises
  With leg raises
  With alternate leg raises
  With arm and leg raises
  With alternate arm and leg raises
- Supine pelvic bracing
- Bridging progression
  Basic position

One leg raised with ankle weights
  Stepping
  Balance on gym ball
- Quadruped
  With alternating arm and leg movements
- Kneeling stabilization
  Double knee
  Single knee
  Lunges, with and without weight
- Wall-slide quadriceps strengthening
- Position transition with postural control
  Abdominal program
    Curl-ups
    Dead bug, supported and unsupported
    Diagonal curl-ups
    Diagonal curl-ups on incline board
    Straight leg lowering
  Gym program
    Latissimus pull-downs
    Angled leg press
    Lunges
    Hyperextension bench
    General upper body weight exercises
  Aerobic program
    Progressive walking
    Swimming
    Stationary bicycling
    Cross-country ski machine
    Running
      Initially supervised on a treadmill

From Frymoyer JW: *The adult spine: principles and practice,* New York, 1991, Raven Press.

REHABILITATION PROTOCOL

Acute, Mechanical Lower Lumbar Pain

Indications	• Symptoms of less than 6 weeks' duration • Prior examination and evaluation to correctly diagnose mechanical low back pain and rule out other etiology	Exercise	• Encourage early ambulation to limit muscular and cardiovascular deconditioning. • Restrict (limited duty) from lifting, climbing, squatting, strenuous physical activity during the initial acute pain period. • Institute the McKenzie back exercise program if available (see p. 377). Some physicians prefer the Williams' flexion exercise regimen.
Bed rest	• We do not recommend bed rest (p. 374). For the occasional patient who has had success with this type of treatment and is adamant about using it, we recommend only 2 days of supine (not lying on the side) bed-rest.		• After the acute pain has subsided (typically within 2 weeks), begin further aerobic conditioning in an effort to improve spine, abdominal, and lower extremity muscular endurance.
Medication	• Give nonsteroidal antiinflammatory medication unless contraindicated. Discuss the risks, warning signs, and possible complications with the patient. • Muscle-relaxant medications may be beneficial, but their use should be strictly time limited (typically 1 week).		• Avoid exercise that places major torsion or flexion forces on the spine (such as rowing). Can use swimming, stationary bicycling, and walking.

Continued

Acute, Mechanical Lower Lumbar Pain

Exercise —cont'd	• Exercise sessions should be at least 20 minutes per session with 3 or more weekly sessions.
Education	• The patient receives instruction on avoiding movements and postures associated with back injury (Fig. 11-11): AVOID: Frequent lifting (25 times/ day) Twisting while lifting Heavy lifting (11.3 kg or more) Improper static postures Forward bending and twisting of the trunk Muscle fatigue

■ *The most deleterious of these motions appears to be simultaneous twisting and forward bending of the trunk. Kelsey et al. report a sixfold increase in back injuries as a result of this motion.*

	• Discuss manual material handling methods, including maintaining the load close to the body and avoiding twisting motions.
	• No scientific evidence supports the assertion that those in poor physical condition are prone to back injury. Despite this, training in strength and fitness should be encouraged, with emphasis on aerobic capacity, endurance, flexibility, musculoskeletal strength, and cardiovascular fitness. The patient may be progressed to a lumbar stabilization program (see p. 383).
Life-style	• Encourage eating-habit modification and proper dieting. Deyo reported that individuals in upper fifth quintile of weight are at greater risk for back pain.
	• The effect of cigarette smoke on invertebral disc metabolism remains unclear. Tobacco-use studies are varied in their findings with regard to the effect of tobacco on acute back pain. One study revealed no relationship, whereas another showed predictive value for future disability in a group of healthy subjects.
Back school	• Formalized back education programs that train patients in manual materials handling, ergonomics, and stress management have had varying results. Back school should be considered for patients whose work environment points to possible benefit from such training.

Rehabilitation After Disc (HNP) Surgery

The postoperative care of patients after disc surgery is dramatically changing. Medical economics and managed care are stimulating a strong movement toward shorter hospital stays and less expense, while minimally invasive surgery is allowing rapid rehabilitation with little or no hospitalization and almost immediate return to work. However, the criteria for the various types of minimally invasive surgery are rigid. Some HNPs require extensive surgical exposure. Postoperative care depends on the pathoanatomic abnormalities, the surgical procedure, and the individual resources of the patient.

Operative procedures with the least amount of tissue disruption are less painful postoperatively, with shorter hospital stays and more rapid rehabilitation. There is, however, a tradeoff between minimal exposure and the ability to identify and correct the pathologic condition. More extensive surgical exposure decreases the likelihood of missed sequestrated disc fragments and unrecognized spinal stenosis. Minimally invasive procedures limit the ability to perform extensive disc nucleus extraction and thorough foraminotomy. Ultimately the long-range results of minimally invasive surgery have not compared favorably with more extensive exposure, despite the fact that it shortens the hospital stay and reduces recovery time.

A patient with a low pain tolerance who is poorly trained and has a high level of psychosocial involvement will have a different rehabilitation process than will a highly motivated, well-trained individual. As with most other musculoskeletal surgical procedures, rehabilitation will be more rapid and more successful for patients who are in good physical condition and who understand how to care for themselves. Patients with disc surgery who have been well trained in body mechanics and are in good physical condition have fewer recurrences of HNP and less likelihood of developing spinal stenosis.

MINIMALLY INVASIVE DISC SURGERY

Minimally invasive disc surgery includes microscopic discectomy, arthroscopic microdiscectomy, laser discectomy, transforaminal discectomy, and epidural discectomy. All of these techniques can be performed with the use of local anesthesia or minimal general anesthesia. Surgical incisions generally are less than 1 inch long, and wound drains or Foley catheters rarely are used. Complications are rare, and patients usually go home the day of surgery. These patients must be carefully educated in body mechanics so that they can avoid recurrent herniation and decrease postoperative pain. Pain is the guide to activity level. As long as the spine can be kept in a balanced neutral position without lumbar flexion, activities can be increased as rapidly as pain allows. Walking a few blocks and attending to normal activities of daily living usually are possible within a few days. Within a week, return to office-level work activities is possible, and within a month, light athletic activities and moderate labor can be resumed. Patients should be given guidance and training through physical therapy, work hardening, or functional restoration as they progress to normal activities.

STANDARD LAMINOTOMY

For decades, a several-inch incision has been used to approach the lamina and perform unilateral or bilateral laminotomy. Such an approach allows fairly extensive exposure through which extensive discectomy, bilateral discectomy, and unilateral or bilateral foraminotomy can be performed with minimal risk of missed pathology. It does, however, require considerably more tissue dissection than the minimally invasive techniques and usually requires the use of a wound drain, which limits the patient's mobility for the first 24 hours after surgery.

Patients with this type of surgery have traditionally remained in the hospital for several days. More recently, education, attitude, and the mental set of the patient has been shown to affect the length of hospital stay. Postoperative hospitalization has been reduced from as long as a week to as short as 1 to 2 days.

Rehabilitation and recovery after standard laminotomy usually require weeks, compared with a few days after minimally invasive techniques. Generally, these patients are not ready for physical therapy and formal rehabilitation until a week or two after surgery. They require assistance for 1 or 2 days in the hospital for ambulation and activities of daily living. With good preoperative education, they can return to light work activities within a week or two, but do not generally return to normal work or recreational activities for at least 1 or 2 months and, frequently, 3 months.

EXTENSIVE LAMINECTOMY AND DISCECTOMY

If considerable spinal stenosis is present in addition to a herniated disc, or if internal disc disruption is suspected in a patient with only back pain, a more extensive laminectomy may be indicated. An entire spinous process and both laminae may be removed, sometimes at two consecutive levels when pain generators at two levels are demonstrated. This type of surgery requires considerably more exposure and more tissue disruption, leading to inflammation, muscle spasm, and wound drainage that keeps the patient in the hospital for several days. Return to functional activities takes weeks to months longer than after a minimally invasive procedure. See box for general principles of care.

General Principles of Rehabilitation After Disc Surgery

Postoperative education and physical and psychologic training are major keys to a successful rehabilitation program.

The patient should progress into safe functional activities as rapidly as pain allows.

Therapists and trainers should be used before and after surgery to assure that the patient is using safe body mechanics during return to normal activities.

A rehabilitation plan should be developed before surgery, and the patient should be committed to follow the plan after surgery.

Before surgery, the patient should be advanced to the highest level of rehabilitation possible within the limits of pain and disease process.

After surgery, the patient should be expected to accomplish reasonable goals commensurate with the underlying condition, the surgery performed, and the general physical and psychologic resources.

Postoperative pain should be controlled to allow rehabilitation.

Patients with chronic pain or psychosocial involvement that inhibits rehabilitation should be placed in a functional restoration or chronic program.

REHABILITATION PROTOCOL

Disc Surgery

In hospital	• Generally, encourage walking on the first day after surgery. • Reinstitute isometric abdominal and lower extremity exercises. • Minimize sitting to lower intradiscal pressure (p. 375). • Progressively increase walking. • When the patient is walking comfortably and pain medication is minimal, the patient may be discharged from the hospital.
At home	• As strength increases, begin gentle isotonic leg exercises. • Allow increased sitting after the fourth week. • Prohibit lifting, bending, and stooping for 6 weeks, and gradually progress after the sixth week. • Do not allow long trips for 3 months.
	• Increase lower extremity strength from the eighth to twelfth weeks.
Return to work	• Allow patients with jobs requiring much walking without lifting to return to work within 4 weeks. • In general, allow patients with jobs requiring prolonged sitting to return within 6 to 8 weeks provided minimal lifting is required. • Heavy laborers return to modified duty in approximately 12 weeks. Patients with jobs that require exceptionally heavy manual labor may have to permanently modify their occupation or seek an occupation with lighter work loads. • Keeping patients out of work for more than 3 months rarely improves pain relief or recovery.

Bibliography

Armstrong J: *Lumbar disc lesions,* ed 1, London, 1958, E & R Livingston CTD.

Basmajian JV: Acute back pain and spasm: a controlled multicenter trial of combined analgesic and antispasm agents, *Spine* 14:438, 1989.

Brown MD, Seltzer DG: Perioperative care in lumbar spine surgery, *Orthop Clin North Am* 22:353, 1991.

Cherkin D, Deyo R, Berg A: Evaluation of a physician education intervention to improve primary care for low-back pain. II. Impact on patients, *Spine* 16:2273, 1991.

Deyo RA: Nonoperative treatment of low back disorders. In Frymoyer JW, editor: *The adult spine: principles and practice,* New York, 1991, Raven.

Deyo RA, Diehl AK: Psychosocial predictors of disability in patients with low back pain, *J Rheumatol* 15:1557, 1988.

Deyo RA, Diehl AK, Rosenthal M: How many days of bedrest for acute low back pain? *N Eng J Med* 315:1064, 1986.

Dimaggio A, Mooney V: The McKenzie program: exercise effective against back pain, *J Musculoskel Med,* p. 63, Sept, 1987.

Dimaggio A, Mooney V: Conservative care for low back pain: what works? *J Musculoskel Med,* p. 65, Dec, 1987.

Dolan P: Commonly adopted postures and their effects on the lumbar spine, *Spine* 13:197, 1988.

Donelson R, Silva G, Murphy K: The centralization phenomenon: its usefulness in evaluating and treating referred pain, *Spine* 15:211, 1990.

Forrsell M: The back school, *Spine* 6:104, 1981.

Frymoyer JW: Predicting disability from low back pain, *Clin Orthop* 279:102, 1992.

Frymoyer JW, Nachemson A: Natural history of low back disorders. In Frymoyer JW, editor: *The adult spine: principles and practice,* New York, 1991, Raven.

Gilbert JR, Taylor DW, Hildebrand A: Clinical trial of common treatments for low back pain in family practice, *Br Med J* 291:791, 1985.

Greenough H, Fraser R: The effects of compensation on recovery from low back surgery, *Spine* 14:947, 1989.

Hart D, Stobbe T, Jaraiedi M: Effect of lumbar posture on lifting, *Spine* 12:138, 1987.

Kellett K, Kellett D, Nordholm L: Effects of an exercise program on sick leave due to back pain, *Phys Ther* 71:283, 1991.

Kelsey JL et al: An epidemiologic study of lifting and twisting on the job and risk for prolapsed lumbar intervertebral disc, *J Orthop Res* 2:61, 1984.

Kjalil T et al: Stretching in the rehabilitation of low-back pain patients, *Spine* 17:311, 1992.

Kopp JR et al: The use of lumbar extension in patients with acute herniated nucleus pulposus, *Clin Orthop* 202:211, 1986.

Liang M, Komaroff M: Roentgenograms in primary care patients with acute low back pain: a cost effectiveness analysis, *Arch Intern Med* 142:1108, 1982.

Lindstrom I et al: Mobility, strength, and fitness after a graded activity program for patients with subacute low back pain, *Spine* 17:641, 1992.

Maigne JY, Rime B, Deligne B: Computed tomographic follow-up study of forty-eight cases of nonoperatively treated lumbar intervertebral disc herniation, *Spine* 17(9):1071, 1992.

McKenzie, RA: *The lumbar spine: mechanical diagnosis and therapy,* Waikanae, NZ, 1981, Spinal.

Micheli LJ, Couzens GS: How I manage low back pain in athletes, *Phys Sports Med* 21, 1993.

Nachemson A: Disc pressure measurements, *Spine* 6:93, 1981.

Nachemson A: Advances in low back pain, *Clin Orthop* 200:266, 1985.

Nachemson A: Newest knowledge of low back pain, *Clin Orthop* 279:8, 1992.

Polatin P: The functional restoration approach to chronic low back pain, *J Musculoskel Med* 7:17, 1990.

Robison R: The new back school prescription: stabilization training, part I. *Spine State Art Rev* 5:341, 1991.

Saal J: The new back school prescription: stabilization training, part II, *Spine State Art Rev* 5:357, 1991.

Shah J, Hampson W, Jayson M: The distribution of surface strain in the cadaveric lumbar spine, *J Bone Joint Surg* 60-B:246, 1978.

Spengler DM et al: Back injuries in industry: overview and cost analysis, *Spine* 11:241, 1986.

Syms J: Stabilization training can help your back patients gain control, *Back Pain Mon* 8:101, 1990.

Waddell G: A new clinical model for treatment of low back pain, *Spine* 12:632, 1987.

Waddell G et al: Objective clinical evaluation of physical impairment in chronic low back pain, *Spine* 17:617, 1992.

White A, Mattmiller A, White L: *Back school and other conservative approaches to low back pain*, St. Louis, 1983, Mosby–Year Book.

Williams PC: The lumbosacral spine, emphasizing conservative management, New York, 1965, McGraw-Hill.

Index

Fracture
    acetabular, 147-150, 152
    ankle, 258-264
        pediatric, 329-330
        stable open reduction and internal fixation of bimalleolar or
            trimalleolar, 259-263
        treatment considerations in, 258-259
    clavicular, 314-315
    elbow, 86-88
    femoral, 155-165
        distal, 163-165
        of femoral neck, 155-157
        of femoral shaft, 160-163
        intertrochanteric, 157
        subtrochanteric, 158-159
    hand, 53-63
        mallet equivalent epiphyseal, 16
        metacarpal and phalangeal, 53-57
        repair before flexor tendon repair, 2
        scaphoid, 58-59
        ulnar collateral ligament of thumb injury in, 57-58
        wrist and, 59-63
    hip, 150-152
        pediatric, 322-326
    humeral, 315-316
    lower extremity
        classification of, 144-145
        delayed union and nonunion in, 146
        general rehabilitation principles in, 146-147
        infection and, 145, 146
        stabilization of, 145-146
    patellar, 165-167
    pelvic, 152-155
    tibial
        distal, 177-178
        pediatric, 327-329
        plateau, 168-171
        of tibial shaft, 171-176
Frontal plane motions of foot, 348
Frozen shoulder, 130-135
Frykman classification of distal radius fracture, 59
Full weight-bearing closed-chain exercises, 147
Functional electrical stimulation
    in Colles' fracture, 62
    in extensor tenolysis, 34
    in flexor tendon injury
        zone 1, 2, or 3, 5
        in zones 4 and 5, 6
Functional plane of motion in shoulder rehabilitation, 95
Functional testing after anterior cruciate ligament reconstruction, 191-194
Functional training in patellofemoral disorders, 232

G

Gait, 351-352, 353, 354
    after total hip arthroplasty, 300
Galloway, DeMaio, and Mangine protocol in epicondylitis, 79-80
Gamekeeper's thumb, 57-58
Garden classification of femoral neck fractures, 155-156
Gastrocnemius
    gait and, 354
    stretching of, 266
Gentamicin, 144
Glenohumeral joint, 92, 93
    pendulum exercise for, 109
    subacromial impingement and, 94
Glide component, 233, 234
Gluteus maximus stretch, 228
Golf program after arthroscopic subacromial decompression, 116
Golfer's elbow, 75-80
Gout, 277
Graft
    in anterior cruciate ligament reconstruction, 185-186
    in reconstruction of ulnar collateral ligament, 72
Great toe taping, 272
Griffin protocol in patellofemoral pain, 236
Grundberg procedure, 23
Gustilo-Anderson classification of soft tissue injury in open fractures,
    144-145

H

Hamilton protocol after ankle ligament reconstruction, 257-258
Hamstring
    graft of, 185
    strengthening exercises for, 308

Hamstring curl, 187-188
Hand, 1-66
    arthroplasty of, 50-53
        for boutonnière deformity, 51
        Eaton volar plate, 51
        interposition and sling suspension, 52
        for joint stiffness, 50
        lateral deviation, 50
        metacarpophalangeal joint, 51
        silastic trapezial, 52
        thumb carpometacarpal joint, 52
        total wrist, 53
    deQuervain's tenosynovitis of, 35-37
    digital nerve repair in, 44
    extensor tendon injury to, 13-34
        anatomy in, 13-14, 15
        basic rehabilitation principles in, 14, 16
        boutonnière deformity in, 18-26
        swan-neck deformity in, 26-31
        in zones 1 and 2, 16-18
        in zones 4, 5, and 6, 31-32
        in zones 7 and 8, 32-34
    extensor tenolysis and, 34-35
    flexor tendon injury to, 2-13
        anatomy in, 3
        decompression of flexor carpi radialis tunnel syndrome and, 13
        delayed mobilization of flexor pollicis longus of thumb and, 11
        early mobilization of flexor pollicis longus of thumb and, 8-10
        Idler early motion program in, 7
        modified Duran protocol in zone 1, 2, or 3 in, 4-6
        modified Duran protocol in zone 4 and 5 in, 6-7
        noncompliant patient and, 8
        tendon healing and, 3-4
        timing of repair and, 2-3
        trigger digit release in, 12-13
        two-stage reconstruction for delayed tendon repair in, 11-12
    fractures and dislocations of, 53-63
        metacarpal and phalangeal, 53-57
        scaphoid, 58-59
        ulnar collateral ligament of thumb injury in, 57-58
        wrist and, 59-63
    intersection syndrome of, 35
    nerve compression syndromes of, 37-43
        carpal tunnel syndrome in, 37-38
        cubital tunnel syndrome in, 40-41
        pronator syndrome in, 38-39
        radial tunnel syndrome in, 41-42
        thoracic outlet syndrome in, 42-43
        ulnar tunnel syndrome in, 40
    nerve injury to, 43
    replantation and revascularization of, 48-50
    splinting for nerve palsies, 43-44
    tendon zones of
        extensor, 14
        flexor, 3
    wrist disorders and, 44-47
        dorsal and volar carpal ganglion cysts in, 44-45
        ligament reconstruction in, 45-46
        rheumatoid arthritis in, 46-47
        scapholunate ligament repair in, 46
Heat therapy, 338
Heel insert, 278
Heel lift, 359, 365
Heel pain, 274-280
    anatomy and pathomechanics of, 274, 275
    etiology of, 275-276
    modified DeMaio and Drez protocol in, 279
    orthosis and, 368
    plantar fasciitis and, 277-278
    signs and symptoms of, 276-277
Heel slide, 207
Heel-strike to flat-foot, 351
Hemiarthroplasty in femoral neck fracture, 155
Hemitransverse fracture, 148
Heparin
    in deep venous thrombosis prophylaxis, 285, 286
    after hand replantation, 49
Herbert screw, 327
Herniated nucleus pulposus, 384-386
Heterotopic ossification in acetabular fracture, 148
High-volt pulsed direct current, 338
Hinton-Boswell method of taping, 251
Hip
    abduction exercises of, 290